THE ENCYCLOPEDIA OF

MIND

BODY

SPIRIT

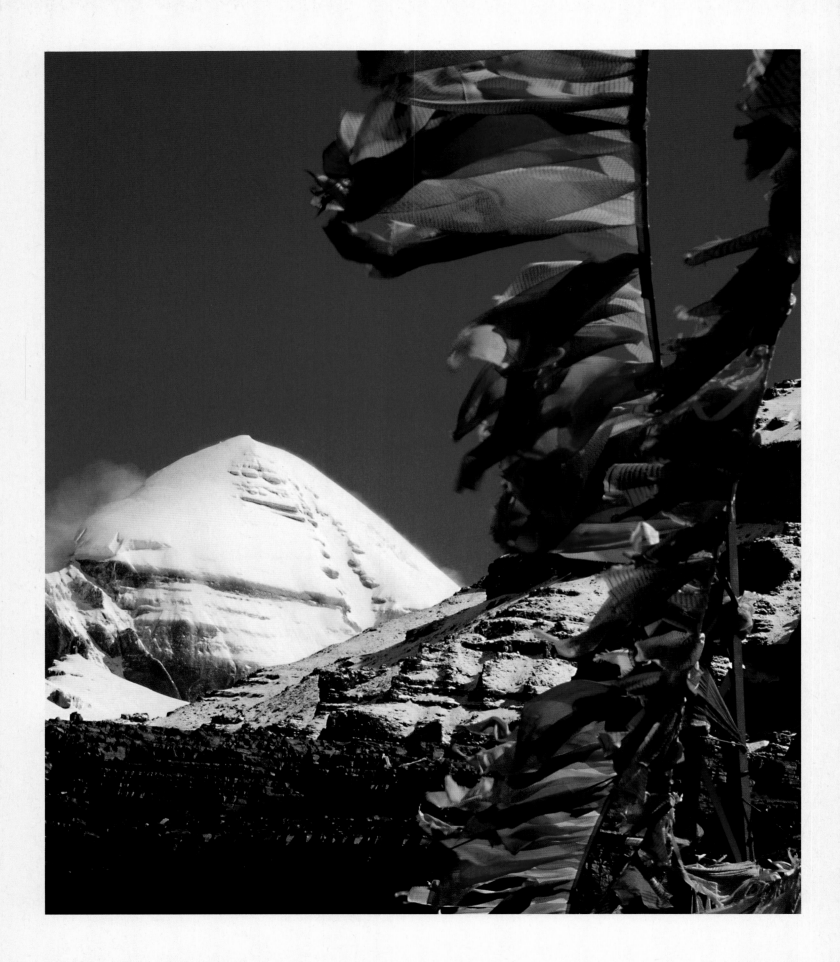

THE ENCYCLOPEDIA OF

MIND

BODY

SPIRIT

THE COMPLETE GUIDE TO HEALING THERAPIES, ESOTERIC WISDOM AND SPIRITUAL TRADITIONS

Consultant Editors
Dr William Bloom, Judy Hall, Professor David Peters

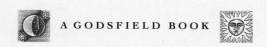 A GODSFIELD BOOK

An Hachette UK Company
www.hachette.co.uk

First published in Great Britain in 2009
by Godsfield Press, a division of
Octopus Publishing Group Ltd
2–4 Heron Quays,
London E14 4JP
www.octopusbooks.co.uk
www.octopusbooksusa.com

Distributed in the U.S. and Canada by Octopus Books USA:
c/o Hachette Book Group
237 Park Avenue
New York NY 10017

ISBN: 978-1-84181-354-7

A CIP catalogue record for this book
is available from the British Library.

Printed and bound in China

10 9 8 7 6 5 4 3 2 1

About the consultants

Healer, teacher and author, **Dr William Bloom** co-founded and directed
the Alternatives Programme, London, a major platform for holistic
perspectives on religion, psychology and healing. He has been on the
faculty of the Findhorn Foundation for over 20 years and teaches and
runs workshops internationally. He is the author of a number of books
including *Solution: The Holistic Manifesto*, *The Endorphin Effect* and was
editor of *The Penguin Book of New Age and Holistic Writing*.

Judy Hall has over 35 years experience in holistic healing and psychic
development, leading workshops, lecturing and teaching in the UK and
throughout the world. A qualified healer and counsellor and expert in
crystals, astrology, past lives, alternative therapies and psychic protection,
she holds a B.Ed in Religious Studies and an M.A. in Cultural Astronomy
and Astrology and has an extensive knowledge of world religions and
mythology. She is the author of the bestselling *The Crystal Bible*, *The
Astrology Bible*, *The Encyclopedia of Crystals*, *Crystal Healing*, *Past Life
Astrology* and many other titles.

Professor David Peters is a qualified medical practitioner and trained
homeopath and osteopath. He practised as a family doctor in one of
the first National Health Service practices to bring conventional and
complementary practitioners together. He is Clinical Director at the
School of Integrated Medicine, University of Westminster, Chair of
the British Holistic Medical Association and chairs the advisory group
for the Prince, a Foundation for Integrated Health.

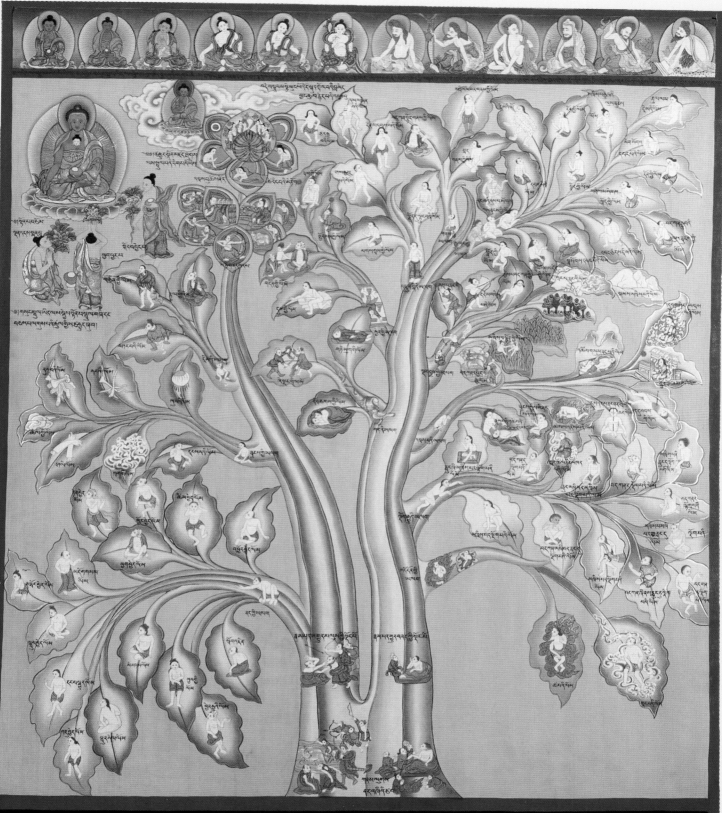

CONTENTS

INTRODUCTION 8

PART ONE 10
MIND

PSYCHOLOGICAL APPROACHES 14
Mind and brain 16
Uncovering the unconscious 18
The collective unconscious 20
Dreams and dream analysis 22
Psychological types 24
Behaviourism and attachment theory 26
Humanistic psychology 27
Cognitive behavioural therapy and mindfulness 28
Hypnotherapy 30
Neuro-linguistic programming 31
Psychosynthesis 32
Creative visualization and guided imagery 33
Mystical and transcendent states 34

PSYCHIC SKILLS AND OTHER DIMENSIONS OF THE MIND 36
Intuition, precognition and premonition 38
Psychic skills 40
Channelling 42
Psychic protection 44
Out-of-body experiences 46
Exceptional human experiences 48
Past lives and past-life therapies 50
Cosmic ordering and abundance 52

DIVINATION 54
Western astrology 56
Chinese astrology 58
Vedic astrology 60
The tarot 62
Runes 64
Numerology 66
Palmistry 68
I Ching 70
Other forms of divination 72

MIND AND BODY 74
Psychoneuroimmunology 76
Meditation 78
Autogenic training and the endorphin effect 80
Breathwork 81
Body-centred therapies 82
Neurobiology of emotion 84
Biofeedback 86
Energy psychology therapies 87

PART TWO 88
BODY

EASTERN APPROACHES 92
Ayurveda 94
Traditional Chinese Medicine 98
Tibetan medicine 102

BODY WORK 104
Yoga 106
Pilates 110
T'ai chi 112
Chi kung 114
Martial arts 116
Alexander technique 118
Swedish massage 120
Thai massage 122
Indian head massage 123
Shiatsu 124
Acupuncture 126
Acupressure 127
Reflexology 128
Chiropractic and osteopathy 132
Craniosacral therapy 136
Feldenkrais method 137
Bowen technique 138
Rolfing 139
Iridology 140
Bates method 141

NUTRITIONAL AND HERBAL APPROACHES 142
Naturopathy 144
Vitamins and minerals 146
Superfoods 147
Food combining 148
Macrobiotics 149
Fasting and detoxing 150
Herbalism 152

ENERGY THERAPIES 154

Aromatherapy 156
Flower essences 158
Homeopathy 160
Colour therapy 162
Sound therapy 163
Healing water 164
Crystal healing 166
Applied kinesiology 168
Polarity therapy 169

BODY AND SPIRIT 170

Chakras and the aura 172
Reiki 174
Spiritual healing and therapeutic touch 176

PART THREE 178
SPIRIT

WESTERN FAITHS 182

Western mystery traditions 184
Judaism 186
The Kabbalah 188
Christianity 190
The Gnostic Gospels 192
Spiritualism 194
Islam 196
Sufism 198
Bahai 200

EASTERN FAITHS 202

Hinduism 204
Hindu sacred texts 206
Buddhism 208
Buddhist sacred texts 210
Tibetan buddhism 212
Zen buddhism 213
Tantra 214
Taoism 216
Taoist sacred texts 218
Confucianism 220
Jainism 222
Sikhism 223

TRIBAL, SHAMANIC AND ANIMIST TRADITIONS 224

Shamanism 226
Australian Aboriginal spirituality 228
Oceania 230
Native American spirituality 232
African traditions 234
Shinto 236
Paganism 238
Wicca 240
Druidry 242

EARTH MYSTERIES 244

Sacred land 246
Feng shui 248
Sacred geometry 250
Megaliths and earthworks 252
Archeoastronomy 254
Earth energies 256
Landscape lines 258
Green spirituality 260

SPIRITUAL, SECRET AND OCCULT SOCIETIES 262

Knights Templar 264
Rosicrucianism 266
The Illuminati 267
Freemasonry 268
Theosophy 270
Rudolf Steiner and anthroposophy 272

ANCIENT MYSTERIES 274

Atlantis 276
Ancient Egyptian wisdom 278
Judaeo-Christian mysteries 280
The Holy Grail 282
Prophecy and Nostradamus 284
Mayan prophecy 285
Mythical creatures 286

PATHS TO OTHER REALMS 288

Angels 290
Fairies 292
The Goddess 294
Alchemy 296
Pilgrimage and retreats 298
Spiritual leaders 300
Energy 302
Contemporary spirituality 304

INDEX 306
ACKNOWLEDGEMENTS 320

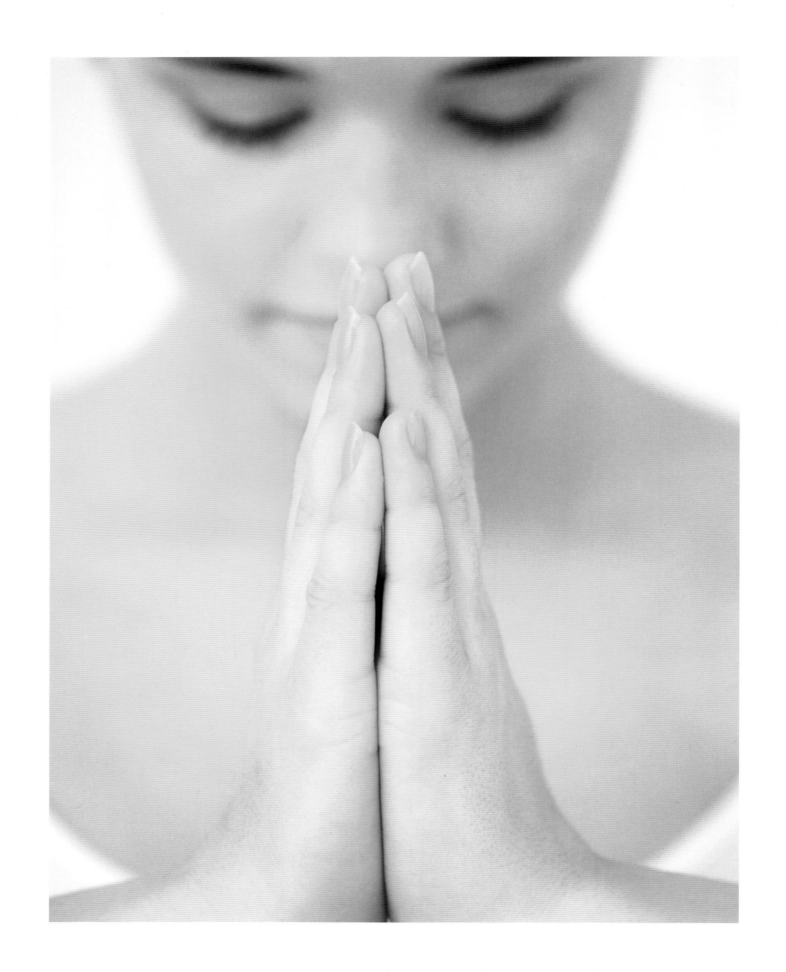

INTRODUCTION

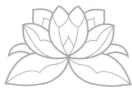 In this book you will discover psychotherapies and psychic skills, bodywork and energy therapies, as well as spiritual traditions, that offer insight and guidance as to how we might lead happier, healthier and more fulfilling lives.

The Mind, Body and Spirit (MBS) movement, also known as the New Age or holistic movement, arose as a social force in the West during the 1960s and 1970s, partly in response to increased access to traditions from a wide range of cultures, and partly due to a disenchantment with traditional Western approaches. Despite this relatively recent flowering, however, many of the approaches within the MBS field are extremely ancient. Yoga, for example, dates back thousands of years and has supported the health of millions of people around the world, while acupuncture has been practised for at least 4,000 years. This book traces the lineage of healthcare and spiritual traditions and the form they currently take, providing a general context for their use today.

In recent years science has also revealed new understandings of how the mind and body influence each other, the nature of energy and vitality, and the interdependence of people and their environment. This book explores the most recent research developments in these fields, including insights concerning mind–body medicine and altered states of consciousness.

How to use this book

The wealth of subjects that come under the MBS umbrella can make it challenging to find information quickly and easily. The encyclopedia has been designed to be comprehensive yet also easy to use, helping you to find key topics readily, as well as tracing the connections between different subjects.

The three parts

The encyclopedia is organized into three parts: Mind, Body and Spirit. Three leading authors and practitioners in the MBS field introduce you to each part. Therapist and specialist in the esoteric arts Judy Hall explores the fascinating complexity of the mind and consciousness, including dreams and dream analysis, hypnotherapy, creative visualization and the divinatory arts. Practising homeopath and osteopath Professor David Peters introduces the wide-ranging approaches to the understanding of our health and wellbeing,

Mind, body, spirit *The therapies, philosophies and spiritual insights discussed here will help to provide you with the inspiration and guidance you need to achieve a sense of inner peace and well being.*

from Traditional Chinese Medicine to Pilates, and from macrobiotics to aromatherapy. Spiritual teacher and activist Dr William Bloom shares the wealth of enriching spiritual insights from a wide range of traditions from all regions of the world, encompassing both the major religions and the more esoteric and shamanic approaches.

Chapters

Within these three main parts you will find chapters written by experts in the field. Each chapter brings together key therapies and approaches under themes such as bodywork and nutritional therapies. The chapters are then broken down into individual entries on specific approaches, for example reflexology and herbalism.

In recognition of the interrelated aspects of so many subjects in this field, each part is linked to the next via a chapter exploring these connections. Therefore, Part 1, Mind, merges into Part 2, Body, with an exploration of the disciplines that reveal how the mind can directly influence our health and wellbeing through such tools as energy psychology therapies. Part 2, Body, is linked to Part 3, Spirit, via body–spirit approaches including spiritual healing and reiki.

Individual entries

Beside the heading for each entry you will find a list of related topics that you may also like to read about, together with the relevant page number. In this way you can trace interconnections between subjects and take your understanding to a deeper level. For instance, the meditation entry will also lead you to cognitive behavioural therapy, hypnotherapy, yoga and the sacred texts of the East.

Each entry can be read on two levels. The opening paragraph functions as a brief definition of the subject so that you can use the encyclopedia almost like a dictionary. Highlighted in bold in the opening paragraph are some of the key aspects of each discipline, which are then expanded on in detail in the text.

The benefits of exploring Mind, Body and Spirit

We are all engaged on a voyage of discovery in our lives, learning about ourselves, our environment and what we most require to enrich us and fulfil our innermost needs.

May this book act as a guide on your journey, providing you with the essential reference points, signposts and waymarkers to lead you to your place of peace and wisdom.

PART ONE
MIND

PSYCHOLOGICAL APPROACHES 14

PSYCHIC SKILLS AND OTHER DIMENSIONS
OF THE MIND 36

DIVINATION 54

MIND AND BODY 74

PART ONE
MIND

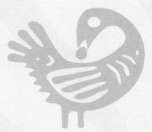

I have been psychic since I was born. I 'saw' what was not there, talked to the dead and had numerous déjà vu experiences. My first near-death experience occurred at five years of age, and I was rarely in my body. So I always knew that I was more than my body and that my consciousness roamed freely, which made it challenging when I entered the academic world in the 1970s as a student who wanted to explore the many facets of religious belief and the soul's journey.

Ever since French philosopher and mathematician René Descartes wrote 'I think, therefore I am' in 1637, mind has been afforded a superior position in the modern world. Descartes didn't invent the idea, but in saying 'I *have* a body' rather than 'I *am* a body' he perpetuated the 'ghost in the machine' concept that created a body–mind split and left out spirit altogether. But the man who also said 'mind is entirely indivisible' would surely have been amazed at how many levels of mind are recognized today and at the number of psychological approaches these have spawned, plus investigations into intuition, parapsychology and consciousness.

Ancient peoples recognized a totality of mind, body and spirit that is, in turn, part of the universe in which we live, move and have our being. This wholeness, or holism, has been revived by the MBS movement. The ancients also believed that *something* – soul, spirit, mind or consciousness – survived death and that this could operate away from the body even before death. It is with this *something*, and its powers and abilities, that metaphysics is concerned. However, near-death and similar experiences of consciousness leaving the body and existing separately are now being referred to by a few enlightened scientists as exceptional human experiences; experiences that enrich, expand and profoundly transform the world-view of the person involved. At last scientific reality is colliding with my metaphysical reality.

Researchers have intensively tested abilities that ancient people took for granted, such as the power to view remote scenes, exchange information through the mind or read the future. However, science requires consistent results that replicate. Intuition and other psychic skills aren't like that. They are capricious, unreliable and unpredictable, and all the more exciting for that, creating an opportunity to open up new dimensions of consciousness or to return to ancient ones as in divinatory and shamanic practices. Scientists have also extensively researched, and hotly debated, the whole concept of mind and consciousness and whether these are indissolubly tied to the brain, but anyone who has been pronounced dead and yet has continued to experience, as I have, can assure them that consciousness continues!

The interconnection of mind and body is used to great effect in energy psychology, and the truly awesome powers of mind are, finally, being glimpsed. One of the greatest contributions of the MBS movement has been in opening up the frontiers of consciousness and recognizing that the mind can move beyond time and space to interpenetrate *everything*, which, in turn, is consciousness. What excites me most is the idea that, as Dr Manjir Samanta-Laughton has pointed out:

> 'This… world is not one devoid of meaning or thought, but one alive with consciousness, where we dance in a field of light imbued with the mind of God.'

Judy Hall

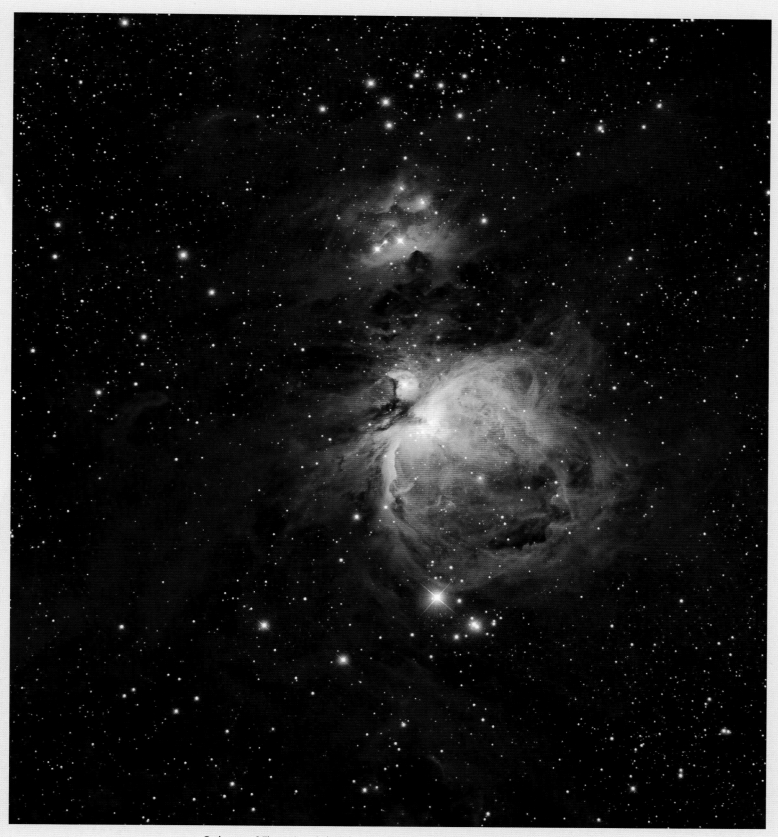

God or man? *The ancients believed in the aphorism 'as above, so below' but even they may have been surprised by 'The Running Man' striding across the outer reaches of our galaxy.*

FLEGMAT

SANGVIN

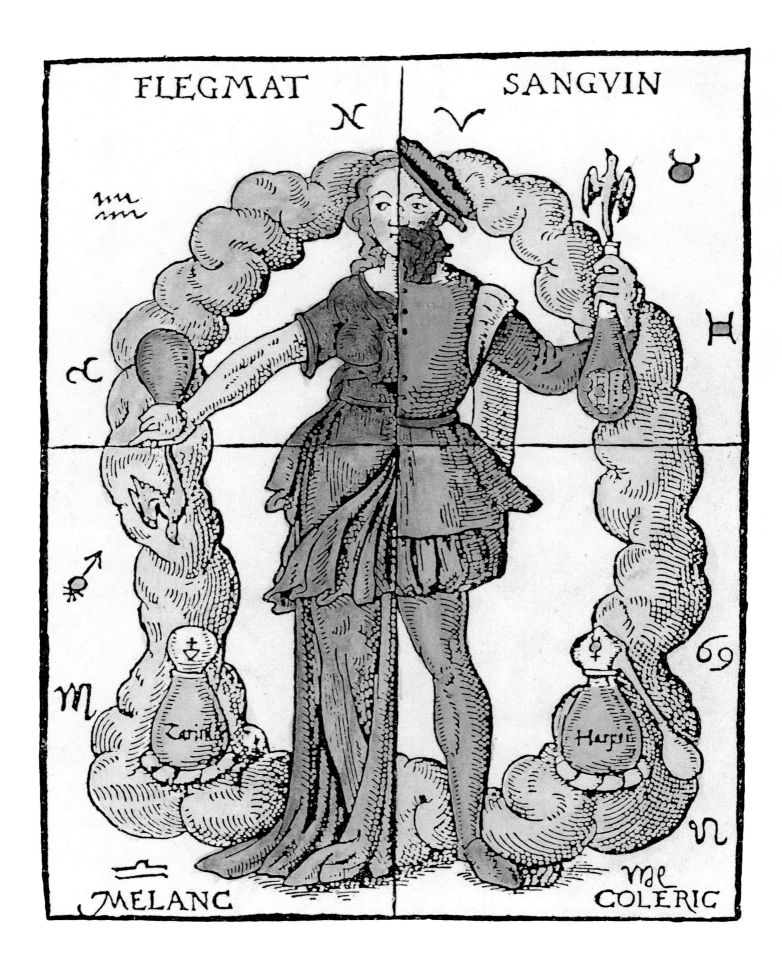

MELANC

COLERIC

PSYCHOLOGICAL APPROACHES

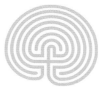

Psychology examines both our mental processes, such as memory, perception and cognition (how we think), and our emotional life and relationships. Although interest in human behaviour dates back to ancient times, and the four basic personality types of choleric, sanguine, melancholic and phlegmatic (the humours) were established very early on, the modern discipline of psychology as a science in its own right is generally considered to have begun with the establishment of the first laboratory for psychological research in Leipzig by Wilhelm Wundt in 1879. Wundt (1832–1920) took a strictly scientific approach to studying the mind, trying to break down human consciousness into identifiable parts, and focused on experimentation to verify his findings. In pioneering work into the study of memory and the process of learning, Hermann Ebbinghaus (1850–1909) was the first to detail 'the learning curve', the process by which skills are gradually acquired. One of psychology's most influential thinkers, Russian Ivan Pavlov (1849–1936), described the process of mental conditioning based on his experiments with dogs. Pavlov's work revealed the extent to which human behaviour is modified by our experience and paved the way for a major movement in psychology, behaviourism.

Exploration of the psyche

But there was another seminal development in modern psychology, one that moved away from experimentation and turned instead to exploring the inner depths of the psyche: the unconscious mind. Psychoanalyst Sigmund Freud (1856–1939) developed the theory of the unconscious as the seat of powerful repressed emotions that needed to be recognized and expressed in order to heal the individual. His contemporary and one-time friend Carl Jung (1875–1961) developed the concept of a collective unconscious where humanity's archetypal dreams and memories reside. Highly influential in their

The four humours Theophrastus (371–287 BCE) based the personality types known as choleric, sanguine, melancholic and phlegmatic on Hippocrates' four humours or bodily fluids: black bile, blood, phlegm and yellow bile. The concept of the humours was popular right up until the 19th century.

own time, the ideas of Freud and Jung continue to resonate with millions of people around the world.

Modern developments

Today psychotherapies such as cognitive behavioural therapy, psychoanalysis and approaches such as art and drama therapy are widely available to help people make sense of emotional problems and resolve past issues. In the past few decades neuroscientists have added to the knowledge of psychologists and have made enormous advances in identifying the parts of the brain associated with particular functions. The use of equipment such as magnetic resonance imaging (MRI scans) and positron emission topography (PET scans) has provided fascinating insights into the brain in action.

The great debate

Yet despite the advances of neuroscience and psychology, the mind has remained stubbornly resistant to our complete understanding of how it works, and the nature of consciousness is a hotly debated subject. As neuroscience has revealed the ever more complex functioning of the brain, further questions have arisen. How is it that these complicated brain cells and chemical transmitters work together so coherently and effectively? How are great artistic works created or profound insights gained? And how do we explain powerful mystical and transcendental experiences? Science has yet to provide the full answer. As English anatomist and biologist Thomas Huxley (1825–1895) wrote:

> *'How it is that anything so remarkable as a state of consciousness comes about as a result of irritating nervous tissue is just about as unaccountable as the appearance of the Djinn, when Aladdin rubbed his lamp?'*

This section explores some of the most important psychological approaches that attempt to explain the nature of the mind, heal emotional problems and harness the mind's amazing abilities. These include the development of personality types, such as the Myers-Briggs Type Indicator (MBTI) and the Enneagram, the development of key movements such as behaviourism and more recent approaches, such as neuro-lingustic programming (NLP), cognitive behavioural therapy (CBT) and hypnotherapy.

MIND AND BRAIN

If you are interested in **Mind and Brain**, you may also like to read about:
- **Exceptional Human Experiences**, pages 48–49
- **Psychoneuroimmunology**, pages 76–77
- **Neurobiology of Emotion**, pages 84–85
- **Psychic Skills**, pages 40–41
- **Channelling**, pages 42–43

The **mind** has been defined as 'the faculty of **consciousness** and thought, a person's ability to think and reason, the intellect'. There is continuing debate as to the nature of the mind as distinct from the **brain** and consciousness itself. Scientists, psychologists and mystics alike all have very differing opinions and viewpoints on what the mind and consciousness is or isn't.

What is the brain?

Science has been able to tell us much about the incredibly complex structure of the brain. We now know that the brain consists of three main blocks that have evolved over millions of years: the hindbrain, midbrain and forebrain. The hindbrain is the oldest part of the brain, responsible for the automatic reflexes that control breathing, heart rate and digestion and coordinate movement and sense perception. The midbrain is more pronounced in primates and humans compared to other animals. It controls temperature and fine movements, and also plays an important part in the limbic system, the part of the brain involved in expressing emotions. The forebrain contains the cerebral hemispheres – the right and left sides of the brain – and is the most recently evolved part. It controls sophisticated cognitive, sensory and motor functions as well as reproductive, eating and sleeping functions and the display of emotions.

Much interest has focused on the role of the two hemispheres of the brain. We know from the results of split-brain surgery performed in the 1960s to control epilepsy that each hemisphere of the brain has quite different functions that need to work together for optimum brain performance. The left hemisphere is associated with analytical, rational and logical processing, whereas the right is associated with abstract thought, non-verbal awareness, visual–spatial perception and the expression and modulation of emotions. By working together the two hemispheres complement each other, each providing missing gaps in information to provide us with a full experience of everyday reality.

So we know much about the anatomy and functions of the brain, but a bigger question looms large for many people. Is the brain more than the sum of its parts? Above and beyond the brain, many people argue there is 'mind'.

What is mind?

Exactly what mind is lies at the heart of the question 'Are we something more than merely a wonderful machine?' Mind has been defined by the *Oxford English Dictionary* as 'the faculty of consciousness and thought, a person's ability to think and reason, the intellect, a person's memory, attention, will and determination'. However, most of us accept that thought,

intellect and reasoning account for only a small aspect of the mind's abilities. The mind's faculties also encompass such disparate skills and dimensions as creativity, intuition, dreams, psychic abilities, mind–body interactions such as the placebo effect (see page 75) and psychosomatic illnesses, and what have come to be called exceptional human experiences – near-death experiences and transcendent or mystical experiences. Many of these latter states have been harnessed by mystics, priests and shamans over thousands of years to explore the nature of reality.

What is consciousness?

Bound up in a definition of the mind is the question of consciousness, our state of awareness and perception. One definition of consciousness suggests that what we are aware of is purely the product of our brain filtered from physical sensory information; another suggests that hormones and emotions play their part in our experience of 'reality'; yet another, the Buddhist perspective, suggests that all life is an illusion created by our mind; while others believe that mind is part of a wider universal consciousness.

Consciousness is defined by the *Oxford English Dictionary* as 'awareness by the mind of itself and the world, one's awareness or perception of something'. This is the definition most often followed by neuroscientists and focuses on the act of being conscious and aware, via sensory perception. However, other research has suggested a broader definition of consciousness. In 1978 British psychophysiologist Cecil Maxwell Cade (1918–1984) published research on different states of consciousness as measured by EEG readings (electroencephalograms) used to record the brain activity of experienced meditators. On the basis of his results he argued that there were five observable levels of consciousness:

1. Dreaming sleep, where we have no awareness of the external world and are focused on the internal world of the imagination.
2. Hypnogogic (between waking and sleeping) and hypnopompic (between sleeping and waking) states, where we have increased awareness of the external world, but have yet to regain full control over our bodies and still have access to the imagery of the dreaming state.
3. Waking state: our everyday level of consciousness.

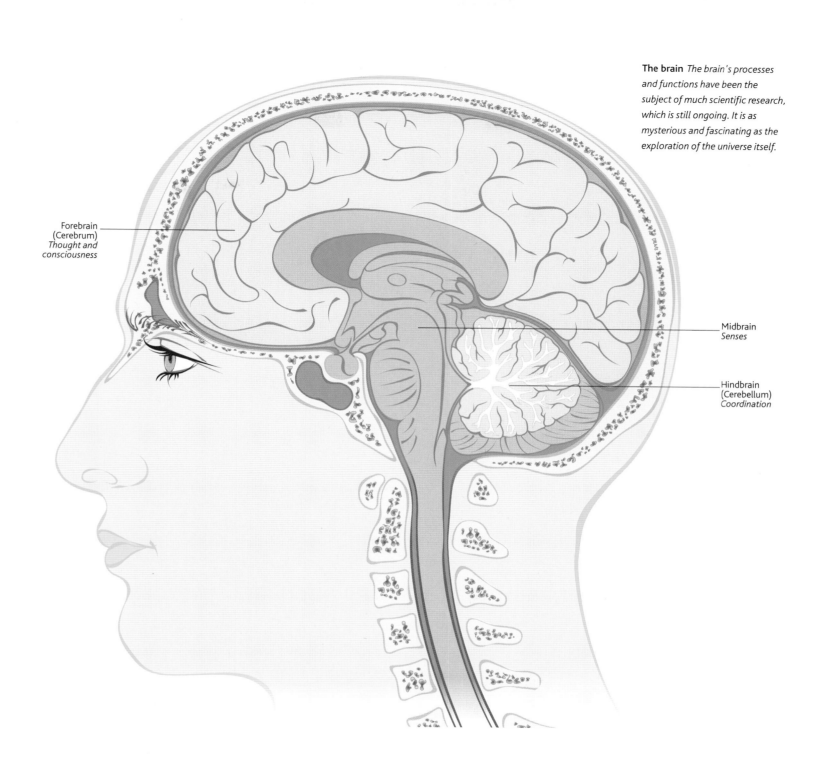

Forebrain
(Cerebrum)
*Thought and
consciousness*

The brain *The brain's processes
and functions have been the
subject of much scientific research,
which is still ongoing. It is as
mysterious and fascinating as the
exploration of the universe itself.*

Midbrain
Senses

Hindbrain
(Cerebellum)
Coordination

4. Meditative state, where we withdraw awareness from the external
environment and focus our attention internally.

5. The 'awakened mind', achievable by Cade's most experienced meditators,
where his subjects were able to maintain both self or internal awareness
and continuous awareness of the external environment. He found that in
this state brain-wave patterns were similar to those seen in the meditative
state but also included beta brain waves associated with higher cognitive
functions, normally seen in the waking state. However, Cade's research also
indicated that the beta wave content was balanced over the two brain
hemispheres, suggesting a balance between left-brain and right-brain
thinking in any state.

These findings suggest there is a continuous spectrum of consciousness
and also that the highest level of consciousness and brain functioning we can
achieve is not our normal waking consciousness.

Metaphysicians, psychics and mystics understand consciousness and mind
more broadly still. From their standpoint, consciousness is immanent within
the universe; it is never distinct or separate, but rather is the energetic glue
that holds everything together.

UNCOVERING THE UNCONSCIOUS

If you are interested in **Uncovering the Unconscious**, you may also like to read about:
- **The Collective Unconscious**, pages 20–21
- **Dreams and Dream Analysis**, pages 22–23
- **Mystical and Transcendent States**, pages 34–35
- **Western Astrology**, pages 56–57
- **Alchemy**, pages 296–297

The **study of the unconscious mind** remains one of the most enduring and influential developments in modern psychology. Although psychologists disagree on the exact nature of the unconscious, for many people **Freud's** concept of it as the storehouse of our strongest needs and desires – so-called **unconscious drives** – which go unrecognized by our normal, alert state, remains a popular and accessible definition. His contemporary **Carl Jung** also recognized the power of the unconscious and explored its influence on the shaping of people's personalities.

Study of the unconscious mind

'The unconscious' in a modern psychological sense could be said to have been first investigated by the Bishop of Lisieux, Nicolas Oresme (c. 1323–1382), a 14th-century mathematician, philosopher and physicist who formulated a theory of 'two attentions': the conscious and unconscious. The unconscious was also noted by Paracelsus (1493–1541) in the 16th century; his clinical and medical research is often considered to be the beginnings of modern scientific psychology. In his work *Von den Krankheiten* he writes about the mind's role in disease: 'Thus, the cause of the disease *chorea lasciva* is a mere opinion and idea, assumed by imagination, affecting those who believe in such a thing.' There is an ongoing controversial debate over the unconscious. In contemporary cognitive psychology, for example, the unconscious is considered merely to be those mental processes not mediated by any sensory awareness.

Freud and unconscious drives

Austrian psychiatrist Sigmund Freud (1856–1939) founded the psychoanalytical school of psychology and was famous for his theories of the unconscious mind, repression as a defence mechanism and the clinical practice of psychoanalysis. He was also renowned for his work on dream interpretation as a source of great insight into the workings of the unconscious, as well as his theory of client 'transference' and therapeutic techniques such as 'free association'.

The key that underpinned Freud's work was the concept that unconscious drives have a profound influence on our lives and that it is only by recognizing and becoming aware of these unconscious wishes that an individual can truly progress in life. He believed that many psychological problems, including anxiety and depression, have their roots in unresolved issues from the unconscious. He was also famous for his work on sexual desire as the basic instinctual, unconscious drive in human beings.

Freud theorized that consciousness consists of the mind's state of active awareness and perception, while the unconscious is a powerful hidden force driving the individual; the place where the individual represses those things that are unwanted, rejected or denied.

Freud's theory of personality was based on the influence of the unconscious. He believed that personality consists of three elements: the id, ego and superego. The id is unconscious and not connected with external reality. It works entirely according to the pleasure principle – seeking pleasure and avoiding pain. The ego is formed as a child grows and begins to experience the limitations of the external world. It tries to continue to be guided by the pleasure principle, but works within the boundaries of consensual reality. The superego is our moral sense, taking into account whether our behaviour is right or wrong. Freud argued that the ego used unconscious methods to distort reality in order to try to meet its needs. According to Freud, anxiety arises when the demands of the id, ego and superego conflict, and repression is one of the most powerful ways in which the ego resolves these conflicts.

Carl Jung's theories

The Swiss psychologist Carl Jung (1875–1961) was an influential thinker throughout the 20th century. He studied the workings of the psyche through philosophy, religion, art, alchemy, astrology and mythology, explored Eastern mysticism and was famous for his theories of the collective unconscious, synchronicity and archetypes. Jung's main contribution to the concept of the unconscious was his development of the theory of the collective unconscious.

Unlike Freud, Jung believed that the holistic health of an individual must include a spiritual dimension in life. In addition, he held that it was essential that we discover our innate potential to become who we are, a process he described as 'individuation'. Jung agreed with Freud that the unconscious was a powerful force in our lives and that our personalities are shaped by its

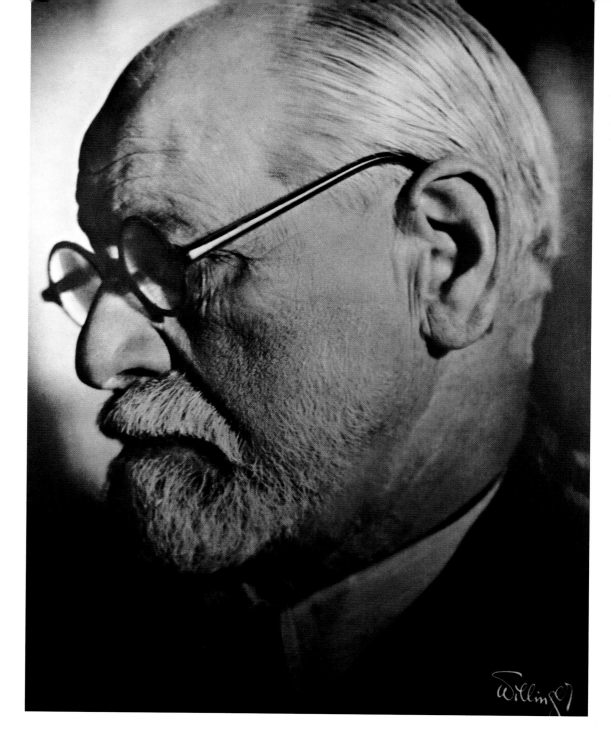

Sigmund Freud *The founder of the psychoanalytic school of psychology, his ground-breaking work on dream analysis and the unconscious mind is still lauded today.*

workings. He believed that our persona is the identity we present to society, but that this often masks the influence of unconscious forces, which include the 'anima', 'animus' and the 'shadow aspect'.

Anima, animus and the shadow self

Jung held the view that society created traditional male and female personas that masked deeper identities. He theorized that the 'anima' embodied the feminine side of the male psyche (emotions), while the 'animus' embodied the masculine side of the female psyche (logic and reason). A third aspect of our identity, he perceived, is our 'shadow aspect', which represents the part of the unconscious where repressed weaknesses, unacceptable qualities and

irrational fears are stored and also provides a link to more primal aspects of ourselves. Jung believed that the less we consciously recognize our 'shadow self', the darker and denser it might be. He also stated, however, that 'in spite of its function as a reservoir for human darkness – or perhaps because of this – the shadow is the seat of creativity' in that we also repress positive feelings such as love, joy and desire.

Our psychological health, Jung believed, is based on the extent to which we recognize and embrace these opposing forces, accepting the 'anima', 'animus' and 'shadow self'. He postulated the idea of 'unconscious collusion', whereby the psyche strives for wholeness by unconsciously attracting people or events in our lives that embody qualities we lack or have denied.

THE COLLECTIVE UNCONSCIOUS

If you are interested in **The Collective Unconscious**, you may also like to read about:
● Taoism, pages 216–217
● Buddhism, pages 208–209
● Cosmic Ordering and Abundance, pages 52–53

The concept of the collective unconscious was developed by psychologist Carl Jung from his psychoanalytic work with patients and from his study of world myths and religions, and is centred on the theory that humanity shares memories and experiences dating far back into prehistory. He concluded that across cultures there were shared explanations for questions such as how the universe began. Jung referred to the contents of this 'reservoir of the experience of our species' as **archetypes** and believed that the concept of **synchronicity** and the study of **mythology** were both keys to understanding this.

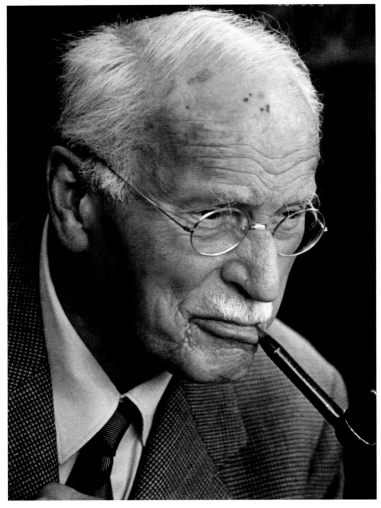

Carl Gustav Jung *Due to his pioneering work on the 'collective unconscious' he is known as the founder of the School of Analytical Psychology.*

Archetypes

Jung believed that the collective unconscious was made up of archetypes. The word 'archetype' means 'original pattern or model' and derives from the Greek word *archetypo*, meaning 'first model' or 'first-moulded'. Jung described these archetypes as the 'great dreams of humanity' and considered them to be embedded in the soul as universal blueprints. Notable Jungian archetypes include the 'shadow self', the 'anima' (the feminine principle in a man's psyche), the 'animus' (the masculine principle in a woman's psyche), the 'hero', 'trickster' and 'child'.

Jung developed the concept of a 'complex' based on his observation that his patients often reacted strongly to mention of important archetypes such as 'mother' or 'father'. He believed that a complex developed when a group of powerful unconscious or suppressed memories or associations centred on an archetype.

Synchronicity

This term describes the experience of events that are not logically or causally related, but occur together in a way that becomes meaningful. Examples of synchronicity could include close friends having had a similar dream, or a chance encounter between old friends who had been thinking about each other. Jung's theory of synchronicity is important in understanding the collective unconscious because it is through the principle of 'meaningful coincidence', or 'synchronicity' as he dubbed it, that the interconnectivity of the universe is revealed, he believed. Jung later called the collective unconscious the 'objective psyche' in that it directs the self through dreams, archetypes and intuition towards what he termed 'individuation', becoming who you are innately meant to be. Therefore, in his view, we should pay close attention to chance events, as this could be evidence of the collective unconscious at work, bringing about events necessary for our personal growth and development.

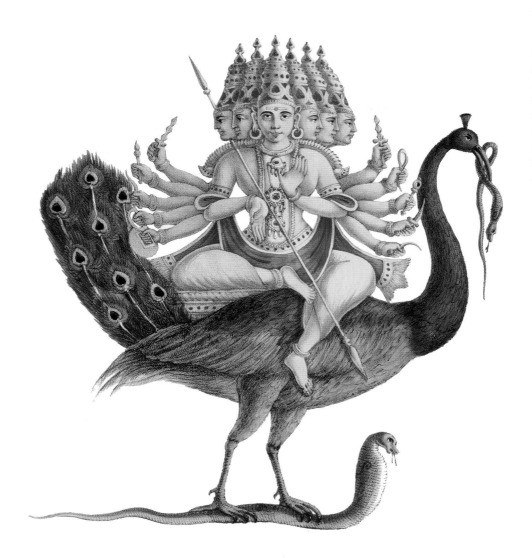

Mythology

Jung believed that myths could also reveal the workings of the collective unconscious, as he considered these sacred stories to be the voices of our ancestors and, consequently, our own inner voice. Through myth we can reconnect to the universal nature of ourselves. No matter how separate we believe ourselves to be as individuals, Jung held that mythology reveals an underlying thread that weaves us into a tapestry of wholeness that is both the collective unconscious and the individual.

Jung identified powerful archetypes present in myths from all cultures. For example, there are father-figure types who can be both nurturing and destructive, such as the Hindu god Shiva and the ruthless Greek god Kronos, who prevents his children from overthrowing him by eating them alive. The mother too is a powerful archetype and is represented in goddesses such as Demeter, who was so overcome with sorrow at the abduction of her daughter, Persephone, that she caused the earth to become barren and unproductive. This myth encapsulates many ideas about the mother role, such as love and protection as well as vengeful destruction.

American writer and professor Joseph Campbell (1904–1987) was strongly influenced by Jung's views on archetypes and myth. Campbell believed that world mythology and religion embodied universal truths that could be uncovered by comparison. In his book *The Hero with a Thousand Faces*, published in 1949, he developed the idea of the monomyth, a basic mythic pattern that encapsulates transcendent truths about the human experience. He argued that the stories of Osiris, Prometheus, Moses, Buddha and Christ all follow the same archetypal pattern and embody the concept of a hero taking up a quest in order to improve the world.

Archetypal psychology

Psychologist James Hillman further developed Jung's ideas to formulate 'archetypal psychology'. This focuses on the soul or psyche, which Hillman believes has been ignored by 20th-century psychology. Hillman has attempted to restore the 'soul' or 'psyche' to what he considers to be its proper place in psychology. His theory, argued in his book *The Soul's Code*, published in 1997, is that we all contain a unique potential for growth, irrespective of our childhood experiences or path in later life. It is up to each individual to reconnect with the soul in order to achieve all that we can be. Hillman sees the soul at work in myth, the imagination and fantasy, and he believes that the multiple gods and goddesses of mythology reveal the myriad aspects of the psyche. For Hillman: 'Psychology shows myths in modern dress and myths show our depth psychology in ancient dress.'

DREAMS AND DREAM ANALYSIS

If you are interested in **Dreams and Dream Analysis**, you may also like to read about:
- **Uncovering the Unconscious**, pages 18–19
- **The Collective Unconscious**, pages 20–21
- **Creative Visualization and Guided Imagery**, page 33
- **Native American Spirituality**, pages 232–233
- **Exceptional Human Experiences**, pages 48–49

A dream is defined as a sequence of sensations, whether mental, visual, aural, imagery, feelings or emotions, occurring during sleep. Of **universal importance**, dreams have been viewed by many cultures as spiritual messages from a divine source. However, during the 20th century dream interpretation was revolutionized by the publication of Freud's *The Interpretation of Dreams* and **Jung's dream theories**, and **contemporary theories** have helped to shed further light on the nature of dreams.

Universal importance

Virtually all cultures have accorded great importance to dreams. The Bible records Joseph's abilities to interpret dreams, while in ancient Greece pilgrims slept at special 'dream' temples in order to incubate a divinely inspired dream. A similar concept was practised by Native Americans in the form of the vision quest where, to mark their path to adulthood, adolescent boys went to a specific site to gain a powerful vision. Their vision was considered to provide guidance on their future direction in life.

The Interpretation of Dreams

Freud's hugely significant work, *The Interpretation of Dreams*, published c. 1900, marked a turning point in psychoanalysis. Freud gave enormous weight to the significance of dreams. He described them 'as the royal road to the understanding of unconscious mental processes' and believed that they revealed the deepest wishes and desires of an individual, desires that might often be rejected by the waking mind. Freud held that dreams allowed these secret wishes to be expressed in a disguised form. He believed that through the technique of 'free association', where an individual is asked to discuss with his or her therapist ideas, feelings or images that come to mind from the dream, the true or hidden meaning could be revealed.

Jung's dream theories

Jung took a more mystical approach to dreams and considered that they reflected the complexity of the entire personal and collective unconscious. He believed that archetypes, such as the 'shadow self', 'hero' and 'warrior', manifested as people or dream symbols and that 'great' or profound dreams come from the deepest level of the collective unconscious, embodying universal ideas. However, Jung also recognized that there could be more personal dreams reflecting the dreamer's unique experience and situation and that dreams should be explored in relation to the client's issues. Rather than embodying wish fulfilment, Jung believed that dreams could help us towards greater psychological health. He postulated that dreams might point

the way or even correct an individual's attitudes, providing balance between conscious and unconscious beliefs.

German psychoanalyst Fritz Perls (1893–1970) expanded on Jung's idea that every character in the dream represents some aspect of the dreamer. He believed that inanimate objects were representative of the dreamer too and are projections of the self that have been repressed or denied.

Contemporary theories

Research from the second half of the 20th century has helped us better understand the nature of dreaming. The rapid eye movement (REM) phase of sleep was discovered by Nathaniel Kleitman (1895–1999) and Eugene Aserinsky (1921–1998) in 1953 at the University of Chicago, USA, and it is generally agreed that this is the phase of sleep when vivid dreaming occurs. Dreaming also occurs during non-REM sleep, and experiments indicate that dreams experienced during this period tend to be verbal, ruminative or intellectual dreams.

Research also suggests that dreaming is vital for our health. Sleep researcher William C. Dement studied dream deprivation in the 1950s and found that subjects deprived of REM sleep would rapidly return to REM sleep when woken from it, and their periods of REM sleep were much longer when they were once more allowed to sleep normally. This suggests that REM sleep and, by implication, dreaming, are vital to our healthy functioning. Later researchers questioned these findings and pointed out the difficulty of distinguishing the effects of sleep deprivation from dream deprivation.

The question of why we dream is open to debate. Neurologist Hughlings Jackson (1835–1911) proposed that dreaming allows us to file the previous day's memories and experiences into those that are unimportant and those of significance. Other researchers suggest that dreams allow the dreamer to make connections between past and present events and act like psychotherapy, or that dreams complete the pattern of an emotional expectation and reduce stress. American dream researcher Calvin S. Hall (1909–1985) considered the dream to be a series of visual representations of

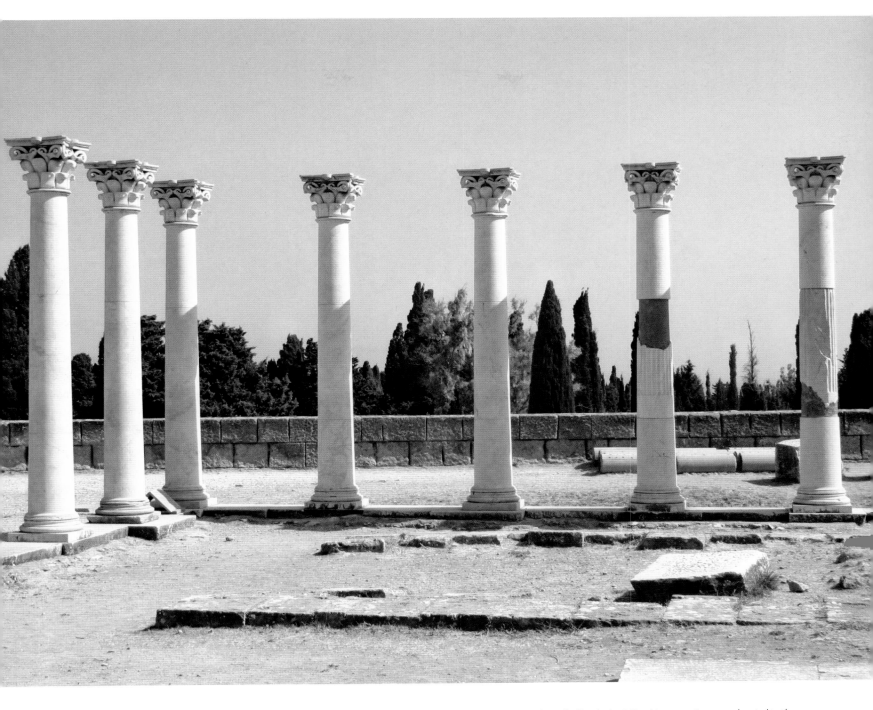

many different thoughts in a sequence that is entirely random but contains metaphors for deeper issues.

Recently, researchers such as William Domhoff at the University of California, Santa Cruz, USA, proposed the 'continuity hypothesis', which suggests that the content of dreams is not remote from our waking reality, but simply continues to display the prominent themes and concerns of the individual as they evolve or change during his or her life. Recurring dreams are frequent dreams that convey the same themes and are common to most people across cultural differences. They include dreams of falling, being chased, flying and sexual dreams.

Asclepion *Healing temples called 'asclepion', like this one on Kos, were devoted to the Greek god of medicine, Asclepius, and were set up for pilgrims to retell their dreams to a priest, who then prescribed them a cure. This is where Hippocrates received his training.*

Lucid dreaming

Lucid dreams, now classed as exceptional human experiences, are dreams in which the individual is aware that he or she is dreaming and can influence the course of the dream, including changing location. Many begin as 'flying dreams', linked to out-of-body experiences. People often describe lucid dreams as being profoundly healing or as providing solutions to problems.

PSYCHOLOGICAL TYPES

If you are interested in **Psychological Types**, you may also like to read about:
- **Western Astrology,** pages 56–57
- **Numerology,** pages 66–67
- **Palmistry,** pages 68–69
- **Ayurveda,** pages 94–97

Analysing personality or character is another aspect of studying the mind. In 340 BCE Plato outlined four character profiles – artistic, sensible, intuitive and reasoning – while the 20th-century philosopher Erich Fromm (1900–1980) described four human orientations – exploitive, hoarding, receptive and marketing. Today **Jung's psychological types**, the **Myers-Briggs Type Indicator** and the current renewed interest in the **Enneagram** are among the most popular tools for understanding personality.

Jung's psychological types

In 1921 Carl Jung published his findings on psychological types. Jung argued that our personalities can be categorized according to the way we deal with the world – how we function – and our attitude. He theorized that there are two key types of attitude: either introverted or extraverted. Introverts are inward-looking, reflective and private, while extraverts are objective, curious and want to engage with the environment. Jung believed that everyone possesses both attitudes, with the unexpressed attitude being hidden in the unconscious and often being its prime motivating force.

In terms of the way we deal with the world, Jung stated that there were four basic functions: sensing, intuiting, thinking and feeling. Sensing describes people who prefer to gather information by means of the five senses, trusting what can be measured and documented. Intuiting types prefer to trust their own intuition and tend to read between the lines and value imagination. Thinkers focus on objectivity and analysis, while feelers make decisions on how much they care about an issue or whether they feel it is right.

Jung concluded that every individual uses all four functions, but each one of us will have a preference for a function that we use most frequently. This is described as the dominant function. Combining function preferences with attitudes produces Jung's eight psychological types: extravert sensing, extravert intuiting, extravert thinking, extravert feeling, introvert sensing, introvert intuiting, introvert thinking and introvert feeling.

Myers-Briggs Type Indicator

Based on Jung's original eight psychological types, the Myers-Briggs Type Indicator (MBTI) was first developed by Katharine Cook Briggs (1875–1968) and her daughter Isabel Briggs Myers (1897–1980) during the 1940s in order to help women decide which jobs they would best be suited to during the Second World War.

The MBTI adds two more possibilities to the personality equation: judgment and perception. The judgment/perception pair define how an individual deals with the world. Judgment types are cautious, decisive and

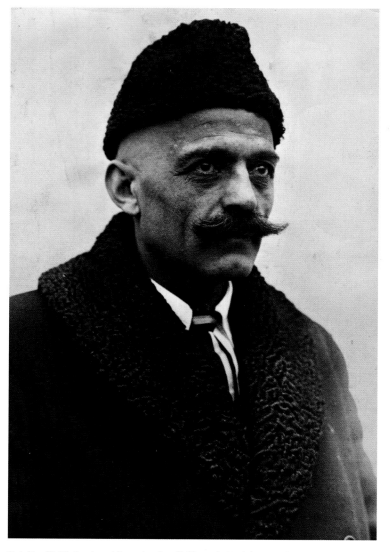

G. I. Gurdjieff *Russian philosopher Gurdjieff popularized the use of Enneagrams through his teaching of 'the Fourth Way', a personality transformation exercise.*

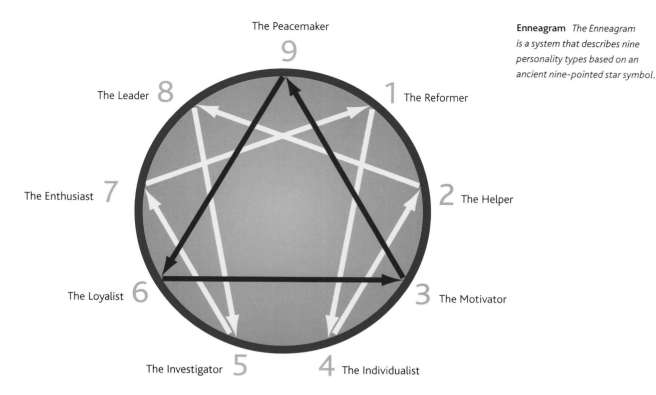

The Peacemaker
9

The Leader 8

1 The Reformer

The Enthusiast 7

2 The Helper

The Loyalist 6

3 The Motivator

The Investigator 5

4 The Individualist

Enneagram *The Enneagram is a system that describes nine personality types based on an ancient nine-pointed star symbol.*

organized; perceptive types are curious, adaptable and open. Adding these elements to Jung's personality types created a total of 16 possible types.

The MBTI questionnaire to determine personality type was first published and made available to the public in 1962. It is still used today to measure psychological preferences in marketing, career counselling, life coaching, marriage counselling, leadership and executive training. The European version is comprised of 88 forced-choice questions, with a choice of only two possible answers, and the USA version has 93 questions.

The Enneagram

Also known as the Enneagram of Personality, the Enneagram is a system that describes nine personality types based on an ancient nine-pointed star symbol. The term derives from the Greek words, *ennea*, meaning 'nine', and *gammon*, meaning 'writ' or 'draft'. The Enneagram also includes the interrelationships between the main personality types numbered between one and nine, and the other facets of the personality connected by the nine points. The Enneagram first came to light in the 1930s when Greek-Armenian mystic G. I. Gurdjieff (c. 1866–1949) began his personality transformation teachings called 'the Fourth Way'. However, it was the Bolivian-born Oscar Ichazo and the Chilean psychiatrist Claudio Naranjo who were really responsible for developing the Enneagram as a personality-type indicator.

Each of the nine personality types is assigned various traits or patterns of behaviour, rather like the 12 signs of the zodiac. With knowledge of where one's primary attention is focused, the Enneagram reveals how the individual can develop a more positive sense of self and become more self-aware and conscious of his or her choices. It is often used as a tool for spiritual development in psychology, psychotherapy, career coaching, education and

business training. A questionnaire is usually carried out to determine the basic personality number, followed by further self-questioning tests to indicate other personality traits which need conscious development.

The Enneagram's personality types
One the Reformer: critical, judgmental, perfectionist, moral
Two the Helper: caring, generous, needy, but competent
Three the Motivator: approval seeker, needing recognition, but industrious
Four the Individualist: emotional, sensitive, artistic
Five the Investigator: objective, calm, knowledgeable
Six the Loyalist: vigilant, fearful, intuitive
Seven the Enthusiast: fun-loving, adventurous, noncommittal
Eight the Leader: dominant, protective, intense
Nine the Peacemaker: compassionate, lacking boundaries and making good mediators and diplomats.

The Enneagram then breaks down into three sub-divisions or 'triads': Feeling, Thinking and Instinctive. These triads make clear an individual's psychological orientation. The Feeling Triad, comprising the Helper, Motivator and Individualist, is oriented towards emotions and self-image; the Thinking Triad, comprising the Investigator, Loyalist and Enthusiast, is oriented towards thought processes and how to find security; and the Instinctive Triad, comprising the Leader, Peacemaker and Reformer, is oriented towards the instincts and how a person relates to the world.

The 'wings' are the two adjacent personality points on either side of the main personality and can colour the individual's main personality. The wing is the second side of an individual's personality, and the merging of the main personality with a wing creates a further 19 sub-types.

BEHAVIOURISM AND ATTACHMENT THEORY

If you are interested in **Behaviourism and Attachment Theory**, you may also like to read about:

● **Cognitive Behavioural Therapy and Mindfulness**, pages 28–29

Behaviourism became the dominant academic approach to psychology for much of the 20th century. The behaviourists sought to prove that human behaviour was controlled by the environment. **Attachment theory**, developed by John Bowlby, focuses on the importance of forming close attachment relationships in early life.

Behaviourism

American John Watson (1878–1958) proposed the concept of behaviourism in an article entitled *Psychology as the Behaviourist Views It*, first published in 1913. Watson had been inspired by the work of Russian psychologist Ivan Pavlov and his 1903 experiments on classical conditioning in dogs. Pavlov found that if he rang a bell just before feeding his laboratory dogs, over time the sound of the bell alone, without the presence of food, would be enough to cause the dogs to salivate. They had been 'conditioned' to expect food.

Pavlov's dogs *Russian psychologist Ivan Pavlov's famous animal experiments on psychological conditioning provided the basis for phobia research and created the term 'Pavlovian response'.*

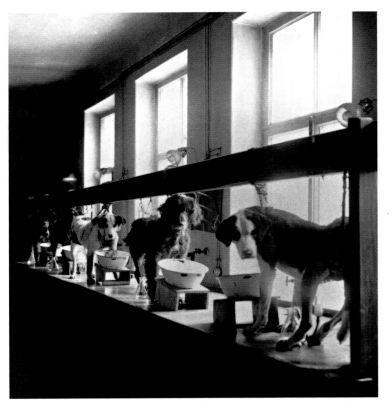

Pavlov applied the same principles to human learning: for example, a child bitten once by a dog might acquire a fear of all dogs and so develop a phobia. The phobia, it was theorized, could be overcome by a process of reverse conditioning, whereby the child was gradually exposed safely to dogs so that he or she learned that most dogs do not bite.

Behaviourism sought to prove that the individual is controlled by external stimuli and that the only measurement valid in psychology is that of observable behaviour. Thus any internal thought processes are irrelevant, as are emotions or subjective motives. Watson rejected all introspective methods such as Freud's psychoanalysis, and tried to restrict psychology to an empirical, reductionist methodology.

B. F. Skinner's (1904–1990) research on 'operant conditioning' made him one of the most influential psychologists of the middle of the 20th century. Operant conditioning describes behaviour that is determined by reinforcements, such as a 'reward' to strengthen behaviour or 'punishment' to weaken behaviour. Other notable behaviourists include Canadian Albert Bandura, who became famous during the early 1960s for his Bobo doll experiment to prove that behaviour in children is learned through imitation. This experiment revealed that children who watched an aggressive adult hit a doll tended to mimic that behaviour and subsequently develop aggressive behaviour themselves.

Attachment theory

Child psychiatrist John Bowlby (1907–1990) formulated attachment theory in the late 1950s and early 1960s. Its principal concept is that humans are biologically hard-wired to form and maintain attachment relationships with the person who is primarily caring for them. These attachments are formed most easily when the child is between three months and three years old and form the basis of intense emotional experiences. Bowlby argued: 'No variables have more far-reaching effects on personality development than a child's experiences within the family.' He believed that insecure or anxious forms of attachment could have lasting effects on a child's ability to form happy and stable relationships throughout his or her life. Attachment theory remains highly influential in contemporary psychology.

HUMANISTIC PSYCHOLOGY

Arising in response to behaviourism, humanistic psychologists refocused psychology away from studying behaviour towards an analysis of the whole person. Humanistic psychology holds that the individual has free will to make choices, and considers personal growth and fulfilment to be a basic human motivation. At the forefront of the Humanistic School of Psychology were Americans **Abraham Maslow** and **Carl Rogers**.

If you are interested in **Humanistic Psychology**, you may also like to read about:
- Neuro-Linguistic Programming, page 31
- Cognitive Behavioural Therapy and Mindfulness, pages 28–29
- Uncovering the Unconscious, pages 18–19
- The Collective Unconscious, pages 20–21

Abraham Maslow

In 1943 Abraham Maslow (1908–1970) published his highly influential paper *A Theory of Human Motivation*. He theorized that people are motivated to seek personal growth and transformation, a process he called self-actualization. He defined a self-actualized person as follows: 'If one expects nothing, if one has no anticipations or apprehensions, if in a sense there is no future... There can be no surprise, no disappointment... and no prediction means no worry, no anxiety, no apprehension, no foreboding.'

Maslow studied individuals that he considered self-actualized, including Albert Einstein, Abraham Lincoln and Walt Whitman, and from their life stories identified 15 needs that had to be met in order for a person to achieve self-actualization. The hierarchy of needs was arranged as a pyramid, moving from the primary needs at the bottom upwards.

Maslow believed that everyone could climb the pyramid and self-actualize, but life experiences such as job losses or marriage break-ups would disrupt this growth. The top two layers were 'being' or growth needs, and led to the individual 'becoming everything one is capable of becoming'. Later, in 1962, Maslow commented that an individual is always in a process of 'becoming' throughout life.

Carl Rogers

Concurring with Maslow's emphasis on personal growth, Carl Rogers (1902–1987) developed what became known as client-centred therapy, where the therapist enters into a more personal relationship with his or her client rather than the traditional doctor/patient model. Rogers believed that behaviour is not simply a function of responding to external reality but arises from the individual's unique personal experience, shaped by the individual's own world view. The therapist's role, as he saw it, was to try and empathize with his or her client in order to better understand their world-view. Rogers identified the importance of the regard of others and self-regard in achieving happiness and personal growth; he was therefore one of the first therapists to recognize the significance of self-esteem.

Maslow's pyramid *Abraham Maslow designed this pyramid to illustrate the needs that have to be met in order for a person to achieve self-actualization.*

SELF-ACTUALIZATION — *Realization of one's potential, seeking of personal growth and self-knowledge, creativity, lack of prejudice, spontaneity, problem solving*

AESTHETIC NEEDS — *Beauty in nature and art, balance, harmony, order*

COGNITIVE NEEDS — *Knowledge, curiosity, sense of meaning, exploration*

ESTEEM NEEDS — *Esteem of others, mastery, self-acceptance, self-esteem*

LOVE AND BELONGINGNESS NEEDS — *Intimacy, affection, trust, acceptance*

SAFETY NEEDS — *Security, law, stability, protection from the elements*

PHYSIOLOGICAL NEEDS — *Food, sex, oxygen, rest*

COGNITIVE BEHAVIOURAL THERAPY AND MINDFULNESS

Rational emotive behavioural therapy, pioneered by Albert Ellis in the 1950s, was based on the assumption that undesirable behaviour, such as anxiety or severe depression, is caused by abnormal thinking processes. A similar approach developed a decade later.

Cognitive behavioural therapy (CBT) combines techniques for changing people's behaviour (behavioural therapy) with a recognition of the importance of an individual's style of thinking in affecting their emotions. In recent years many CBT therapists have become interested in **mindfulness**, an approach derived from Eastern traditions.

If you are interested in **Cognitive Behavioural Therapy and Mindfulness**, you may also like to read about:
● **Buddhism**, pages 208–209
● **Meditation**, pages 78–79
● **Psychological Types**, pages 24–25

Rational emotive behavioural therapy

American psychologist Albert Ellis (1913–2007) theorized that we all have specific assumptions unique to us as individuals. However, some people develop irrational assumptions and then react in irrational ways, thus limiting their chance of success or happiness. For example, irrational assumptions could include: 'I should be competent at everything'; 'I should be loved by everyone'; 'If life isn't how I want it to be, then it's a disaster'. Ellis used a technique known as the ABC Technique of Rational Beliefs, designed to help people reach a more reasonable belief about their experiences. In this system 'A' represents the activating agent or event that causes anxious or depressed thoughts, 'B' is the person's belief that arises from the event and 'C' is the consequence of these thoughts or beliefs. So if John, for example, is miserable because he failed his driving test, then the activating event is the failed driving test, the belief is that to fail means that John is useless/unworthy/ not good enough and the consequence is that he feels he has let himself or something/someone down. The therapist then 'reframes' the irrational belief so that John can see that failing the driving test does not 'prove' he is unworthy or useless. Rather it is his assumption or belief that needs to be addressed and changed to a positive belief.

Cognitive behavioural therapy

Aaron T. Beck's cognitive behavioural therapy, developed in the 1960s, is more therapeutic in approach than Ellis's rather harsh, teacher-like stance with the client. CBT also uses behavioural techniques to bring about practical changes in a person's daily life.

In CBT people are encouraged first to become aware of their negative thoughts and then to challenge them with more positive thoughts. At the same time they are encouraged to change their behaviour, which might also

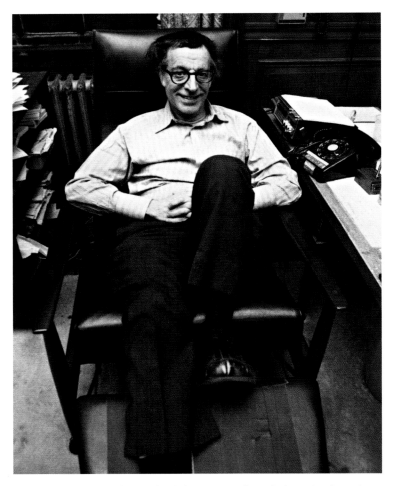

Albert Ellis *Seen here reclining at his desk in 1970, Dr Ellis worked on rational emotive behavioural therapy and the ideas of irrational assumptions, paving the way for CBT.*

be contributing to a negative cycle of unhappiness or distress. So, for example, a person who suffers social anxiety and shyness might be encouraged to attend a party in order to make a change to their usual, more retiring behaviour; at the same time they would be encouraged to challenge their negative thoughts and expectations about how they might behave at the party and how people will react towards them. Clients are asked to keep diaries to record their own thoughts, feelings and behaviour in order to monitor ways in which their negative thinking affects their emotional state, which might in turn affect their behaviour negatively. The challenge is to break the negative cycle of unhappy thoughts leading to negative feelings, leading to behaviour that might cause unhappy thoughts.

CBT has been used successfully in treating depression, addictions, mood disorders and other panic and anxiety disorders.

Mindfulness

Modern psychology has increasingly become interested in many ancient approaches to wellbeing in order to help people in a therapeutic setting. Recently the Buddhist practice of mindfulness or Sati has been taught as a technique to overcome depression and anxiety.

Mindfulness is described as being aware of the present moment and paying attention to the here and now. In fact it is a practice of 'self-awareness' and a realization that one's thoughts are simply thoughts, one's sensations simply sensations, and an understanding that we are not merely our thoughts or sensations. In this way it is similar to CBT's challenge to question negative thoughts and feelings. Mindfulness observes negative thoughts without any self-criticism, judgment or emotional investment in those thoughts. If we pay attention to the moment, we do not get caught up in the past or future. Instead of dwelling on what has been or worrying about what will be, we can see these thoughts for being only that, thoughts.

Through mindfulness the individual can release any attachment, particularly to negative agendas and repeating patterns of assumptions and scripts. Once we observe the many narratives going on in our head, even when walking or running, washing the dishes or waiting for a bus, then we are free to disassociate from these judgmental perceptions. If an individual chooses to be in a mindful state, there is a realization in that choice that you are more than your thoughts. For example, while waiting for a bus, you might be thinking, 'Why won't it hurry up? I'm bored waiting, I should have gone in the car, what will they say at the office if I'm late?' These are all judgmental perceptions of the event or experience.

Mindfulness is to go beyond those running commentaries or thought sequences and see them for what they are, simply thoughts. It has been proved to help clients with depression so that they can see more clearly the patterns of the mind, learn to recognize negative thinking and work on attending to the moment rather than worrying about the future or the past. It has also been a key component in Gestalt therapy, where it is known as self-awareness, and is often used as a psychotherapeutic tool in cognitive behaviour therapy, acceptance and commitment therapy, dialectical behaviour therapy and stress management.

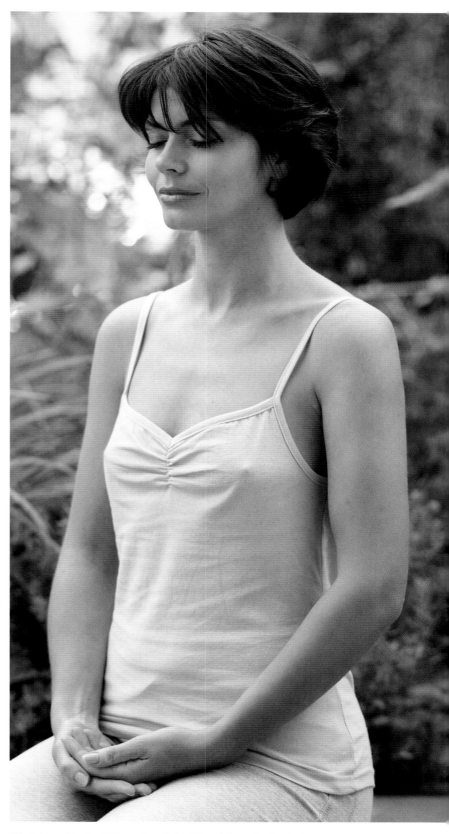

Mindfulness *The Buddhist practice of mindfulness brings attention to the present moment and can be useful for combating negative thoughts, which can lead to anxiety, depression and other psychological problems.*

HYPNOTHERAPY

If you are interested in **Hypnotherapy**, you may also like to read about:
● **Meditation**, pages 78–79
● **Creative Visualization and Guided Imagery**, page 33
● **Neuro-Linguistic Programming**, page 31
● **Past Lives and Past-Life Therapies**, pages 50–51

In **hypnotherapy** clients are guided into a state of focused relaxation to help with stress and emotional or behavioural problems. Under **hypnosis** the mind is brought into an **altered state of consciousness** that helps the client access deeper levels of awareness and become more open to beneficial suggestions.

Undergoing hynopsis

A hypnotherapist begins by helping the client enter the hypnotic state, a process called hypnotic induction. This may involve asking the client to relax by closing their eyes and breathing deeply or focusing their attention on a particular image. As the client begins to enter a state of deep relaxation, the therapist will begin to make positive suggestions about changes in behaviour or attitudes, or will explore the causes of difficulties. Therapists may treat a range of problems from stress to help with quitting smoking. Some individuals are found to be more 'suggestible' than others, meaning that they enter the hypnotic state more easily. However, an increasing body of research indicates that a wide range of people can benefit from hypnotherapy.

The development of hypnotherapy

In 1843 the Scottish neurosurgeon James Braid (1795–1860) coined the term neuro-hypnotism (sleep of the nervous system) after studying 'mesmerism',

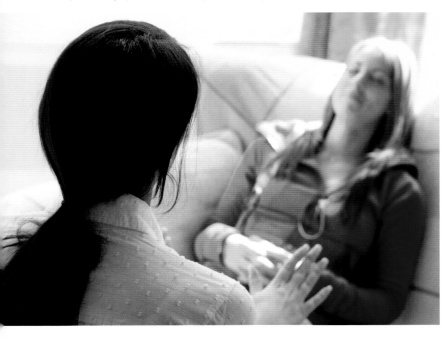

Hypnotherapy *Hypnosis is now almost universally acknowledged as a positive treatment for a variety of ailments including stress, anxiety and a number of addictions.*

a form of therapy in which the subject was induced into a trance-like state. Although mesmerists claimed that their results were based on the effects of what they termed 'animal magnetism', Braid observed that the subjects were in a different state from normal consciousness or real sleep. His work subsequently influenced a French doctor, Ambroise-Auguste Liébeault (1823–1904), who along with French neurologist Hippolyte Bernheim (1840–1919) established the Nancy School of Psychotherapy. Liébeault was later acknowledged as the founder of hypnotherapy. Visitors to the school included Sigmund Freud and Emile Coué (1857–1926), a notable French psychologist who introduced a self-improvement therapy called 'optimistic autosuggestion' which was popular in the 1920s.

One of the most notable and influential contemporary hypnotherapists was the American psychiatrist Milton Erickson (1901–1980). Erickson had great faith in the creative powers of the unconscious mind and believed that hypnosis was an important tool for working with the unconscious. His view was that we all slip into trance or hypnotic states readily and frequently throughout the day, for example while waiting for a bus or gazing out of a window. Erickson developed an indirect form of hypnosis where he encouraged the client to choose to enter a trance-like state. He also believed that authoritarian suggestions would be rejected by the client and encouraged 'artfully vague' suggestions that the client's unconscious mind could shape to his or her own needs.

Altered state of consciousness

There has been much debate as to the nature of the hypnotic state. Although many people believe that under hypnosis an individual accesses the unconscious mind, the latest research argues that the hypnotic state is a calm, relaxed, yet alert state of focused attention, free from external distractions. However, these two viewpoints are not mutually exclusive. In many ways this state seems similar to the meditative state where the mind is alert, yet calm. Recently researchers at Imperial College, London, have measured the brain activity of individuals under hypnosis using magnetic resource imaging (MRI) scans. The team found that highly suggestible individuals showed significant brain activity in the area of the brain responsible for detecting and responding to errors and evaluating emotional outcomes, as well as higher-level cognitive processing.

NEURO-LINGUISTIC PROGRAMMING

If you are interested in **Neuro-Linguistic Programming**, you may also like to read about:
- **Uncovering the Unconscious**, pages 18–19
- **Psychological Types**, pages 24–25
- **Hypnotherapy**, page 30

Nowadays referred to simply as NLP, neuro-linguistic programming is the practice of understanding how each individual organizes their thinking, behaviour and language into their own **mental map**. NLP enables an individual, group or even corporation to follow a method that **models** the effectiveness of experts in their chosen field.

Mental maps

Pioneered by John Grinder and Richard Bandler at the University of California, Santa Cruz, USA, in the early 1970s, NLP grew out of their curiosity as to why certain people are geniuses or good at what they do. The key concept behind NLP is that we all form internal mental maps of the world, and each map is unique to the individual. Our maps are formed by the way we take in information from the world around us, using our five senses. Some people have a preference for processing information visually, while others are more focused on processing information via touch or the kinesthetic sense, for instance. We make sense of our world via the language we use and this also gives clues as to how we prefer to take in information. For example, a person who uses a lot of 'touch' metaphors, such as 'I can't get a grip on that' or 'I need to get a handle on this', might have a preference for perceiving the world kinesthetically. By observing a person's preferences for how they process information we can learn to communicate more effectively.

Modelling

In NLP terms, this is the process of replicating the language and behaviour of someone who excels at any given activity. Grinder and Bandler studied the Gestalt therapist Fritz Perls, the family systems therapist Virginia Satir (1916–1988) and the psychiatrist-hypnotherapist Milton Erickson, all working in the therapy field and, as such, agents of change. NLP practitioners consider themselves to be likewise agents of change. The modellers, Grinder and Bandler, selected aspects of the behaviour and language of the three 'geniuses' and coded this information into language-based models, such as the Milton Model based on Erickson's approach and the Meta Model based on the approach of Perls and Satir. The Milton Model entails building rapport with another person by the use of 'artfully vague' terms, distracting the conscious mind and accessing unconscious resources; the Meta Model by contrast aims to identify deletions, distortions and generalizations in the language people use in order to clarify meaning.

People's subjective experience is integral to NLP. As each person's reality is unique to them, so the NLP practitioner must work with that person's sense of reality. NLP practitioners believe that people have the means necessary for change, whether consciously or unconsciously, and the mind is willing to change, or improve itself, once it knows how.

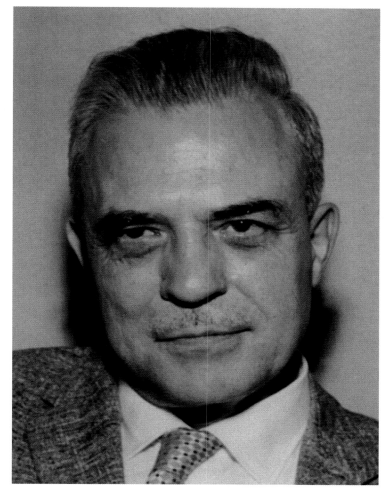

Milton Erickson *This picture, taken in 1965, shows US psychiatrist and hypnotherapist Milton Erickson. NLP's Milton Model was based on his language and behaviour.*

Currently NLP is a lucrative business; there are numerous workshops, teachers, books and exercises, but there are also different standards of training and considerable disagreement among practitioners as to which models are correct and which are not. NLP can be applied in many diverse fields, whether business, corporate, leadership, education, marketing or personal development.

PSYCHOSYNTHESIS

If you are interested in **Psychosynthesis**, you may also like to read about:
- Humanistic Psychology, page 27
- Creative Visualization and Guided Imagery, page 33
- Cognitive Behavourial Therapy and Mindfulness, pages 28–29

Psychosynthesis was founded by Italian psychiatrist **Roberto Assagioli** (1888–1974) in the early part of the 20th century. Psychosynthesis aims to heal and integrate all aspects of the human experience, from early traumas through to issues of identity and purpose, emphasizing the achievement of **self-realization** and contact with the **superconsciousness** or higher consciousness.

Roberto Assagioli

Assagioli originally trained as a psychoanalyst and was a contemporary of both Freud and Jung. Although he recognized the importance of uncovering past trauma, he believed that psychoanalysis failed to acknowledge the significance of the spiritual realm or what is now usually referred to as the 'transpersonal' in an individual's growth to happiness. He believed that this missing realm includes inspiration, love, wisdom and spiritual belief. He considered that psychoanalysis delved into the 'basement' of the psyche, while psychosynthesis looked after the whole of the psyche's 'building'.

Self-realization

Today psychosynthesis is understood more as a general approach to understanding ourselves rather than as a therapy that employs specific techniques to achieve its goals. Consequently, a wide range of methods can be used by practitioners to assist this personal growth and integration, including dreamwork, visualization, art therapy and drama therapy as well as approaches from cognitive behavioural therapy (CBT) and family therapy. It is recognized that each client has individual needs and that the techniques used should reflect the individual's preferences and interests. Unlike other 'therapies', psychosynthesis has no premise as to what someone 'should' be like. Rather we become who we are or wish to be. As a form of transpersonal psychology, psychosynthesis helps with the crisis of meaning that is so common in Western culture. It works on the healing of these crises by harmony and synthesis of the self.

If psychoanalysis is 'separation of something into its different parts to understand its nature and function', psychosynthesis goes further and puts these parts back more harmoniously to create an integrated whole. Therefore psychosynthesis is a holistic therapy that includes physical, mental, emotional and spiritual wellbeing.

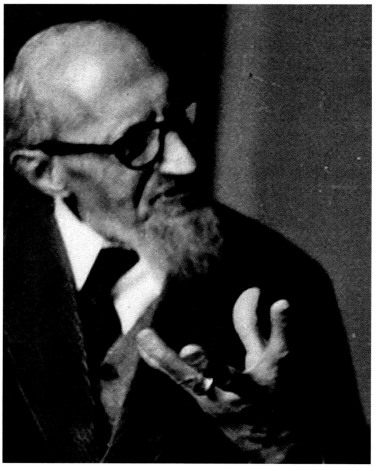

Roberto Assagioli *Italian Roberto Assagioli developed psychosynthesis in the early part of the 20th century as a comprehensive approach to self-realization and to help people discover their spiritual nature.*

The superconscious

One of the most important aspects of psychosynthesis is its identification of the superconscious or higher consciousness. Assagioli believed that this is a realm where all our finest impulses originate – artistic and spiritual insights, altruism and humanitarian acts, and a sense of meaning and purpose. He held that repression of this aspect of our identity is just as harmful as repression of past trauma. Many techniques in psychosynthesis aim to make contact with the higher consciousness and access its wisdom.

CREATIVE VISUALIZATION AND GUIDED IMAGERY

Creative visualization, also known as guided imagery, uses the **mind's power** to visualize scenes and experiences in order to bring about positive changes in thoughts and feelings.

Visualization techniques and guided imagery aim to encourage the individual to focus on positive images in order to bring about healing and as an aid to relaxation.

If you are interested in **Creative Visualization and Guided Imagery**, you may also like to read about:
- **Past Lives and Past-Life Therapies**, pages 50–51
- **Meditation**, pages 78–79
- **Buddhism**, pages 208–209
- **Psychoneuroimmunology**, pages 76–77
- **Hypnotherapy**, page 30
- **Colour Therapy**, page 162

The mind's power

The power of visualization is believed to relate to the fact that we use mental images to make sense of our world long before we can use words. Images are therefore viewed by many psychotherapists as being at the heart of our unconscious mind. Images shape our view of who we think we are and what we believe we deserve, and so actively developing positive imagery can work powerfully with our unconscious mind to bring about change.

Clinical observations have shown that the mind often finds it difficult to distinguish between actual events and events taking place in the imagination. In experiments, individuals asked to remember a traumatic event have been seen to experience physiological symptoms such as increased pulse rate, perspiration and raised blood pressure, which all suggest that the mind is signalling to the body that there is real danger physically present. These observations seem to indicate that evoking calming or healing images in the mind would have a correspondingly calming and healing effect on the body. Visualization and guided imagery have rapidly grown in popularity for the treatment of a range of common ailments and problems. These include stress reduction, pain management and coping with bereavement and grief.

Visualization techniques

When practising visualization the individual begins by entering a relaxed state, as this is considered to help the mind become more receptive to the imagery. He or she is then encouraged to enhance the power of visualization by involving all the senses in the creation of the image. For example, if the person is working on building a positive image for a forthcoming meeting, he or she would try to imagine the smell of the room, the feel of the chair and any relevant sounds to make the image as powerful in their mind's eye as possible. Once the scene is fully imagined, they may be asked to rerun it in their mind, bringing in positive elements and their desired outcome.

Visualization *Visualization techniques involve the participation of all the senses, whether the colour of the sky, the sound of lapping waves on a shore, or the smell of the sea.*

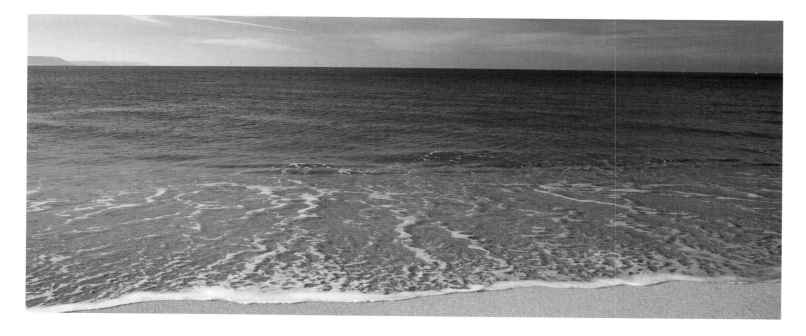

MYSTICAL AND TRANSCENDENT STATES

A mystical or transcendent state is a conscious awareness of another reality, or a sense of being at one with the universe, God or a spiritual truth. It is the goal of many **spiritual practices** including meditation and yoga. In the 1960s **Timothy Leary** introduced the West to the possibility of reaching altered states via hallucinogenic drugs.

If you are interested in **Mystical and Transcendent States**, you may also like to read about:
- **Western Mystery Traditions**, pages 184–185
- **Exceptional Human Experiences**, pages 48–49
- **Shamanism**, pages 226–227
- **Sufism**, pages 198–199
- **Hinduism**, pages 204–205
- **Tantra**, pages 214–215

The link between transcendence and religion

Transcendence means 'going beyond oneself' or 'outside of oneself'. A mystical experience is a state of self-transcendence in which the 'self' or 'ego' is left behind or abandoned. People may feel that they have become one with

Baba Ram Dass *This former Harvard researcher set up the Psilocybe Project with Timothy Leary to promote the use of hallucinogens.*

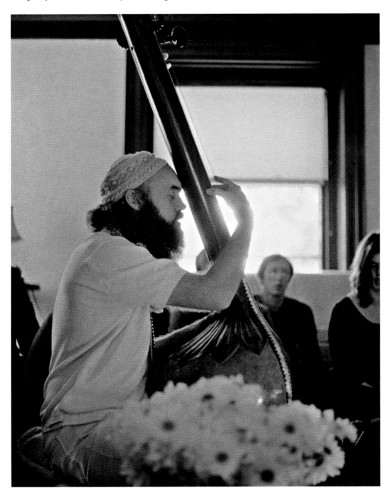

the universe or God. Everything is seen in a new perspective and may seem 'real' for the very first time.

Mystical states are common goals of religions, esoteric beliefs and spiritual practice, but they can be achieved or experienced in different ways. The term 'mysticism' derives from a Greek word *mystikos*, the name for an initiate of a mystery religion. Thus a mystical state is sometimes described as 'initiating the self into the divine'.

Mystical experiences and spiritual practices

In both Buddhism and Hinduism practices such as meditation aim eventually to achieve a transcendent state described as 'nirvana'. Nirvana is considered to be a state of mind free from craving, anger and suffering. The individual is in a state of perfect peace, free from the cycle of rebirths. Some traditions also believe that nirvana is linked to a radically altered state of consciousness where the individual is aware of the empty nature of phenomena and experiences a kind of 'luminous consciousness'. In the collection of sacred Buddhist texts known as the *Tipitaka*, the *Nibbana Sutta* or Nirvana Sutra defines the attributes of nirvana as follows:

> 'There is that dimension where there is neither earth, nor water, nor fire, nor wind; neither dimension of the infinitude of space, nor dimension of the infinitude of consciousness, nor dimension of nothingness, nor dimension of neither perception nor non-perception; neither this world, nor the next world, nor sun, nor moon. And there, I say, there is neither coming, nor going, nor stasis; neither passing away nor arising: without stance, without foundation, without support. This, just this, is the end of stress.' (translated by Thanissaro Bikkhu)

This state is similar to that described by mystics from other traditions. St Teresa of Avila (1515–1582) experienced periods of religious ecstasy, which she described in her autobiography. She reached the conclusion that there are four stages in the ascent of the soul, the final stage being 'the devotion of ecstasy or rapture'. In this state, which is described as a passive one, awareness of the physical body disappears, and memory, consciousness and the imagination are all united with God into a sense of unity or feeling of wholeness.

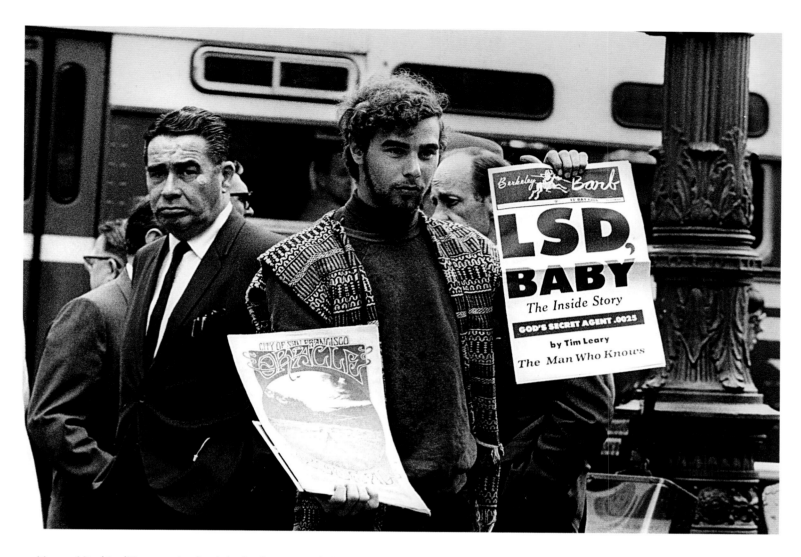

Many spiritual traditions use ritual to help the devotee reach this transcendent state. Chanting, meditation, silence and seclusion are common to many traditions. In Sufism the remembrance of Allah is performed in the form of the music and dance ceremony known as the *sema*. In this ceremony dervishes whirl in a circle around their sheikh, who in turn whirls within his own axis. In virtually all shamanic traditions, mystical states were attained through drumming or chanting, or by taking preparations of psychoactive plants. Within these cultures the taking of such preparations was strictly controlled as a ritualized experience. In the 20th century Western researchers became fascinated by the mind-altering properties of these substances.

Timothy Leary and psychedelics

The word 'psychedelic' was first coined by psychiatrist Humphrey Osmond (1917–2004) in 1957, but it became popularized by American writer and psychologist Timothy Leary (1920–1996) in the 1960s. In Leary's 1964 book *The Psychedelic Experience*, based upon the Tibetan Book of the Dead, he wrote: 'A psychedelic experience is a journey to new realms of consciousness... its characteristic features are the transcendence of verbal concepts, of space-time dimensions, and of the ego or identity.'

Psychedelic drugs *The mind-altering effects of drugs such as LSD were considered to be of spiritual value by advocates such as Timothy Leary and his followers in the 1960s.*

Leary argued that taking psychedelic drugs was a route to this new realm of consciousness. He first sampled *Psilocybe mexicana*, a psychedelic mushroom, during a visit to Mexico in 1960. His experiences convinced him that psychedelic drugs were of both spiritual and therapeutic value, and later that year he and Richard Alpert, subsequently known as Ram Dass, set up the Harvard Psilocybe Project to promote the use of mushrooms and other hallucinogens. Leary was dismissed from his lecturing post at Harvard University in 1963, but remained a key counterculture figure in the USA up until his death in 1996. In *The Psychedelic Experience* Leary makes it clear that drugs were not an end in themselves, but simply a key to another dimension of the mind, and he noted that other approaches such as yoga, meditation and religious devotion could also lead to this transcendent state.

Considerable research is now being undertaken into the effect of psychoactive (etheobotanic) plant substances, traditionally used by shamans, and endogenous (naturally occurring) neurochemicals in the brain and their links to mystical experiences and the multi-dimensions of consciousness.

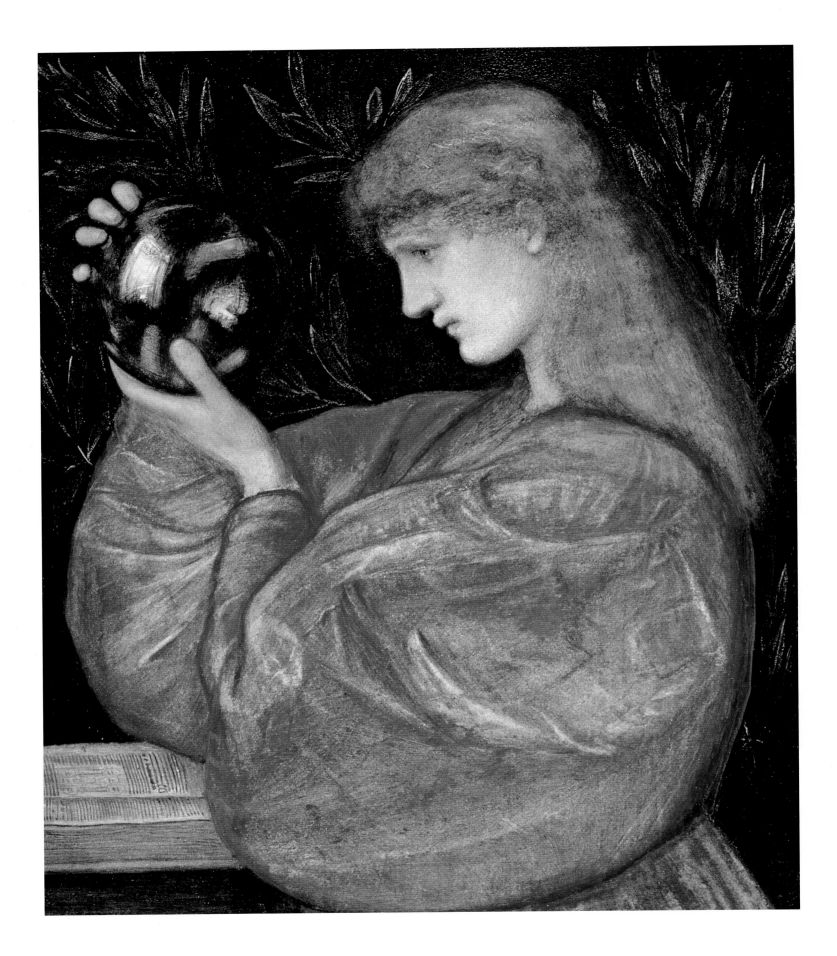

PSYCHIC SKILLS AND OTHER DIMENSIONS OF THE MIND

Psychology and its earlier antecedent, the philosophy of the mind, aimed to understand the mind through observation and experimentation. However, throughout history many disparate societies and cultures have also celebrated highly unusual mental abilities that, while difficult to test or measure, have always been accorded enormous respect. Astrologers, seers, prophets and shamans were all considered to possess an 'unknown power', and ancient Hindu texts describe in some detail *siddhis* – attainments or accomplishments of psychic abilities, including levitation, teleportation, telepathy and divination. Famous examples of individuals with special abilities of the mind include the priests of Ra in ancient Egypt; Pythia, the high priestess who presided over the oracle at Delphi; the French seer Nostradamus (1503–1566); and more recently the 20th-century American psychic Edgar Cayce (1877–1945). But just what were the abilities that these individuals possessed?

Psychic sense

Today the term 'psychic' has become an umbrella description for people possessing a wide range of skills, including clairvoyance, intuition, telepathy and channelling, and it may be applied to shamans as well. They are generally considered to be able to perceive things not normally perceptible by the five senses, unlock hidden knowledge and provide information on the state of others as well as themselves. Someone who is 'psychic' normally, but not necessarily, connects with the living rather than the dead, and this is generally considered to be the distinction between psychics and mediums. On the other hand, mediums and shamans, who receive messages and communicate with 'spirits' or those who have 'crossed over', can be psychic.

Einstein and relativity

How can we explain psychic phenomena? We know that Eastern traditions recognize a universal energy flowing in and through all life, described as 'chi'

Astrologia *This 19th-century Pre-Raphaelite painting by Sir Edward Burne-Jones shows a lady gazing into a crystal ball.*

or 'prana'. Modern physics has supported this concept, great scientists such as Albert Einstein (1879–1955) stating that all matter consists of energy. If this is so, it is suggested, the sensitive person can become aware of and tap into this universal energy or consciousness; they can access other people's energy fields and become sensitive to their thoughts and experiences beyond the restrictions of time and place. Furthermore, Einstein's Theory of Relativity also argued that space and time are not absolute concepts. Many people before Einstein had realized that an object in space can only be defined relative to some other object. Einstein, however, argued that time was also relative because light needs time to travel from an event to the observer. Normally this time is so short that we have the impression that events happen instantaneously, but this is in fact an illusion. Many laboratory experiments have been able to confirm that when particles are moving almost at the speed of light, time is relative. If space and time are relative, then perhaps modern physics – and particularly the quantum variety – provides a framework for understanding how a sensitive person might be able to see both past and future, as well as things at a physical distance from them. Psychics and mystics would simply say that consciousness is everywhere, there is no division and it can be accessed at any point.

Attainment

Eastern philosophers and sages have always had a concept of the relativity of space and time; they have argued that these concepts are creations of the mind and when our consciousness is expanded, the limitations of our view of reality are revealed. An ancient Buddhist text, *Madhyamika Karika Vritti*, states:

> *'It was taught by the Buddha, oh Monks, that the past, the future, physical space and the individuals are nothing but names, forms of thought, words of common usage, merely superficial realities.'*

Is it possible, then, for us all to attain psychic powers? A Hindu text describing the unique spiritual and psychic powers or *siddhis* provides an intriguing answer that is claimed to have come from Lord Krishna himself:

> *'For a sage who has conquered his senses, breathing and mind, who is self-controlled and always absorbed in meditation on Me, what siddhi could possibly be difficult to achieve?'*

INTUITION, PRECOGNITION AND PREMONITION

If you are interested in **Intuition, Precognition and Premonition**, you may also like to read about:
- **Psychic Skills**, pages 40–41
- **Uncovering the Unconscious**, pages 18–19
- **Dreams and Dream Analysis**, pages 22–23
- **The Tarot**, pages 62–63
- **Past Lives and Past-Life Therapies**, pages 50–51

Intuition describes an innate or instantaneous understanding of a situation, object or person beyond the powers of reasoning. Often used interchangeably with the term 'the sixth sense', intuition also includes the experiences of **premonition**, **precognition** and **déjà vu**. Einstein said, 'the only really valuable thing is the intuition'.

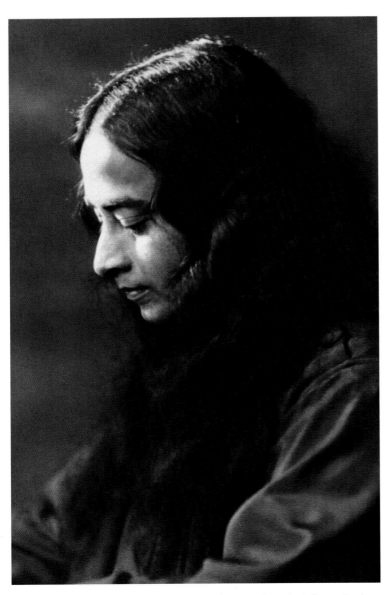

Paramahansa Yogananda *This photograph from the 1950s shows the Indian yogi and guru Paramahansa Yogananda, who taught his followers to listen to their intuition.*

Intuition

The word 'intuition' comes from the Latin *in* meaning 'at' or 'on' and *tueri*, 'to look at' or 'watch over'. Intuition can be defined as a sudden awareness of complete 'knowing' or 'certainty' about a person or situation that may occur almost instantly. How intuition actually manifests is a controversial subject. Experimental psychologists and neurologists explain it as a process involving the right side of the brain (see page 16), the hemisphere associated with visual and musical skills, creativity and feelings. When the right side of the brain processes events, it is argued, emotions are strongly involved and so the individual powerfully 'knows' that his or her behaviour or interpretation of an event 'must' be correct, beyond the bounds of ordinary reasoning. Yet however it manifests, intuition appears to 'watch over' us, as a deep, mysterious capacity for knowing.

Another explanation of intuition is that it makes an instant connection to our unconscious, tapping into what many New Age theorists describe as 'the universal storehouse of knowledge' or 'higher consciousness'. Alice Bailey (1880–1949), an early 20th-century esoteric writer, believed that intuition was an external divine power that is received by an individual and works through the individual.

However it manifests, intuition is universally recognized as a powerful force. Indian yogi and guru Paramahansa Yogananda (1893–1952) described intuition as: 'like a light, a flame of knowledge, that comes from the soul. It possesses all-sided power to know all there is to be known.' And Swiss psychiatrist Carl Jung (1875–1961) said: 'Intuition is that aspect of consciousness that allows us to see round corners.'

Sixth sense

Extra-sensory perception (ESP) is the ability to receive information by a sense other than the known five senses. ESP is also referred to as 'intuition', 'the sixth sense' and more popularly as 'a hunch', 'a feeling' or 'a gut instinct'. The term 'the sixth sense' was coined by Charles Richet (1850–1935), the Nobel Prize-winning French physiologist in his 1928 publication *Notre Sixième Sens*. He concluded that there must be a sixth sense sensitive to specific vibrations that none of the other senses could process. Most psychic skills such as

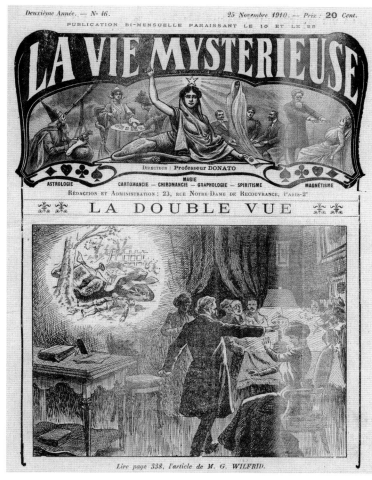

Clairvoyance *This publication reports how a French clairvoyant described a car accident involving her cousin while in a trance. It was later discoverd that this accident had actually occurred that night.*

precognition, clairvoyance and telepathy involve some kind of ESP, none of which has yet been explained by scientific means.

A great deal of research into ESP and intuition has been carried out by scientists and psychologists throughout the last century. In the 1930s, Joseph Rhine (1895–1980) and his wife Louisa developed psychic research into experimental psychology. To avoid associations with mediums, ghosts and spirits, they called it 'parapsychology'. Throughout the 1940s and 1950s, Rhine and other psychologists from Colorado University and Hunter College, New York, USA, carried out independent tests and experiments, and reported significant results to suggest that ESP is an identifiable phenomenon, but they could not actually explain how it occurs. Rhine insisted that further research was needed into unconscious processes and the human personality, a challenge that was taken up by researchers during the decades that followed and still continues today.

Precognition

Derived from a Latin word meaning 'foreknowledge', precognition describes the experience of direct knowledge of the future occurring mostly in dreams,

but also in waking visions or thoughts. It can be induced through channelling, divinational trance and mediumship. Precognition has been extensively studied by scientists throughout the 20th century. British aeronautics engineer J. W. Dunne (1875–1949) discovered through his own experiences and research that precognitive dreams are more common than we realize. One theory put forward to explain precognition is that psychokinetic energy is unleashed when the individual experiences precognition. This in turn sets off a chain reaction in the universe so that the foreseen event then happens.

Premonition

Often confused with precognition, premonition derives from the Latin word meaning 'a forewarning'. A premonition can be described as a warning that something is going to happen, but the individual does not know exactly what. The person cannot put a name to it, but has a gut feeling, usually while awake, of a future event or experience not to be welcomed. Psychologists suggest this is because we are more sensitive to things that make us feel anxious rather than happy. This, however, does not explain why or how we actually experience this 'forewarning'.

Déjà vu

This has been referred to as 'remembering the future'. A strangely paradoxical effect, the French phrase *déjà vu* means 'already seen', and was coined by French philosopher Emile Boirac (1851–1917), who was noted for his book on psychic research, *L'Avenir des Sciences Psychiques*, which was published in 1917. When experiencing déjà vu, the individual senses that he or she is either repeating something that has already happened or recognizes something about the moment as if witnessing themselves doing something a split second before doing it or reliving a familiar event from the distant past. It feels both familiar and yet strange, as if, in the paraphrased words of the poet T. S. Eliot, you return to the place you started from and know yourself for the first time.

Historically, déjà vu has been the subject of much fascination. For example the 14th-century Japanese monk, Yoshido Kenko, wrote, 'It has happened on various occasions that I have felt, just after someone has said something or I have seen something, or thought something, that it has occurred before. I cannot remember when it was, but I feel absolutely sure the thing has happened. Am I the only one who has such impressions?' On the other hand, 'jamais vu' describes a familiar situation that is not recognized by the observer, even though rationally they know they should recognize it. People who experience 'jamais vu' comment on a similar eerie or strange feeling, but in this instance not of being aware of the past, but rather as if the experience of familiarity has yet to happen.

Many scientists and psychologists have tried to prove déjà vu to be merely a neurological fault between short-term and long-term memory (the short-term memory records events in the present, while long-term memory records events in the past). Other kinds of déjà vu have been coined as *déjà vécu* – already lived, *déjà senti* – already felt, and *déjà visité* – already visited, as well as paramnesia – false memory syndrome.

PSYCHIC SKILLS

If you are interested in **Psychic Skills**, you may also like to read about:
- **Western Astrology**, pages 56–57
- **The Tarot**, pages 62–63
- **Other Forms of Divination**, pages 72–73
- **Chakras and the Aura**, pages 172–173

Specific psychic skills and techniques include **clairvoyance**, **psychometry**, **telepathy** and **psychokinesis**. Individuals who possess these skills are considered to be able to access other dimensions of time, space and matter. These skills are often thought to be innate, but can also be acquired through practising specific techniques.

Clairvoyance

From the French word *clairvoyant* dating back to the 13th century, meaning 'seeing clearly', clairvoyance is often known as having 'second sight' or seeing with the 'third eye' or 'inner eye'. This is the ability to be acutely aware of other people through extra-sensory perception (ESP). It is also called 'the sixth sense'. Clairvoyants are believed to be able to retrieve information about people, experiences and events, find missing objects or reveal hidden information, see a person's aura and communicate with spirits.

Clairaudience

This term comes from the French words *clair* and *audience*, meaning 'clear' and 'hearing' respectively, to imply 'clear listening' in an extra-sensory way.

The clairaudient person is sensitive to sounds, tones and even music, but not through the usual aural means, and can also hear voices or thoughts of the living as well as spirit voices.

Clairsentience

The word 'clairsentience' comes from the French *clair* for 'clear' and *sentience* for 'feeling'. A strong feeling rather than a mental image is felt by the clairsentient person, enabling them to 'feel' or sense something about that person or situation. This method is used by many psychics to sense the energy of other people, as well as their moods, emotions and feelings. Other psychic senses associated with clairvoyance are 'clairgustance' (tasting) and 'clairalience' (smelling).

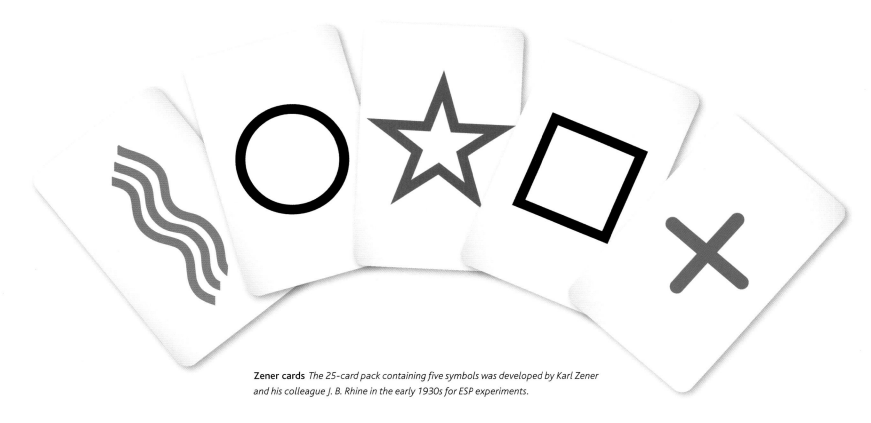

Zener cards *The 25-card pack containing five symbols was developed by Karl Zener and his colleague J. B. Rhine in the early 1930s for ESP experiments.*

Claircognizance

This is another form of ESP rooted in the French words *clair*, meaning 'clear', and *conoissance*, meaning 'knowledge'. This term describes an individual receiving psychic knowledge about other people without knowing why or how they actually know it.

Psychometry

From the Greek words *psyche* – 'soul', and *metron* – 'measure', psychometry describes the psychic retrieval of information about someone through contact with their belongings, such as a watch or piece of clothing. The term was coined by Joseph Rhodes Buchanan (1814–1899) in the 1840s. Psychometry became the basis of a popular stage act where members of the audience would offer up an object for analysis. After handling the object, the psychic would be able to tell the audience members something that no one else present could know about their life.

Telepathy

From the Greek words *tele*, meaning 'distant', and *patheia*, meaning 'to be affected by', telepathy is the transference of thoughts, feelings or ideas between two or more individuals via ESP. Classical scholar Frederick W. H. Myers (1843–1901), the founder of the Society for Psychical Research, coined this word in 1882 as a replacement for the original term, 'thought-transference'. Ancient Hindu texts also describe telepathy. It is one of the five *siddhis* or accomplishments of yoga and meditation.

Parapsychologists of the 20th century devised experiments to test for telepathy in individuals with Zener cards, which use five very specifically different symbols. One person, the 'sender', is asked to concentrate on one card at random and visualize it, while another person, the 'receiver', attempts to receive the information via ESP. Distance has no effect on telepathy; the astronaut Edgar Mitchell conducted Zener telepathy experiments from the moon in 1971. In what is known as a ganzfeld experiment, the sender is placed in a location far away from the receiver, the latter being situated in a controlled, electromagnetically blocked environment deprived of any sensory input. The sender must then telepathically relay information to the receiver, either simultaneously or after a time delay.

Silva Method

This self-help programme was devised by José Silva (1914–1999) in the 1940s and eventually marketed in the 1960s. It claims to be able to raise people's IQs and enhance psychic awareness by teaching them how to use their right side of the brain. By practising the art of positive thinking, visualization techniques and meditation, the individual can learn to tap into a psychic source. According to Silva, this method puts the individual in touch with an underdeveloped sense that is innate. In addition, the person can learn to project his or her mind for a specific purpose, such as viewing distant objects or locations and connecting with a higher intelligence for guidance. The Silva Method is often grouped with other therapeutic techniques known as the Human Potential Movement, akin to humanistic psychology.

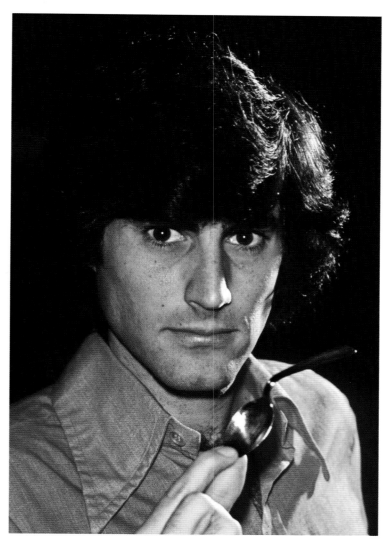

Uri Geller *Israeli-born Uri Geller claims to be able to bend spoons psychokinetically, using just the power of his mind.*

Psychokinesis

From the Greek *psyche*, meaning 'soul' or 'animating spirit', and *kinesis*, meaning 'motion', this term was coined by writer and publisher Henry Holt (1840–1926) in 1914 to describe how the mind or 'soul' has the power to move physical objects without physical influence. Self-levitation, shape shifting, teleportation, thought-form projection and object deformation (such as magician Uri Geller's bending of spoons) all come under the general umbrella term of psychokinesis. This word was later introduced to the psychological community by parapsychologist Joseph Rhine in 1934. Ancient Hindu texts also describe teleportation as a *siddhi* or accomplishment that it was possible for an adept to achieve.

Telekinesis is more specifically the movement of objects or matter by means of ESP. This term was originally coined by Russian psychic researcher Alexander N. Aksakof (1832–1903) in 1890, and at the time referred to the movement of objects by ghosts, spirits or supernatural powers, such as poltergeist cases.

CHANNELLING

This is a New Age term for a specific kind of mediumship. The channeller connects to a 'higher source' in order to access information and relay this information to the client. This can be achieved using various **chanelling methods**, but is usually done through **spirit guides**, **ascended masters**, **the 'grid'** or even the channeller's 'higher self'.

If you are interested in **Channelling**, you may also like to read about:
- Theosophy, pages 270–271
- Meditation, pages 78–79
- Native American Spirituality, pages 232–233
- Spiritualism, pages 194–195
- Sacred Geometry, pages 250–251

Methods of channelling

There are several ways to channel. One is by means of psychic communication with a spirit guide; another is when the channeller enters a trance-like state and willingly allows the spirit guide to talk through them, often with a very different voice or language. The person literally becomes a 'channel' or 'conduit' for communication. Trance channelling was performed by Native American shamans, ancient Egyptian priests and by the priestesses who revealed the Delphic oracles. Trance channelling was also the preferred method used by mediums in parlour seances, which became popular at the end of the 19th century. However, the main difference between channelling and mediumship is that mediums contact the spirits or souls of the departed, while channellers usually search out and communicate with a highly evolved spirit teacher or master.

Spirit guides

These are considered to be entities who watch, teach, heal and help the channeller on their journey into greater awareness. The number of spirit guides an individual has varies within that person's experiences. Teaching spirits can go by many names and connect with more than one person at a time. Sometimes spirits come to the channeller for a specific purpose, such as for healing, spiritual development or resolving problems. Popular and well-known channellers include Jane Roberts (1929–1984) and her spirit guide Seth; Margaret McElroy and Maitreya; and J. Z. Knight and Ramtha.

Ascended masters

Many New Age channellers communicate with guides who are termed ascended masters. These are individuals who are believed to have undergone

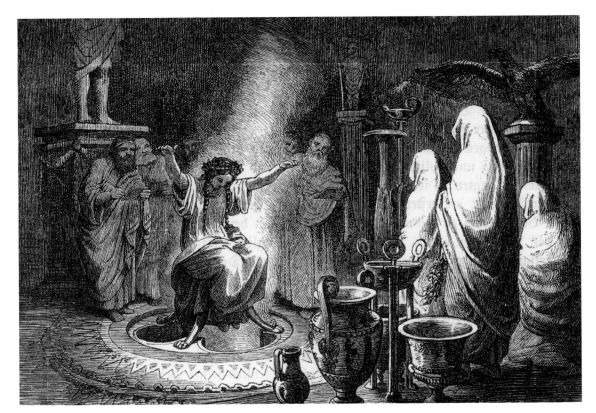

The Oracle of Delphi *This illustration shows the Pythia, the high priestess of the Oracle at Delphi, entering a trance-like state to channel messages and interpret omens from the gods.*

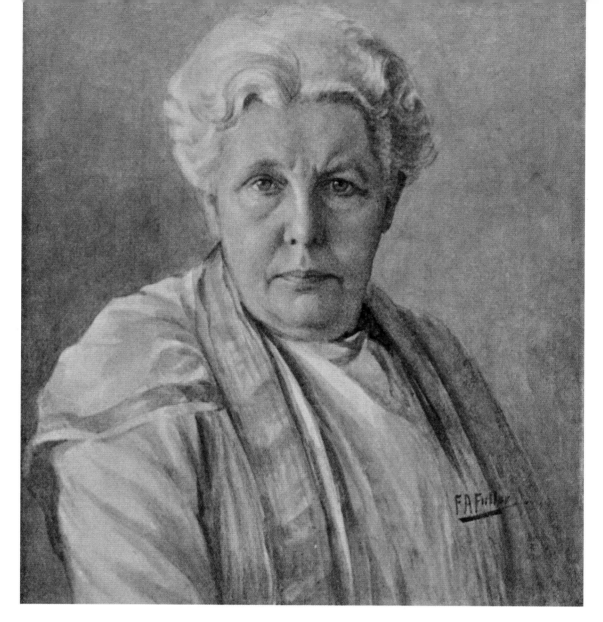

Annie Besant *President of the Theosophical Society, Annie Besant was a firm believer in past lives and described in detail the past lives of ascended masters such as St Germain.*

a process of 'ascension' whereby they have reached a higher state of spiritual awareness and have offered themselves in service to humanity from their divine place in heaven. Spiritual figures such as Jesus and the Virgin Mary are considered by many to be ascended masters.

In the 19th century, Madame Blavatsky (1831–1891), the founder of Theosophy, brought attention to the existence of ascended spiritual leaders when she channelled messages from masters she called 'Mahatmas', highly evolved beings who lived in the Himalayas. She commented: '... from them we have derived all theosophical truths'. Her well-known spirit guide was Koot Hoomi or Kuthumi.

Blavatsky's successors in the Theosophical Society, Annie Besant (1847–1933) and Charles W. Leadbeater (1854–1934), developed the idea of ascended masters and described in detail their past lives. One of the best-known examples is St Germain, also known as The Master Rakozi or Master R, believed to have ascended after his final incarnation as Sir Francis Bacon. His previous incarnations included a high priest of Atlantis, Merlin and Christopher Columbus.

Ascended masters, according to Theosophical teachings, remain attentive to the spiritual needs of humanity as a whole. In this they can be compared to the Bodhisattvas of Buddhism or the saints of Christianity.

The popularized concept of spiritual evolution and 'ascension' is well covered in James Redfield's Celestine series, beginning with the 1993 novel, *The Celestine Prophecy*.

The 'grid'

Another New Age approach used to access information is termed reading the 'crystalline grid', an idea developed from the principles of sacred geometry. This 'grid' is considered to be similar to a switchboard that connects everyone and everything in the universe and that vibrates to certain frequencies. When a person channels, they are tapping into (or rather plugging into) the frequency of the 'grid'. For example, an individual wishing to channel a specific spirit can attune to their frequency signature and listen to their message. It's like tuning into a radio: each 'station' vibrates to a specific frequency, which is considered to correspond to colours, chakras, auras and occult symbolism.

PSYCHIC PROTECTION

Psychic protection harnesses the power of the mind and intention to enhance an individual's energies and environment. It is believed to provide **subtle protection** from negative energies, ill-wishing, spirit attachment, psychic attack, geopathic stress and the like, using rituals, **visualizations, cleansing techniques**, crystals, psychic-strengthening activities and **closing down**. Psychic protection arises from inner calm, balance and a **positive attitude**.

If you are interested in **Psychic Protection**, you may also like to read about:
- Out-of-Body Experiences, pages 46–47
- Yoga, pages 106–109
- Chakras and the Aura, pages 172–173
- Crystal Healing, pages 166–167
- Cosmic Ordering and Abundance, pages 52–53

Subtle protection

People using intuition or psychic skills also often practise psychic protection to keep their energy field clear and to ensure that they are working in a safe space. Psychic protection is considered essential if practising channelling or inducing out-of-body experiences, to avoid the absorption of entities. Psychic protection is the means by which a person is considered to be able to prevent or resist psychic attack, ill-wishing or absorption of negative energies from the external world. It also allows an individual to develop protection from his or her own inner fears and negativity. Being well grounded in the body is recommended as the best form of protection, assisted by breathing deeply into the belly and being aware of a deep connection into the earth.

One of the easiest ways to ensure safety is to carry a cleansed and suitably programmed crystal such as a black tourmaline, amber or smoky quartz, which should be cleansed with running water at the end of each day.

An absence of fear, sensible working practices and a clear energy field are useful forms of psychic protection, but it can also be achieved by using rituals, psychic-strengthening activities, specific beliefs and cleansing techniques such as yoga or chakra work, and by understanding how the energy fields of other people, situations and places interact with the individual's own subtle energy field.

Visualization

This entails using the power of the mind to create images in the mind's eye. It isn't, however, necessary to actually 'see' anything to use the power of visualization. Having the intention to be protected and feeling oneself in the bubble of light as described opposite, for instance, will be sufficient to establish the protection. It is also possible to visualize a guardian angel, animal ally, a sword providing protection, or a bright white light sweeping out the space surrounding oneself to clear negativity from the area. Visualization techniques help to focus on a process, whether this is literally 'seeing' the right image in one's mind or using strong thoughts about that image in a positive way.

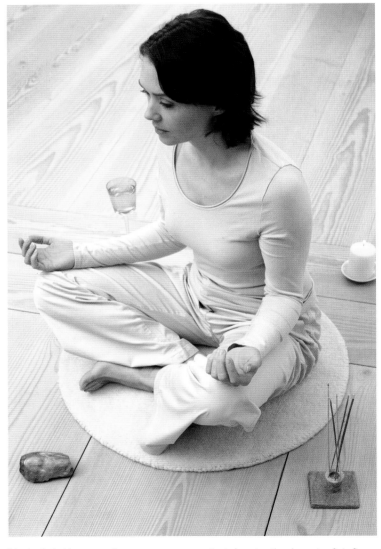

Magic circle *You can easily create your own magic circle, using the elements of air, fire, water and earth. This is a powerful form of protection.*

The protective light bubble

This universal psychic protection device uses the power of the mind to create a protective field around the individual. It is recommended that the bubble be visualized at the start of the day. The following exercise describes the process.

Close your eyes and breathe gently and easily. Focus your attention at arm's length in front of you. Picture a bubble of bright light that slowly expands and surrounds you so that you are sitting in the middle of the bubble of light. It will pass under your feet and above your head, around your back and in front of you. Feel the energy of this protective bright light gently washing over you, cleansing and strengthening your aura. Then allow the outer edges of the bubble to become hard and crystalline, like the surface of a crystal. This bubble will protect you wherever you go.

Cleansing techniques

There are many traditional cleansing techniques, such as taking a salt bath or placing salt on the doorstep; smudging (blowing smoke) with sweetgrass, sage or incense or burning essential oils; or sounding a bell, Tibetan singing bowl or *tingshas* (finger cymbals). Breath has historically been used to cleanse the body, as described in the exercise below.

Stand with your feet firmly on the floor and slightly apart, knees relaxed and springy. Put your hands over your navel in a 'V' shape. Now breathe deeply into your belly, pulling the cleansing air down into the space beneath your hands. Hold it for a moment. Let all your breath out with a big sigh. Feel all your negative energy, destructive feelings, stress and tension leaving your body with the breath. Wait a moment and then take another big, deep-cleansing breath right down into your belly. Pause and then let it all whoosh out again, cleansing your energy still further. Repeat at least four more times.

Now, as you breathe in, imagine bubbles of light flooding in with your breath, filling all the spaces of your being with joyful, bright energy. As you breathe out, hold this light within yourself.

Closing down

Knowing how to close down psychic connections is considered as important as learning how to open them in the first place. One popular method is to stamp a foot on the ground to symbolize the end of the session. It is also considered helpful to visualize each of the chakras (see page 172) closing like flower petals at dusk.

A positive attitude

Fear and negative beliefs or repressed feelings are common problems when it comes to feeling safe. Negative thoughts and feelings are considered to attract negative events and therefore, for effective psychic protection, it is recommended that individuals cultivate a positive attitude and focus on joyful feelings and positive beliefs. For example, think of the happiest you have ever been in your life, then think and believe you can now recreate that exact feeling again within you.

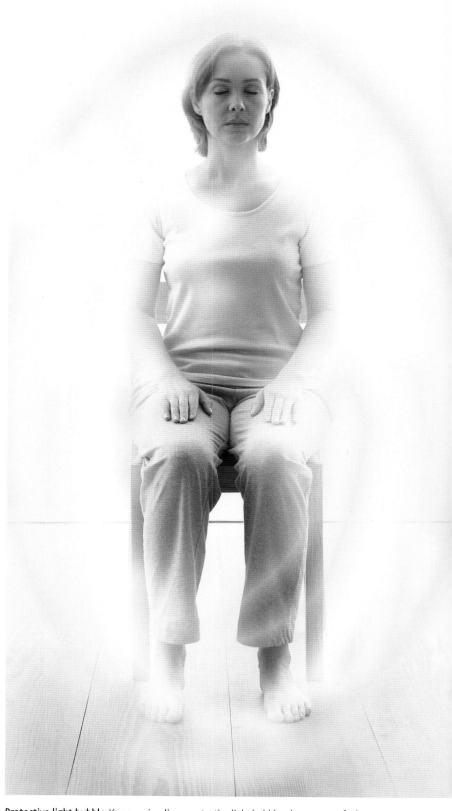

Protective light bubble *You can visualize a protective light bubble whenever you feel the need for protection.*

OUT-OF-BODY EXPERIENCES

The out-of-body experience (OBE) describes a person's sensation of being separate from his or her physical body, and the mind operating independently of the body. These experiences can occur unconsciously or be **induced** by various means. A closely related, spiritual state is that of **astral projection**, while **remote viewing** is a psychic ability enabling the viewing of one's physical body from a place outside it.

If you are interested in **Out-of-Body Experiences**, you may also like to read about:

- Exceptional Human Experiences, pages 48–49
- Dreams and Dream Analysis, pages 22–23
- Mystical and Transcendent States, pages 34–35

When and why they occur

In general, out-of-body experiences seem to occur when the person is on the verge of sleep, entering or leaving the rapid eye movement (REM) phase of sleep, or in a lucid dream state, and can be either highly disturbing or deeply moving. People who have claimed that they have had out-of-body

Visionary picture *This picture was drawn by Dr Susan Blackmore after her own out-of-body experience in 1970. It shows the tunnel of trees she saw during her experience.*

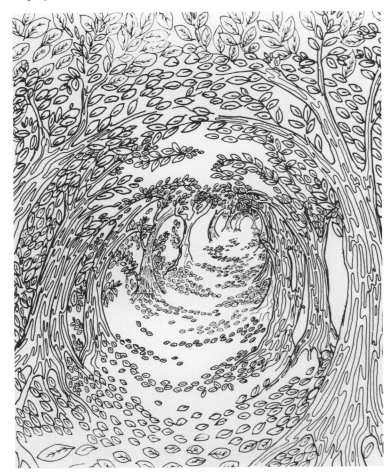

experiences have either willed themselves out of their bodies, been dragged out by some unknown force or have suddenly realized that they are outside their bodies. One simple explanation is that OBEs are exactly that – human consciousness separating from the human body and travelling unhindered by any physical form in the physical world.

Neuroscience explains out-of-body experiences as being due to the stimulation of various parts of the brain. Lecturer and writer Susan Blackmore believes that during an out-of-body experience the person loses contact with sensory input from the body. The world that the individual views is not generated by sensory information, but by the brain's ability to create replicas of the physical world as it does every night in our dreams. However, this theory does not explain how an individual can describe events and people at a considerable distance from their physical body, which appears to be a feature of many OBEs.

Induced out-of-body experiences

There are many different ways of consciously entering into an out-of-body state, such as the forearm 'trick' used by writer and OBE pioneer Sylvan Muldoon (1903–1969). Muldoon held his forearm perpendicularly above him in bed as he drifted off to sleep. The arm would fall as he lost consciousness, restoring his mind to an alert state. This deliberate attempt to stay on the edge between wakefulness and sleep induces a trance-like effect that can help to set off the sensation of an out-of-body experience. Other methods to induce OBEs include lucid-dreaming practice and deep trance and visualization work. Visual imagery includes sensations of floating, or projecting thoughts of one's mind into the air.

Psychologists and scientists have used and researched extensively many other mechanical inductions of out-of-body experiences, such as magnetic stimulation of the brain, sensory deprivation, sensory overload and brain-wave synchronization. Out-of-body experiences can also be induced through hallucinogenic drugs such as ketamine or DMT (dimethyltryptamine). Neuroscientist Michael Persinger in the USA and, more recently, Henrik Ehrsson in the UK have both conducted studies and experiments to prove that there are normal neurological reasons why individuals have OBEs.

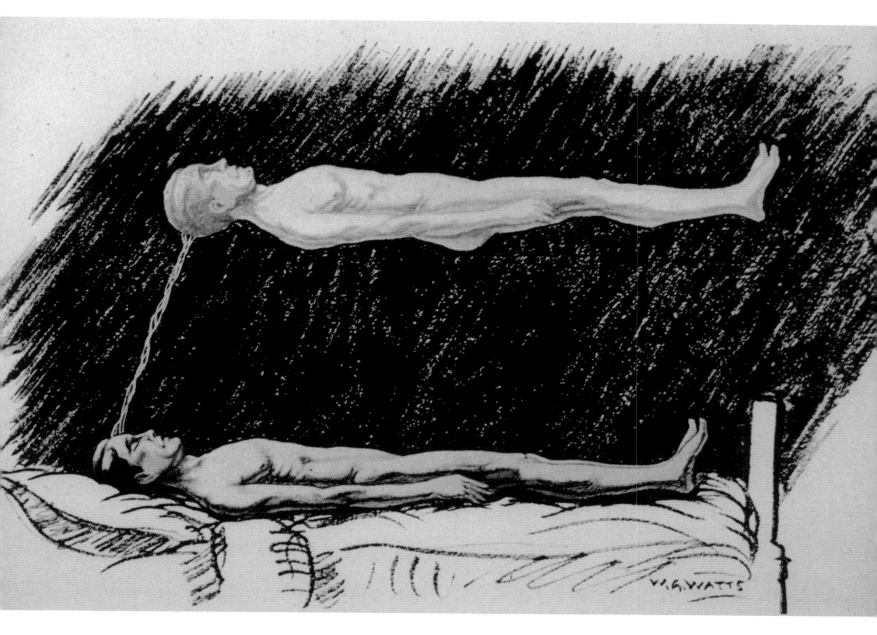

Astral projection

The concept of astral projection differs slightly from the out-of-body experiences described opposite in that it is a belief that the individual has a separate spiritual body capable of travelling to non-physical realms. These realms or planes are termed astral, etheric or spiritual. Thus the experience is described as that of the 'astra' or spirit of the body leaving to travel in this plane. In astral projection consciousness can travel almost without limitation. It therefore perceives not the physical objects, but their astral counterparts and beings in other dimensions. This state was described by Native Amercian shamans, and is also recorded in ancient Hindu texts.

Remote viewing

In 1974 the term 'remote viewing' was coined by physicists Russell Targ and Harold Puthoff to describe a method of collecting information about a

Astral projection *This illustration drawn by Sylvan Muldoon in 1929 shows an astral body lying above a physical body. The two states are connected by a cord.*

distant object that is hidden from view. The skill is rather like dowsing for water with rods, but using the mind instead. It can be applied to anything from finding a lost ring and spying on secret meetings to viewing a distant planet. Remote viewing gained wider awareness in the 1990s after the controversial US government's Stargate Project became public knowledge. A similar project was carried out by the Russians. The Stargate Project used psychics such as Joe McMoneagle to reveal secret information. The project was officially shut down in 1994 as a result of controversy concerning its validity. Currently there are many websites claiming to teach the secret of remote viewing based on increasing or changing the alpha wave levels of the brain.

EXCEPTIONAL HUMAN EXPERIENCES

If you are interested in **Exceptional Human Experiences**, you may also like to read about;
- **Dreams and Dream Analysis**, pages 22–23
- **Out-of-Body Experiences**, pages 46–47
- **Meditation**, pages 78–79
- **Mystical and Transcendent States**, pages 34–35

An exceptional human experience has a variety of specific **characteristics**, but can generally be described as a life-enriching, spontaneous 'experience of transcendence' that takes an individual out of his or her body and everyday consciousness, and that induces profound realizations, usually accompanied by transformative aftereffects. These include **near-death experiences**, UFO encounters and other psychic experiences.

Characteristics of exceptional human experiences

While researchers have studied lucid dreaming, near-death experiences and out-of-body experiences for many years, exceptional human experience is a comparatively recent umbrella term coined by Rhea A. White (1931–2007), one-time research fellow at Duke University Parapsychology Laboratory in Durham, North Carolina, USA, who was more interested in the transformative aftereffects of anomalous experiences than in whether the process was hallucinatory, neurological or brain-induced, or whether a near-death experience subject was clinically dead – the usual focus for researchers. Anomalous experiences cannot be explained away by psychology, neurology or physics. They open what White called 'a window with a new view'. Some exceptional human experiences occur during surgery, meditation, psychic work, psychedelic drug experiences or hypnosis. Strictly speaking, an out-of-body experience or near-death experience is classed as an exceptional human experience only when there have been profound repercussions in the life of the subject, but it is becoming a blanket term for all such experiences.

White identified certain characteristics of exceptional human experiences, as follows, although there is debate over their validity, and it can be questioned whether or not they can be anomalous once the subject has learned to induce an out-of-body experience or lucid dream.

- Spontaneous occurrence
- Physiologically and spiritually heightened state of being
- Transcendent, out-of-body consciousness
- A sense of inter-connectedness to other dimensions of the self and the universe; no separation
- Sense of who the subject is expands beyond its former boundaries: opens the way for a new reality, a different world-view
- Initiates a continuous process of consciousness expansion, and life becomes 'charged with meaning'

Near-death experiences

Most subjects report having these experiences during major surgery, traumatic events such as car accidents, near-drownings and heart attacks, but they have been reported throughout history. One of the earliest accounts is

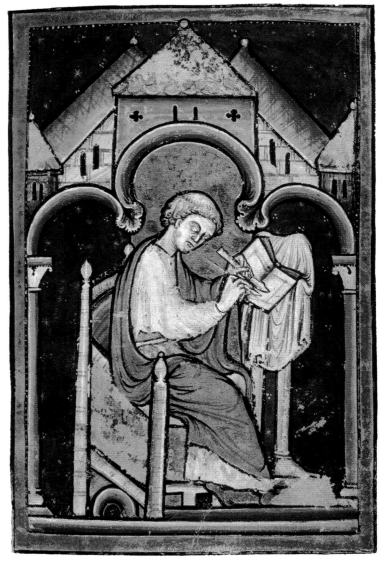

The Venerable Bede *Shown here in a late 12th-century manuscript, the Venerable Bede produced the earliest English account of a near-death experience in his 8th-century work* Historia ecclesiastica gentis Anglorum.

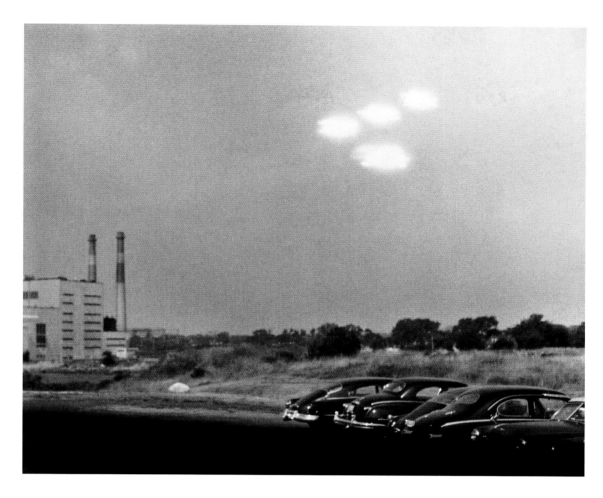

UFOs *This photograph shows four brightly glowing, unidentified flying objects, which appeared in the sky at 9.35 a.m. on July 15, 1952 over a car park in Salem, Massachusetts.*

from a 'drowned man' in Plato's *The Republic*, written c. 380 BCE; and the Venerable Bede, an 8th-century English monk, recorded the story of a Northumbrian man who 'rose from the dead and related the things he had seen, some exciting terror and others delight'.

John C. Wheeler, a more recent near-death-experience subject, drowned and was certified dead, only to revive the next day. In his published account he reported that he could describe everything that had happened, including the recovery of his body. Stating that the thought of returning to his body was repugnant, but that he was forced to return, he sums up the life-changing effect of a near-death experience: 'Up to the time of that experience I had been an agnostic... but my whole outlook on life was changed. I never since have had a shadow of a doubt with regard to a spiritual state of existence. Man is dual and the physical body is the lesser part of him. I don't speak of a future state as a possibility, but as a fact. To me it is knowledge.'

People who have near-death experiences often talk of the feeling that they still have a 'body', but of a very different nature to the one they left behind. Commonly, they glimpse the spirits of relatives and friends who have already died, approach some sort of barrier or border representing the limit between earthly life and the spirit world. They are usually overwhelmed by intense feelings of joy, love and peace, although not everyone has a tranquil experience. If a blind person has a near-death experience, they are able to see quite clearly, describing colours and the appearance of people who tend their physical body.

As from 2008, a three-year research programme is being undertaken to study near-death experiences in selected UK hospitals by Dr Sam Parnia of Southampton University.

Reports of near-death experiences tend to feature classic characteristics, such as those listed below:

- Physical body is typically deeply unconscious or 'dead'
- Consciousness leaves the body suddenly, without premeditation
- Infused with a deep feeling of peace
- Subject passes up a tunnel of light
- Subject is met by a being radiating love, often a religious figure
- Deceased relatives may appear
- Subject hears beautiful music, sees wondrous surroundings
- Soul undergoes a life review experienced intensely and with great feeling
- Subject identifies on-going lessons and processes
- Subject may be offered a choice or is told to return

There is considerable debate about near-death experiences. Rick Strassman, an associate professor of psychiatry, has made the controversial suggestion that endogenous (naturally occurring) DMT (dimethyltryptamine) facilitates consciousness leaving the body. Dr Peter Fenwick, a respected British consultant neuropsychiatrist who has examined over 300 near-death-experience cases, states: '... we are left with a real scientific problem... it looks as if mind and brain – if the data is correct – are separate'.

PAST LIVES AND PAST-LIFE THERAPIES

If you are interested in **Past Lives and Past-Life Therapies**, you may also like to read about:

- **Hypnotherapy**, page 30
- **Creative Visualization and Guided Imagery**, page 33
- **Buddhism**, pages 208–209
- **Hinduism**, pages 204–205
- **Native American Spirituality**, pages 232–233

Past lives and past-life therapies centre on a belief in **reincarnation**, and the concept that an individual has experienced a previous life which can be used to help them understand their purpose in 'this life'. Past lives are a key theme in spiritual movements such as Tibetan Buddhism. There is a growing number of past-life therapies available, such as **past-life regression**, **life-between-lives regression** and **past-life readings**.

Past lives

A belief in past lives is based on a belief in reincarnation. In other words, the essence or soul of the individual is born again into the flesh of a different body. Reincarnation is an ancient concept and has been at the core of many religious traditions. In India, for example, reincarnation was an essential element in the sacred texts called the *Upanishads*, dating back to c. 800 BCE. Many other cultures and traditions, for instance the ancient Greeks, Norse, Inuit and other Native Americans, Sufis, Hindus, Tibetan Buddhists and some forms of modern-day Spiritualism all embrace the idea that the essence of an individual is born again after death and incarnates into another human body. This essence can be referred to as the 'soul', 'spirit', 'divine essence', 'chi' or 'the higher self'.

Reincarnation

The Buddhist belief in reincarnation is slightly different from New Age or Hindu-based religions in that there is no separate, eternal 'soul' that reincarnates, but rather a universal energy that takes on a new form. In most views, the individual 'soul' takes up residence in one body, and when that body dies, the soul is eventually 'reborn' in another body. Many modern pagans, certain African traditions and followers of esoteric and mystical philosophies believe that the soul must pass through some spiritual level or dimension to enable it to travel from one life to the next. A belief in 'future lives' is based on past lives; to reincarnate into another life we must have had a past life in the first place in order to do so.

One of the main tenets of reincarnation is that of 'karma', the idea that how we act in one life will have an effect on the next life. The concept of karma (the Sanskrit word for 'action') is wide-ranging; it is a process in which everything ('good' or 'bad') has consequences and is put in motion from moment to moment.

Past lives lie at the core of movements such as Anthroposophy and Scientology. Rudolf Steiner (1861–1925), Anthroposophy's founder, believed that the 'soul' gained new insight and experience in each incarnation, and would not limit itself to one culture or race. He believed that the future and the past were constantly in conflict and it is this tension that creates the present. Between the events of the past and those that are to come is the space for an individual's free will to make choices and thereby create his or her own destiny.

Many famous individuals have believed themselves to have past lives. Henry Ford (1863–1947) was convinced that he was a soldier killed at the battle of Gettysburg; General George S. Patton (1885–1945) believed that he was the reincarnation of the Carthaginian Hannibal; while John Lennon (1940–1980), the former Beatle, held that he was the reincarnation of Napoleon and that Yoko Ono had been Napoleon's wife Josephine.

Past-life therapies

The three main past-life therapies available are past-life regression, life-between-lives regression and past-life reading. One of the first pioneers of life-between-lives regression was the American hypnotherapist Michael Newton in the 1980s, with sessions lasting up to four hours. Past-life regression therapy has been more extensively developed since the early 1950s and written about by key authors such as Helen Wambach (1925–1986), Brian Weiss, Roger Woolger, Judy Hall and Andy Tomlinson.

Past-life regression

This is a technique whereby therapists use guided imagery, bodywork or a light state of hypnosis to activate memories of the past life of the client. Past-life regression is often used to resolve emotional or psychological problems or to bring about a spiritual awakening through recollection of a past life. Most clients have past-life stories that provide clues as to why they have problems in their current lives. For example, a fear of commitment in intimate relationships in a current life could be the result of being serially betrayed in a past life. Past-life regression therapists claim that unresolved wounds from a past life (the soul's 'karma') are responsible for present psychological problems, but can be healed by 'reframing' or other methods.

Life-between-lives regression

In this technique, therapists use hypnosis to regress the individual to the place between two lives, in other words to reconnect to the soul, spirit or

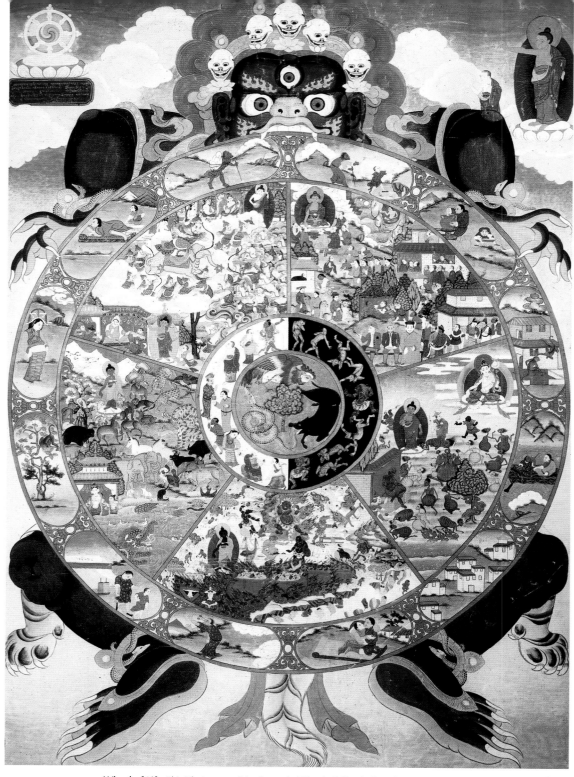

Wheel of Life *This Tibetan mandala shows the Wheel of Life which is often used in Buddhist meditation and depicts the concept of reincarnation.*

divine essence in the 'interlife'. This is also called spiritual regression. Many life-between-lives clients have similar experiences or 'memories', such as remembering the departure of the past life and how they passed through the spirit world. During their regression to their in-between life, subjects can review a past life assisted by spirit guides or evolved souls, plan their next life and choose past-life strengths to help them improve their current life.

Past-life reading

Therapist readers focus on one past life, one distinct period of time in that life or move through several lives, pausing at certain time frames and focusing on important events. Unresolved emotional issues that are carried from one life to another can be seen as either a useful guide for living in this life or as blockages that are holding the individual up on their journey.

COSMIC ORDERING AND ABUNDANCE

If you are interested in **Cosmic Ordering and Abundance**, you may also like to read about:
- **Mind and Brain**, pages 16–17
- **Cognitive Behavioural Therapy and Mindfulness**, pages 28–29
- **Hypnotherapy**, page 30
- **Creative Visualization and Guided Imagery**, page 33

Today there is a great deal of interest in **the power of positive thinking** as a way to change our lives for the better, but its life-changing potential has been recognized for centuries. Cosmic ordering is the power of positive thinking taken one step further. Its basic principle is that if an **order is placed with the universe**, the cosmos will manifest it.

The power of positive thinking

In recent years there has been an explosion of interest in positive thinking movements, such as cosmic ordering and the law of attraction – the principle that thoughts can have an energy that attracts like energy in the cosmos and can manifest themselves as reality – which offer pathways to an abundance of success and happiness.

Rhonda Byrne *Australian writer and producer Rhonda Byrne sold more than four million copies of her book* The Secret *in the first six months after publication .*

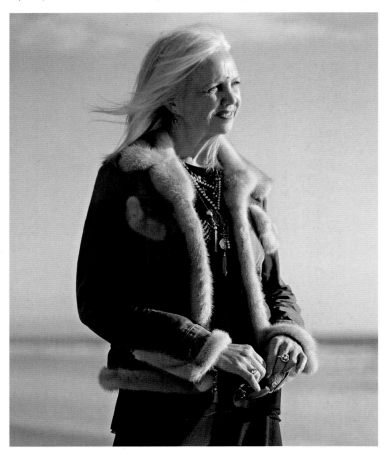

Positive thinking is an attitude that determines how a person perceives and interprets their world. Positive thinkers see the world in the best light, and are optimistic about people and events.

Proponents claim that positive thinking is a key component of happiness, health, wealth and success. Contrary to popular belief, positive thinking does not mean viewing the world in an over-optimistic light and ignoring the negative. Rather than denying the negative, they choose to focus their energies on the other side of the coin – the potential for the positive. They register the problems, such as a rainy day, a bad experience at work or an upset with a loved one, and then, instead of becoming drawn into a spiral of despondency, take action to resolve these issues or, if that is not practical, to change the way they think about them.

Positive thinking through the centuries

There is evidence from archeology and historical writings to suggest that people have been aware of the power of positive thinking in every century. The concept can be found in writings recorded in stone around 3000 BCE, in the precepts of the so-called Emerald Tablet of Hermes Trismegistus (see page 185), and in ancient civilizations such as those of the Babylonians, Egyptians and Greeks. It can even be found in the Old Testament. For example, in Proverbs 23: 7 we are told, 'For as a man thinks within himself, so shall he be...' Elements can be identified in all the world's major religions, including the Hermetic traditions, Hinduism, Judaism, Christianity, Islam and Buddhism. 'All that we are is the result of what we have thought. The mind is everything. What we think we become...' stated Prince Gautama Siddhartha (c. 560–483 BCE), the founder of Buddhism.

Some of the world's great thinkers have explored the power of positive thinking to dictate not just a person's state of mind, but the direction of his or her life. Psychologists such as Albert Ellis (1913–2007) and Aaron Beck have done much to reveal the role of mental attitudes in shaping our feelings and experiences. Over the last century a number of popular writers – beginning with Napoleon Hill (1883–1970) and *Think and Grow Rich*, 1937, and Norman Vincent Peale (1898–1993) with *The Power of Positive Thinking*, 1952, and more recently with James Redfield and *The Celestine Prophecy*, 1993, a novel

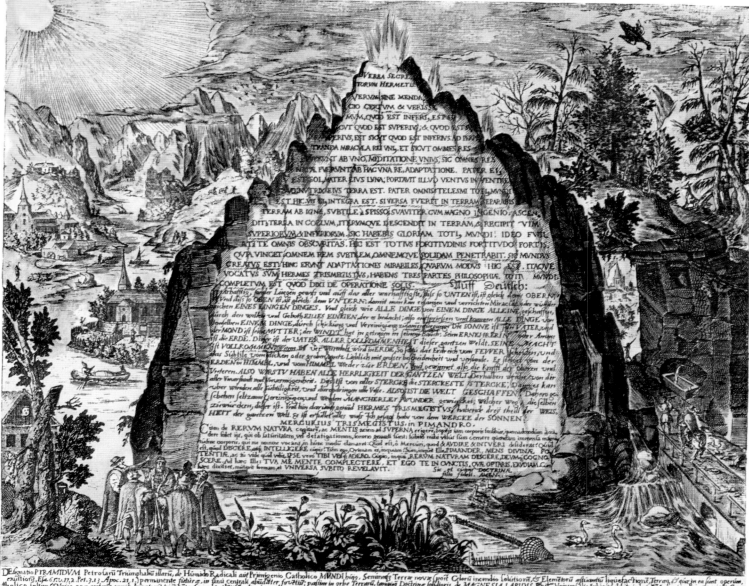

that has since been made into a film, and Rhonda Byrne with *The Secret*, 2006 – have brought the concepts of positive thinking to a mass readership.

Placing an order with the universe

Cosmic ordering is the power of positive thinking taken one step further. The basic principle is that an order is placed with the universe and the cosmos will manifest it. The theory originated in a book by Bärbel Mohr called *The Cosmic Ordering Service: A Guide To Realizing Your Dreams* (2000). Mohr insists that there is more to achieving your wants and desires than just positive thinking. The basis of Mohr's theory is that at the most fundamental level we are all connected to what some people call the 'unified field' or the matrix of the universe.

The Emerald Tablet *This illustration of The Emerald Tablet is taken from the 1602 edition of Heinrich Khunrath's* Amphitheatrum Sapientiae Aeternae. *It reveals one of the keys of cosmic ordering and the laws of attraction: 'as above, so below'.*

Followers of cosmic ordering believe that quantum physics has brought science and spirituality to a place where common ground is being found. Particles influencing each other over immeasurable distances, particles existing simultaneously in two different places and the fact that simply observing events can change them are all seen as mysteries that provide some support for the 'unified field' theory, although such contentions are not generally supported by the scientific community. It is now possible to place your cosmic order over the internet.

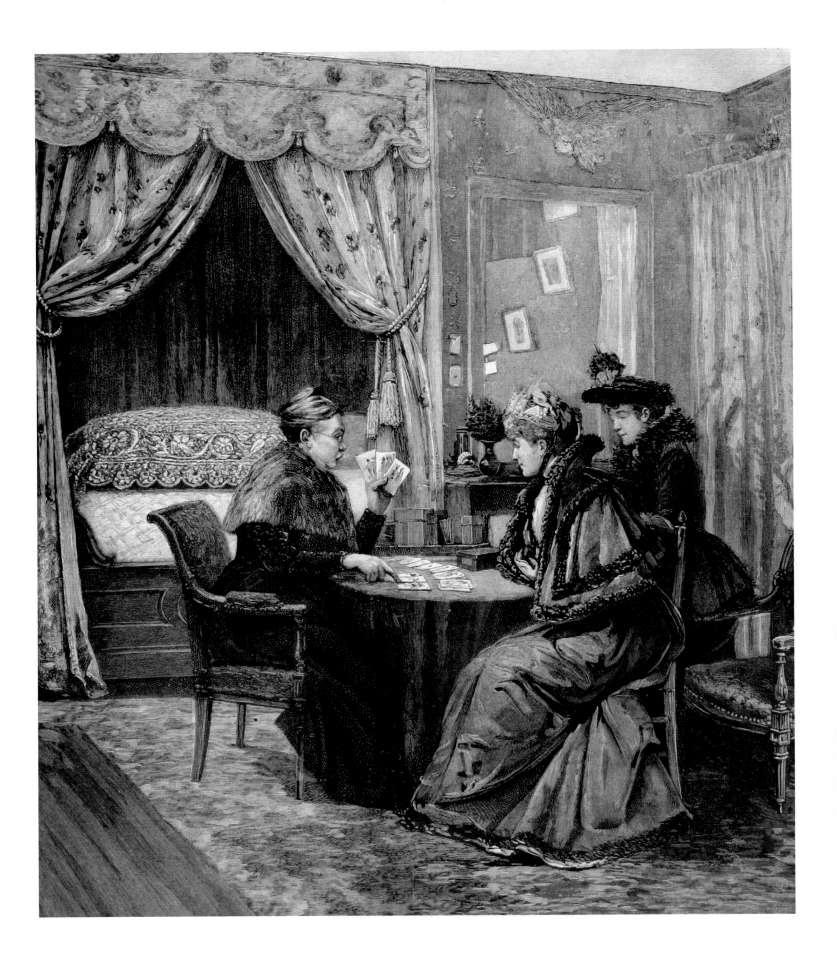

DIVINATION

 We have always wanted to know what the future will bring, regardless of the age in which we live. It is, it would seem, part of human nature and is a very strong need in many people. Even though the precise details of our questions may change according to our individual circumstances, their essence remains the same: will we be happy, will our loved ones be safe, will we have enough money, will everything work out in the way we want? But where do we find the answers?

One option has always been divination. Our ancient ancestors cast animal bones, gazed into water and studied the movements of the heavens, among other forms of divination. In the Ancient Egypt of biblical times, dreams were taken very seriously and Joseph was so successful in interpreting the dreams of the Pharaoh that he was made viceroy over Egypt. In Ancient Greece, people would satisfy their curiosity about the future by visiting the Delphic Oracle, who was said to be in contact with the god Apollo. Periods of adversity, such as wars, famines and earthquakes, would increase the need to know that the future would be more settled. Many methods of divination were performed with items that were easily available but also ephemeral, such as animal entrails, the flight of birds, the drift of rising smoke and the patterns made by salt crystals when they are thrown on the ground.

Today we have a wider range of divination tools to choose from, many of which are described in the following section. Each of them has unique characteristics, but they all help us to gain greater insight into what our future holds. These techniques vary from the comparatively simple to the highly complex. Some of them, such as astrology and the tarot, help us to understand the circumstances in which we find ourselves. They also enable us to gain valuable insight into the motivations and emotions of the other people who are involved in our situations. Other techniques, such as palmistry and face reading, remind us that our characters play an integral part in dictating our future, and that who we are is inextricably linked with

Tarot reading *This 19th-century French illustration shows a fortune-teller at work in a Parisian parlour. Private readings of this type became increasingly popular amongst the middle and upper classes during this time.*

where we are heading in life: character is destiny. In this way, all the divination techniques can be a focus for meditation and guidance as well as a form of oracle.

Psychic influences

If divination can successfully predict the future, the question arises of how this is possible. To give the tarot as an example, if the cards are shuffled and then dealt out in an apparently arbitrary order, how is it that they can describe a person's past and current situation so accurately, and provide insight into the future as well as predict what will happen? Is this always a coincidence? Or is some special psychic force at work? This is a conundrum that has intrigued many people over the centuries. Swiss psychologist Carl Jung (1875–1961), for instance, studied many aspects of the occult and was particularly fascinated by astrology and the *I Ching*. He believed that these two disciplines were examples of what he called 'synchronicity', in which there is a significant relationship between two or more events taking place at the same time.

The role of energy fields

The concept of energy fields has gripped science for many years, and these may also be involved in divination. They might also help to explain the existence of psychic phenomena. When someone reads the tarot cards, is the energy that they transmit while thinking of the question they wish to ask somehow absorbed by the cards, so that the 'right' cards are dealt out to provide the answer? The English biologist Rupert Sheldrake has spent many years developing and exploring his theory of what he calls 'morphogenetic fields', which he believes impose specific patterns on what would otherwise be random patterns of activity. Are these energetic fields at work when the tarot cards are read?

Unexplained aid

Although science has yet to come up with any definitive answers about how divination works, this in no way detracts from its effectiveness and accuracy, and its ability to offer advice, reassurance and hope in times of trouble.

WESTERN ASTROLOGY

If you are interested in **Western Astrology**, you may also like to read about:
- **Chinese Astrology**, pages 58–59
- **Vedic Astrology**, pages 60–61

Many people think of Western astrology as concerning only sun or star **signs**, although there is much more to it than this. Astrology also studies the effects of the **planets**, as well as other features of **astronomy**. When interpreted, an **astrological chart** set for someone's time and date of birth can reveal the innermost workings of their personality. But there are various **different forms of astrology** for other, specific divinatory purposes.

Astrology and astronomy

Humans have been watching the night sky and noticing the correlation between celestial events and those around them for millennia. The people of Sumeria are known to have practised astrology in 4300 BCE, although its origins may lie in the earliest part of the Stone Age. The Greek astrologer and astronomer Ptolemy (c. 100–170 CE) wrote the *Tetrabiblos*, considered to be the first complete surviving astrological textbook, in the 2nd century. Astrology was especially popular in medieval Europe, where astrologers made many astronomical discoveries. At the time, little distinction was made between the two sciences, unlike today.

Astrology grew out of direct observation of the skies overhead and the way that picture changed on a day-to-day basis. Therefore it takes a geocentric or Earth-based view, regardless of the fact that the Earth actually revolves around the Sun (a fact that appears to have been known by at least some ancient astrologers). In the earliest Sumerian astrology no differentiation is made between the fixed stars, the planets and the luminaries – the Sun and Moon – which were all regarded as gods. Gradually the five visible-to-the-naked-eye planets (Mercury, Venus, Mars, Jupiter, Saturn) and the luminaries became known as 'the planets'. As new planets (Uranus, Neptune, Pluto) were discovered and their effects observed, these were added to the astrological lexicon of 'planets'. (Most astrologers still consider Pluto to be a planet, despite its demotion to a dwarf planet by the International Astronomical Union in 2006.) Astrology is calculated using solid astronomical fact: the position of the Sun, Moon and the planets, fixed stars and asteroids as they travel along the annual path – known as the ecliptic – of the Sun against a band in the sky that intersects the celestial equator (a projection of the Earth's equator) at an angle of just over 23 degrees.

Western astrology uses the tropical zodiac, in which the path of the ecliptic is divided into 12 equal sections, each measuring 30 degrees. These sections, referred to as the signs of the zodiac, are named after 12 constellations: Aries, Taurus, Gemini, Cancer, Leo, Virgo, Libra, Scorpio, Sagittarius, Capricorn, Aquarius and Pisces. However, because of a phenomenon known as the precession of the equinoxes (recognized by astrologers from before the time of Ptolemy), they no longer exactly correlate with the astronomical positions of these constellations.

Astrological charts

Astrologers work with charts (sometimes called horoscopes) that are one-dimensional representations of the positions of the planets for a precise moment in a precise place, identified by its latitude and longitude. Until recently, these charts were calculated by hand, in a lengthy process that involved mathematics and logarithm tables. Today most astrologers use computers for calculation, but they still interpret the charts themselves.

The signs, planets and houses

Each of the 12 signs of the zodiac is assigned to one of the four elements – fire, earth, air and water – and one of the three modes – cardinal, fixed and mutable – and it also has a planetary ruler. This means that no two signs have the same element and mode, and each is therefore unique.

Each planet has a particular meaning and exerts its own specific influence. At any time, each planet as it appears to orbit the Earth occupies one of the 12 signs, and is affected by the nature of that sign. For instance, the Moon might be in Aquarius, which means that the instinctive nuturing qualities of the Moon are expressed in a humanity-orientated Aquarian way.

A chart is usually divided into 12 segments, known as houses, into which the planets fall. Each house rules a different sphere of life, which shows where the influence of the planet, in its particular sign, will be experienced.

In addition, a chart will show other important factors, such as the angles and the aspects, all of which help to build up a complex and detailed picture of the characteristics of whatever that chart describes.

The different forms of astrology

One of the most popular uses for astrology is to study people's birth charts. The astrologer analyses all the different components of the natal chart,

A NATAL CHART

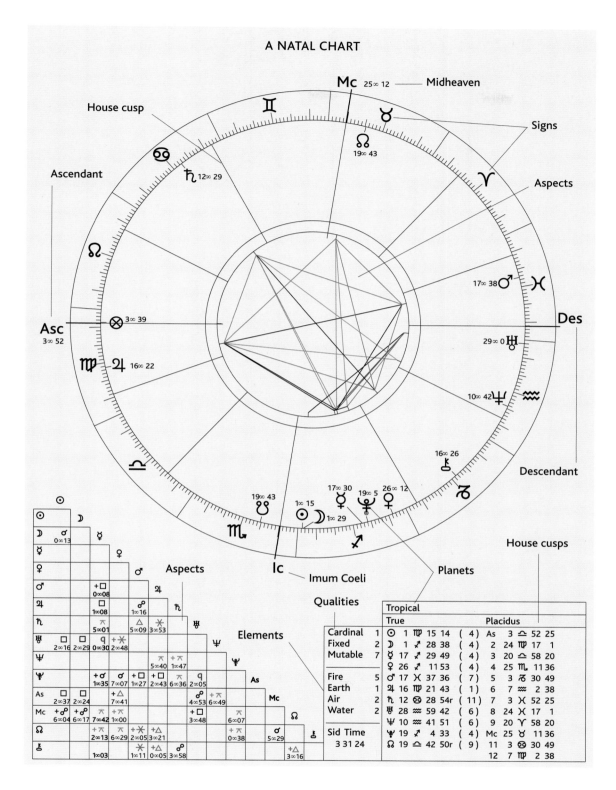

Natal chart for 11:22 p.m., 23 November, 2003 *On this day the new Moon was eclipsed in 1° Sagittarius. The Ascendant is in Virgo and the Midheaven in Taurus. The panel at the bottom left gives the aspects (geometric relationships that the planets make to one another), as well as the size of the orb between them. The coloured lines in the centre of the natal chart show these aspects. An astrologer would be able to analyse this chart to determine the character and life path of the person concerned.*

some of which may contradict one another, and pays particular attention to repeated themes. The astrologer will also examine the chart, using a variety of techniques, to see what the future will bring for their client.

Astrology can also be put to other uses. Electional astrology involves selecting exactly the right time for a particular event or enterprise, such as a marriage or the start of a business. Horary astrology involves the astrologer casting a chart in order to answer a client's question. Decumbiture charts are cast for the beginning of an illness and are interpreted to discover both its cause and its cure. Mundane astrology studies world events, as well as the ingresses of the planets into new signs. Synastry compares two or more charts, especially when exploring the astrological connections between two people. Past life astrology studies previous-life carry-overs.

CHINESE ASTROLOGY

The origins of Chinese astrology can be traced back over 4,000 years, and it has continued to attract millions of devotees. The vivid images of the **12 animal signs** have captured the imagination of many millions of people too. But what may seem at first to be a simple system is in fact much more complex, with its interwoven **two cycles** of elements and signs and associated **modifications**.

If you are interested in **Chinese Astrology**, you may also like to read about:
- Western Astrology, pages 56–57
- Vedic Astrology, pages 60–61
- I Ching, pages 70–71
- Taoist Sacred Texts, pages 218–219
- Confucianism, pages 220–221
- Feng Shui, pages 248–249

The origins of Chinese astrology

Legend has it that the 12 signs of the Chinese zodiac – Rat, Ox, Tiger, Rabbit, Dragon, Snake, Horse, Sheep, Monkey, Rooster, Dog and Pig – are named after the 12 animals that travelled to the bedside of Buddha when he was dying. He was so grateful to them for being the only creatures to make the journey that he named the 12 signs after them. In fact the system was developed even earlier by Emperor Huang Ti or Huangdi, who reputedly reigned from 2497 to 2398 BCE, and as it evolved it was enriched with the philosophies of Confucius (c. 551–479 BCE) and Lao Tzu (604–531 BCE).

The 12 animal signs

Unlike Western and Vedic astrology, where someone's birth sign is determined by the day and month in which they were born, in Chinese astrology their sign is determined by the year in which they were born. Each sign begins at the Chinese New Year, which falls at some point between late January and mid-February. In Western astrological terms, this is the time of the new moon in Aquarius. This means that for births in January and February it is always advisable to check the exact day on which the Chinese New Year falls. The Chinese animal signs are believed to be a reflection of the universe itself and therefore have deep philosophical connections.

The names of some of the animal signs can vary. The Ox is sometimes called the Water Buffalo, the Rabbit can also be the Cat, the Sheep can also be called the Goat and the Pig is also known as the Boar. The difference in the names does not affect the meaning of the signs.

The two cycles

Chinese astrology is based on two interconnecting cycles that meet once every 60 years. One cycle concerns the animal signs themselves, collectively known as 'the 12 earthly branches', and is therefore a 12-year cycle. The other cycle concerns the five elements, also known as 'phases': wood, fire, earth, metal and water. They always run in this order, with two years being assigned to each element, thereby forming a ten-year cycle. These are collectively known as 'the ten heavenly stems'. Although these cycles run concurrently, they only meet once every 60 years, when the start of a new

animal cycle, which always begins with the Rat, coincides with the start of a new elemental cycle, which always begins with wood. The current cycle began in February 1984 and will end in January 2044.

It is these two cycles that determine the precise nature of each of the annual animal signs within the 60-year cycle. This gives subtle but important differences between the same animal signs. For instance, someone born in August 1946 is a Fire Dog, while someone born in the same month 12 years later is an Earth Dog.

Another important factor is yin and yang, which are believed to influence every single thing in the universe. Yin is feminine and cool, while yang is masculine and hot. The animal signs alternate between being yin and yang, starting with the Rat, which is always yang.

Other modifications

Even this simple level of Chinese astrology will provide an in-depth character analysis and a guide to a person's compatibility with the other signs. It also gives an indication of how each person's sign will fare from year to year, since each year is assigned to one of the 12 signs and five elements. Calculations based on a person's exact date and time of birth will add further layers of information. Each month in the year is assigned to one of the 12 signs, as is each day of the month and every hour of the day. The hour of birth is especially important because it reveals what is known as 'the secret animal': the innermost personality. The hours are arranged in 12 groups of two hours each and refer to the position of the Sun in the sky, which may differ from local time because of adjustments for summer time or daylight saving time. Other factors can be calculated too, including the 12 palaces (or houses) in which over 100 stars fall.

This body of information helps to build up a very detailed picture of a person's character, since most Chinese birth charts will contain a considerable mixture of signs and elements. The combination of signs and their individual balance of yin and yang have great significance in feng shui, the ancient Chinese art of arranging objects in order to create a balanced flow of energy through an individual's personal environment, helping them to attune their personal chemistry with the wider world.

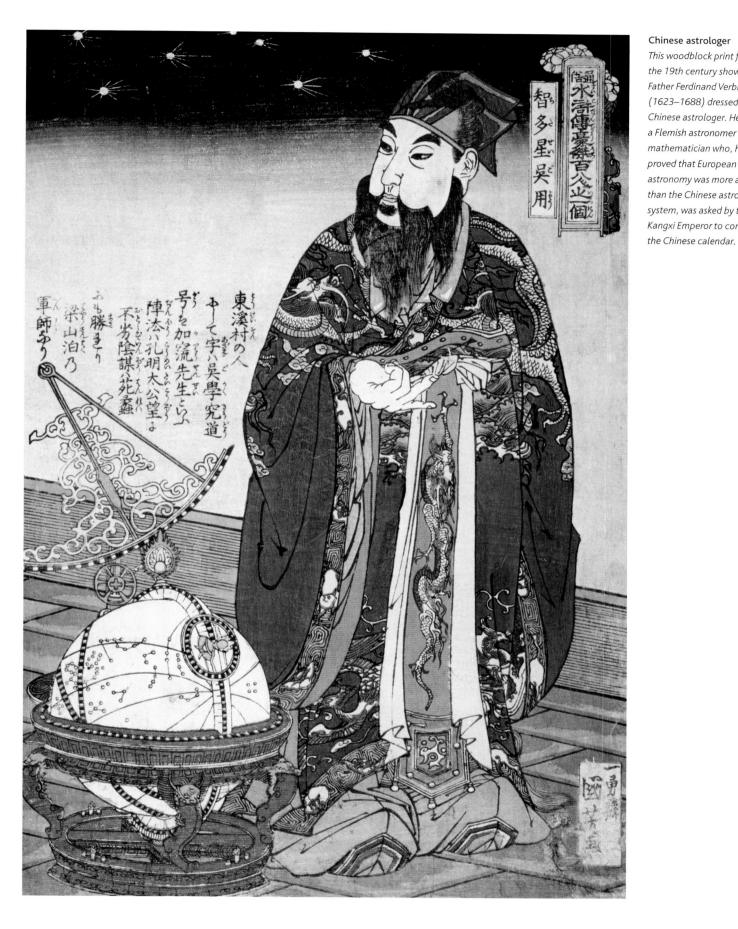

Chinese astrologer
This woodblock print from the 19th century shows Father Ferdinand Verbiest (1623–1688) dressed as a Chinese astrologer. He was a Flemish astronomer and mathematician who, having proved that European astronomy was more accurate than the Chinese astronomical system, was asked by the Kangxi Emperor to correct the Chinese calendar.

VEDIC ASTROLOGY

If you are interested in **Vedic Astrology**, you may also like to read about:
- **Hindu Sacred Texts**, pages 206–207
- **Ayurveda**, pages 94–97
- **Western Astrology**, pages 56–57

This Indian system of astrology has ancient **origins**, and therefore many close links with Indian philosophy and spirituality. **The law of karma** is a very important component of it. Based on **the sidereal zodiac**, Vedic astrology analyses the positions of the **planets** in the signs, with particular emphasis on the Moon.

The origins of Vedic astrology

Vedic astrology has always been treated with great respect in India. It stems from the four Vedas – Hindu sacred texts – and therefore has a deep basis in Indian philosophy that dates back thousands of years. Tradition states that Brahma, the creator, gave Vedic astrology to the world through the *rishis* (sages) who taught it to their students. At first it was passed by word of mouth, before Maharishi Parashara wrote what is widely believed to be the first Vedic astrology text, *Brihat Parasara Hora Shastra*, over 5,000 years ago.

Brahma *In Hindu sacred texts, Brahma, the creator of the universe, inspired the first Vedic astrological text, the* Brihat Parasara Hora Shastra.

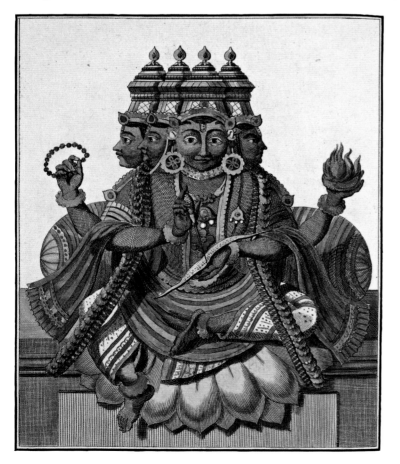

The law of karma

One of the precepts of Vedic astrology is that this life is only one of many, and that we are reincarnated time and again until we are spiritually ready to break this endless cycle and achieve *moksha* (enlightenment). Before this happens, we have to deal with many different forms of karma. These include *sanchita karma*, which is the accumulation of immutable karma from our previous lives and our current one; *prarabdha karma*, which is the immutable karma we have gathered from our present life; and *kriyamana karma*, which we can change by taking the right actions in our current life. Vedic astrology is also known by its Sanskrit name of *Jyotish*, which means 'eye of light', and one of its main purposes is to help people avoid future difficulties and reduce the amount of negative karma they are accumulating in their lives through the study of their birth charts.

The sidereal zodiac

Although Western astrology and Vedic astrology have many similarities, they have different rules and methods. Vedic astrology is centred on the sidereal or star zodiac. This means that it shows the relationship between the planets and the stars as they are seen in the sky now, unlike Western astrology where there is no longer an exact correlation between the signs of the zodiac and the astronomical positions of the constellations after which they are named. The sidereal zodiac of Vedic astrology takes into account a wobble in the axis of the Earth that leads to a phenomenon known as the precession of the equinoxes, in which the point where the celestial equator bisects the path of the ecliptic (the Sun's annual path around the Earth) moves backwards by one degree every 72 years. This means that there is currently a mathematical difference, known in Vedic astrology as the *ayanamsa*, between the sidereal and tropical zodiacs of about 24 degrees, and therefore a planet that is assigned one sign of the zodiac in Western astrology may occupy the previous sign in Vedic astrology.

The planets and constellations

Vedic astrology studies the positions of nine planets, known as the *nava grahas*. These are the seven traditional planets, visible with the naked eye, also used by Western astrology, plus two symbolic astronomical positions that serve as planets. The traditional planets are Surya (the Sun), Chandra (the Moon), Budha (Mercury), Shukra (Venus), Mangala (Mars), Brihaspati (Jupiter) and Shani (Saturn). Each of these rules one or more zodiac signs. The other two planets, known as *chayya grahas* (shadow planets), are Rahu and Ketu. These are the nodes of the Moon: the points on the path of the ecliptic where the Moon's orbit intersects that of the Sun. They are always close to the Sun and Moon during eclipses, which have tremendous significance in astrology, and represent the relationship between the Sun, Moon and Earth. Ketu (the south node) describes karma from the past and Rahu (the north node) describes karma from the present and future. At any time, each of these nine planets occupies a particular sign of the zodiac.

One unique facet of Vedic astrology is the use of the 27 constellations, known as the *nakshatras*, each of which spans 13 degrees 20 minutes of the zodiac. These combine the Indian lunar and solar zodiacs, and are considered to be essential in the evolution of the soul. They have much more significance than the 12 signs of the zodiac. The position of the Moon in its *nakshatra* is of primary importance.

The houses

An astrological chart is divided into 12 *bhavas* (houses). Some of these houses are considered to be auspicious and others are malefic or even *marakas* (killers). Each of them has a lord (planetary ruler) that ameliorates or worsens the effects of the planets in the houses.

Vedic tools

One of the most notable areas of Vedic astrology is the practice of balancing what are seen as negative sections of the *rasi* or birth chart (such as planets being placed in malefic houses) with corrective practices and objects. These can include specific gemstones, mantras and small actions.

Uses for Vedic astrology

Vedic astrology is used especially for ensuring astrological compatibility between two people before they marry. Another popular technique is *mahurata*, where an auspicious time is chosen for a particular event.

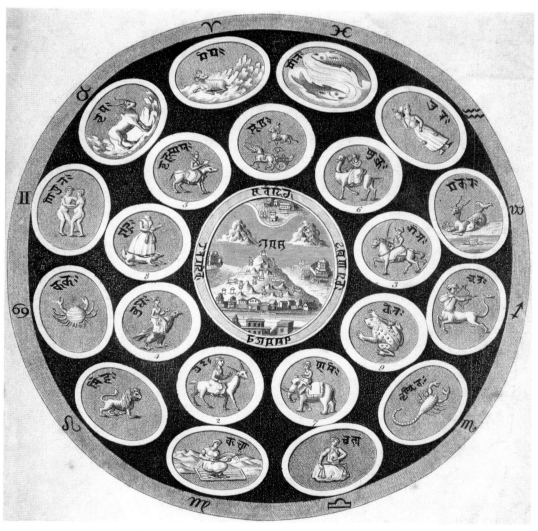

Indian zodiac *This early 19th-century print shows the Indian zodiac. The 12 signs are arranged around the outside of the zodiac wheel, running anticlockwise from Aries at the top.*

THE TAROT

With a **history** dating back more than 600 years, the tarot has been associated with various mystical beliefs and esoteric interests as well as **psychological interpretations**, resulting in a range of **card designs**. There are 78 cards in a tarot deck, divided into the 22 cards of the **Major Arcana** and the 56 cards of the **Minor Arcana**. Together, when shuffled and dealt into a **spread**, they become a method of divination.

If you are interested in **The Tarot**, you may also like to read about:
- **The Collective Unconscious**, pages 20–21
- **Western Astrology**, pages 56–57
- **Alchemy**, pages 296–297

History

The origins of the tarot are still a matter of debate, since there is no conclusive information about where and when it began, but it is generally considered to have developed in Italy in the early 15th century. At this stage, however, the tarot may have been a simple card game, with some Major Arcana cards, also known as 'trump' cards, added to an ordinary deck of playing cards, which, slightly expanded, became the Minor Arcana.

The tarot's role as a means of divination was first publicized in late 18th-century France. It gathered momentum in the middle of the 19th century as it was gradually adopted as a vehicle for different forms of mystical beliefs.

The tarot and psychology

In the late 19th century, the divinatory aspects of the tarot began to be overlaid with psychological interpretations and images, most notably in the Rider-Waite deck that was first produced in 1909. Many of the illustrations on the cards were drawn from mythology, astrology and alchemy. In the early 20th century, the Swiss psychologist Carl Jung (1875–1961) became interested in the tarot, identifying many of the images in the Major Arcana as archetypes of transformation – symbols drawn from the collective unconscious.

The Major Arcana

This section of the tarot deck consists of 22 cards, which are generally believed to depict our journey through life. The exact order of the cards can vary from one deck to another, according to the esoteric beliefs of that deck's designer. For instance, Strength sometimes comes before Justice, while in other decks their order is reversed. The cards of the Major Arcana are always fully illustrated.

The Minor Arcana

This section of the tarot deck comprises 56 cards, which are divided into the four suits of Wands (or Staves), Pentacles (or Disks), Swords and Cups. Each suit consists of ten 'pip' cards, numbered from the ace to ten, plus the four court cards of King, Queen, Knight and Page. The Minor Arcana deals with the detailed situations that we encounter in life, as well as some of the people (signified by the court cards) that we can meet. These cards are fully illustrated in some decks, while others only bear the symbols of the suit to which they belong.

Card designs

The interest in tarot grew so rapidly in the closing decades of the 20th century that there are now many different decks. They range from the classic to the completely innovative, drawing on images that are historical, esoteric or that cater for a particular interest, such as cats or fairies.

Reading the tarot

Tarot cards can be read by an individual for him or herself or for someone else. There is no limit to how often the cards can be read, although continual readings for oneself will eventually result in confusing messages from the cards, signifying the need for a break from them.

At the beginning of a reading, the cards must be shuffled, partly to mix them up and partly to align the energy of the cards with that of the person seeking the reading. While doing this, the person keeps the question they want to ask the cards at the forefront of their mind. The next step is to lay the cards out in a specific pattern known as a spread, either by dealing the cards face down off the top of the deck or by selecting them at random from the entire deck.

Tarot spreads

These vary considerably in complexity, from those using multiple cards, such as the 21-card Bohemian spread or the ten-card Celtic Cross spread, to the simplest involving only one card. In each case, the cards are laid out in a precise pattern, each position within that pattern having a specific meaning. Some spreads involve choosing a significator – a card that represents the person having the reading. If any of the cards are reversed (upside down), some tarot readers assign them special meaning, while others ignore their reversed state. The tarot reader has to interpret each card according to the position it occupies in the spread, and this is where the greatest proportion of the skill in tarot reading lies.

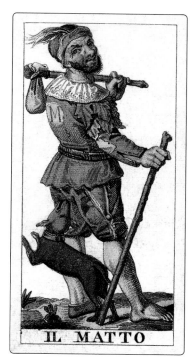

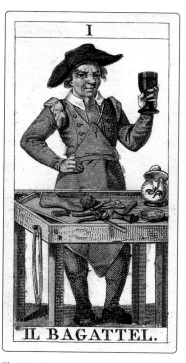

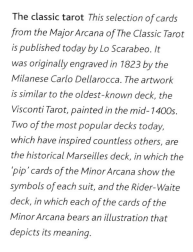

The Fool *Beginnings, often undertaken with great hope and expectation. These may be wise moves, or they may turn out to be foolhardy.*

The Magician *An influential person who may not be reliable. Alternatively, the card is a reminder of a person's many talents and abilities.*

The High Priestess *A good time for an individual to trust their instincts and intuition, and also to pay attention to dreams and spiritual matters.*

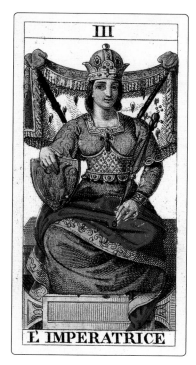

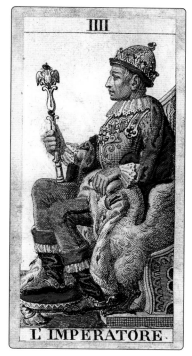

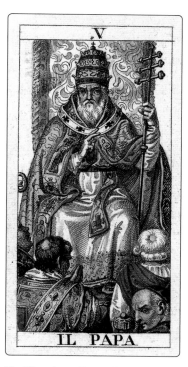

The Empress *A very fertile and creative phase, whether literally or figuratively. The card often signifies the need to be surrounded by nature.*

The Emperor *Increased power, and possibly the need to go into battle over an issue. Sometimes the card describes a helpful authority figure.*

The Hierophant *The need to do things in a traditional, conservative and cautious manner. Sometimes it indicates an increased spiritual need and purpose.*

RUNES

Of all the methods of divination, runes are possibly the most mysterious, partly because of the complexity of their meanings. They originated as a Scandinavian **ancient alphabet** and it was only later that they were used to divine the future, when they became known as **the Elder Futhark**. Today runes are available in a variety of materials, including wood, stone and plastic, and can easily be made at home. They are normally kept in a fabric bag or pouch when not in use. In addition to **interpreting the runes** through various **methods of casting**, they can be used as **talismans**.

If you are interested in **Runes**, you may also like to read about:
● The Tarot, pages 62–63
● Meditation, pages 78–79
● The Collective Unconscious, pages 20–21

An ancient alphabet

The Norse legend about the origin of the runes underlines their power and allure. According to the legend, Odin, the god of magic and the underworld, impaled himself with a spear and hung by his feet from a branch of Yggdrasil, the Tree of the World, for nine days and nights. His search for enlightenment was rewarded when he discovered the runes lying on the ground below him.

The more prosaic explanation of how runes originated is that they began life as an ancient Germanic alphabet. Over time, the letters were used for divination, each one being carved on a small piece of wood. Casting the runes – a process in which the runes were scattered on a cloth – was a solemn ceremony, carried out by the local priest or the male head of the family.

The Elder Futhark

The original Germanic alphabet has gradually evolved and expanded, and should not be confused with the runes, which are used for divination. Traditionally, there are 24 of these, and they are collectively known as the Elder Futhark. The word 'Futhark' is composed of the first six runes, just as the word 'alphabet' is composed of *alpha* and *beta*, which are the first two letters of the Greek alphabet. The Elder Futhark is divided into three categories, or *aettir*, of eight runes each. Each *aett* has a particular significance and atmosphere. The first *aett* is ruled by Freya, the goddess of creation, and describes the basic areas of life. The second *aett*, known as Haegl's *aett*, is the dominion of the ninth rune, Hagalaz, which rules hail. This *aett* is therefore associated with situations that are beyond our control. The final *aett* is named for Tyr, the god of justice and war, and describes transformation.

Recently, there has been much debate about the validity of a 25th rune, sometimes called Wyrd, which is blank. It appears in some sets of runes, but not in others. It represents a turning point in life.

Each rune is drawn with straight lines because these were easily etched on wood or painted on stone. Some of the runes look the same whether they are upright or reversed, and are called non-invertible runes. These have only one meaning. The runes that look different when inverted have two meanings, one for their upright position and one for their reversed position.

Interpreting the runes

Runes do not foretell the future in the same clear-cut manner as the tarot. Instead, they describe situations in broader terms that require careful analysis. They can also prompt much inner reflection. For instance, Uruz is the rune connected with wild oxen, which were dangerous creatures. Therefore it can be interpreted as the power and strength that is used to herd these oxen, or the need to control our own aggression. When inverted, Uruz describes energy that is wild and out of control.

Methods of casting

The runes can be cast in several ways. One is for the individual to place them face down on a flat surface and select a specific number, and then arrange these in a particular pattern, known as a spread. Another method is to place all the runes in a bag or cup and then to throw them on to a special cloth. The runes that land face up are interpreted, and the rest are ignored. A simpler method is for the individual to place the runes in their pouch, shake it while concentrating on a question or the circumstance about which they are seeking help and then to draw one rune, which can be read either as a comment on their situation or as guidance about how to deal with it.

Sigils as talismans

Another way to use runes is as talismans. An individual can translate his or her name into the runic alphabet and use the resulting sigil as a form of protection. A different option is for a person to carry a particular rune so that he or she can draw on its power. An appropriate rune can also be selected as a focus for meditation.

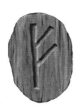 **Fehu** *The need to concentrate on whatever most nourishes you, whether emotionally, spiritually or physically.*

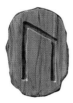 **Uruz** *Strength of character, strength of will and physical strength. Also, the importance of taking responsibility for your actions.*

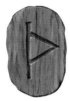 **Thurisaz** *Disruptive and chaotic situations are likely, but there is a reason for them. A time for weathering storms that come out of the blue.*

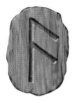 **Ansuz** *A good time for all forms of communication, whether asking for advice, listening to someone's reminiscences or sharing your wisdom with others.*

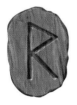 **Raido** *Journeys of all kinds, whether physical, mental, emotional or spiritual. Also, the need to move forward in your life.*

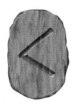 **Kaunaz** *The importance of shedding light on your life in order to understand it better and to see the way ahead.*

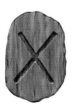 **Gebo** *Love in all its forms. It also represents gifts and generosity, in addition to working for a higher purpose to the benefit of all humanity.*

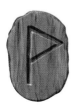 **Wunjo** *The joy that comes from a happy relationship, and from the ability to be content with your lot.*

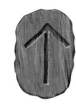 **Hagalaz** *Situations that are out of your control, in which all you can do is take each day at a time and draw on your moral courage.*

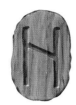 **Nauthiz** *A sense of need, whether for something physical, emotional or spiritual. It can also warn of friction between people.*

 Isa *Something has become blocked or stagnant, so it is difficult to make any progress. It can also describe a longing to cling to the status quo.*

 Jera *The wisdom that comes with time and experience. This rune is also linked with karma.*

 Eihwaz *The importance of being strong in the face of difficulties and challenges. Eihwaz is also linked with all forms of inheritance.*

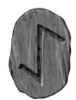 **Perth** *The mysteries of life, especially when you are caught up in something that you cannot explain or understand.*

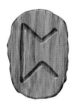 **Algiz** *The importance of taking care of yourself, in every way. This rune is believed to offer powerful psychic protection during meditation or when giving healing.*

 Sowelu *Confidence, optimism and vitality. Difficult situations will improve, so this is an encouraging rune in times of trouble.*

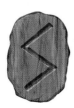 **Teiwaz** *Determination, strength of purpose and the ability to soldier on when times are hard. It also indicates successful business dealings.*

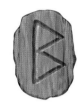 **Berkana** *Associated with all forms of birth, this rune encourages taking care of things that have recently come to life.*

 Ehwaz *This rune is connected with all forms of travel, and also with the importance of establishing a cooperative relationship with others.*

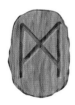 **Mannaz** *The need to be aware of your behaviour and how it affects the people around you. Also, the ability to use your intelligence.*

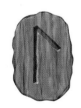 **Laguz** *A good time to connect with your unconscious, whether by using your intuition or by analysing your dreams. Sometimes it describes the need to cleanse your life of someone or something.*

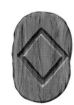 **Inguz** *The ability to live in harmony with nature and the seasons. It also describes fruitfulness in all its forms.*

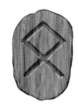 **Othila** *The rune associated with the home and with all forms of inheritance, whether of possessions, personality traits or genes.*

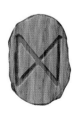 **Dagaz** *Change and fresh starts; the end of one cycle and the beginning of another. This rune can also refer to all forms of enlightenment.*

NUMEROLOGY

If you are interested in **Numerology**, you may also like to read about:
- **Western Astrology**, pages 56–57
- **Western Mystery Traditions**, pages 184–185

Numerology is both a form of divination and a method of understanding the significance of names and numbers. Usually based on the **Pythagorean system**, and involving simple **calculations**, it claims that each **number** has a particular **meaning** and energy, giving us insight into every aspect of our lives, including our psychology and our relationships. Using this knowledge, we can alter our names to align them more closely with our goals and personalities.

The Pythagorean system

Although there are other forms of numerology, the Pythagorean system, developed by the Greek mathematician Pythagoras (c. 580–500 BCE), is the most popular because it is easy to use and understand. Pythagoras believed that the universe is ruled by numbers, and he is reputed to have stated that 'number is the ruler of forms and ideas, and the cause of gods and demons'. In the system he devised, each letter of the alphabet was equated with a particular number, and each of these numbers was assigned a meaning. In this way, anything with a name or number can be analysed using numerology.

Using the Pythagorean system, each letter of the alphabet is assigned a particular number between 1 and 9, as follows:

1	2	3	4	5	6	7	8	9
A	B	C	D	E	F	G	H	I
J	K	L	M	N	O	P	Q	R
S	T	U	V	W	X	Y	Z	

The numbers assigned to each letter of the alphabet are added together. Numbers consisting of two or more digits are then reduced to a number between 1 and 9 by adding up the separate digits. For instance, 17 is reduced to 8: $1 + 7 = 8$. More complex forms of Pythagorean numerology can use multiple-digit numbers. It is quite common for numerologists to keep 11 and 22, known as master numbers, as whole numbers, which cannot be reduced any further.

The resulting number provides the numerological meaning of dates of birth, people's names, business names, the coming years, places of residence and many other things besides.

Some numbers are compatible, while others tend to work against one another. At the simplest level, it is believed that even numbers go well together, as do odd numbers, but they can cause friction when combined.

Number meanings

1. The number of beginnings. Creativity, independence, innovation, originality and leadership
2. Harmonious partnerships and the ability to get on well with others
3. Good communication skills, with a positive, sunny outlook
4. Stability, practicality, with a need for structure and the status quo
5. The number of travel. A need for flexibility and mental stimulus
6. Love for others and for the home. The need to be of service to others
7. Intuitive, mystical and sensitive, but can seem slightly emotionally detached and withdrawn
8. Financially adept, businesslike, ambitious and with strong links to the material world
9. Humanitarian, loyal, energetic and impatient, with a strong spiritual slant
11. Idealistic, with psychic gifts. Determined and inspirational
22. Capable and highly talented, but also a perfectionist

Numerology calculations

Numerology is principally used to examine the meanings of several numbers that are calculated from a person's date of birth and the name they most commonly use.

The destiny number, which is derived from a date of birth, is especially important because it is the one number that a person is born with and cannot legally change. It is calculated by adding up the numbers in a birth date, using the number of the month of birth: for instance, 1 November, 1962 is written as $1 + 1 + 1 + 1 + 9 + 6 + 2$, which, when added together, gives 21 and is then reduced $(2 + 1)$ to give a destiny number of 3.

Another important number is that of the day of the month on which a person is born, such as the 6th or 19th. Once again, any double numbers are reduced to a single number. This number gives further insights into an individual's personality.

Three numbers are calculated from a person's name. This is the name by which they are usually known, including any nicknames or pet forms of their

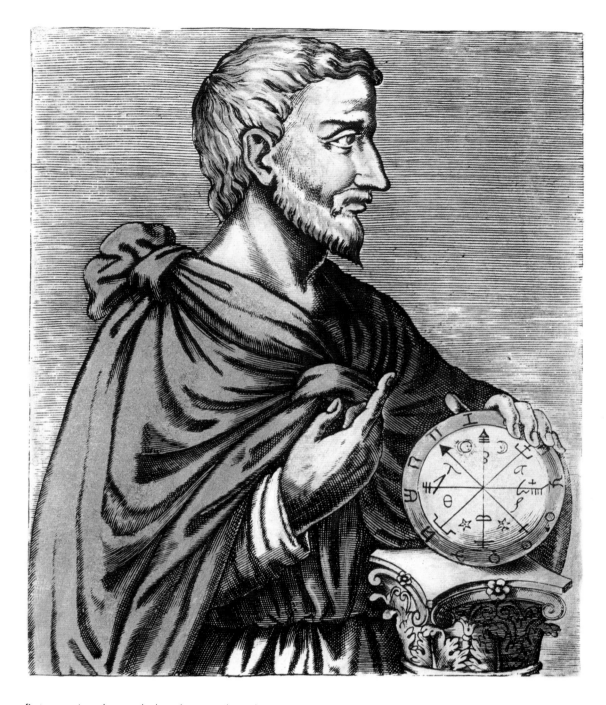

first name. In order to calculate these numbers, the name is written down and each letter is allocated its appropriate number. The vowels in the name are written above the name and the consonants below it. Although 'Y' is not a vowel, it is generally treated as such if it appears in a name in which there are no other vowels. Some numerologists treat 'Y' as a vowel if it sounds like one, as in the name Sally; others prefer to treat it as a consonant.

The first step is to add up the numbers representing the vowels and to reduce the result to a single number between 1 and 9. This number is called the heart number and describes a person's deepest wishes and desires.

The next step is to add up the numbers representing the consonants in the name. Once again, the result is reduced to a single number, which is called the expression number and describes the image that the person presents to the world.

Finally, the heart number is added to the expression number to give the personality number, which consists of all the numbers in the name. This describes the person's natural abilities, as well as revealing their strengths and weaknesses.

Each of these numbers is held to give important insights into the fundamental nature of an individual. Still more information is gained by comparing the numbers. Ideally, they should all complement one another. If they do not, the person has the option of altering the spelling of their name in order to improve its numerological meaning.

PALMISTRY

If you are interested in **Palmistry**, you may also like to read about:
● **Western Astrology**, pages 56–57
● **Other Forms of Divination**, pages 72–73

An ancient tradition, palmistry in all its **different forms** involves **studying the hands** in their many aspects. The shape and texture of the hands, the length and position of the **fingers and thumbs**, and the quality of the **lines on the palms** are all examined in order to analyse a person's character as well as to **foretell the future**.

An ancient tradition

Palmistry began in the East thousands of years ago before it finally spread to the West in the Middle Ages. A few books were written on the subject, but it only really came into its own in the 19th century. Among the famous early palmists were Marie Anne Adelaide Lenormand (1772–1843), who was frequently consulted by Napoleon Bonaparte in the early 1800s, and Count Louis Hamon (1866–1936), who practised under the name Cheiro in the early 20th century.

The different forms of palmistry

In the past, palmistry was divided into two sections: chirognomy, which is the art of analysing someone's character from the shape and size of their hands; and chiromancy, which analyses the lines on the hands. Today there are two further sections: dermatogylphics, which studies the skin patterns on the hands; and body language, which analyses a person's movements in order to understand their character. In practice, most contemporary palmists combine all these disciplines when reading palms.

In recent years medical science has begun to investigate palmistry, and there is now a significant body of work on the subject in which the shape of the hands and lines are studied in great detail to diagnose illnesses. However, this is a very specialized branch of palmistry that calls for a great deal of medical knowledge.

Studying the hands

Classic palmistry begins by studying someone's hands. Their shape and size as well as the texture of the skin are examined closely, because these all provide clues to the person's character and temperament. Traditionally, hands were divided into seven different shapes, including conic, psychic and philosophic. Many contemporary palmists prefer to work with four different hand shapes: fire, earth, air and water. Although these have links with Western astrology, they do not necessarily correlate with an individual's sun sign.

Fingers and thumbs

After assessing the shape of the person's hand, the palmist examines the individual fingers and thumbs, including the fingernails. The thumbs are particularly important, as they represent a person's will – or lack of it. The shapes of the fingertips are considered too, as they add more information to that provided by the basic hand shape. The gaps between the fingers and the position of the thumb on the side of each hand are also assessed. All these factors are believed to provide useful information about the personality.

Palm-reading *This 1560 drawing by Andrea Tricassus illustrates the basic principles of palmistry, including the mounts at the base of the fingers.*

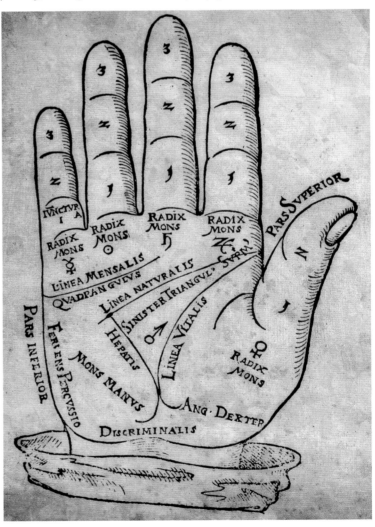

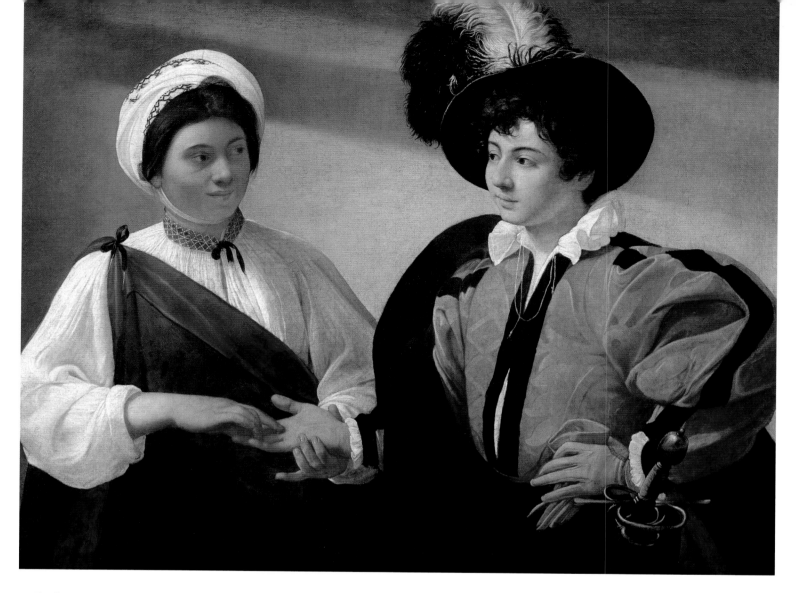

The fingerprints, which belong to the branch of palmistry known as dermatoglyphics, are scrutinized to determine whether there is a majority of whorls, loops or arches. Skin markings on the palms are also noted.

The mounts of the hand – the fleshy pads below the fingers and thumbs – are studied, and their absence can say as much as their presence.

Lines on the palms

For many people, one of the most fascinating aspects of palmistry is the study of the lines on the palms of the hands (chiromancy). These are divided into major and minor lines. The major lines are the life line, which curves around the base of the thumb; the heart line, which sits at the top of the palm; the head line, which crosses the middle of the palm; and the fate line, which runs up the palm from the base of the wrist. All four major lines can normally be seen on the hand, although sometimes the head and heart lines are replaced by a single line, known as the simian line. The minor lines, which still provide useful information but are less significant than the major lines, include the girdle of Venus, which sometimes spans the top of the hand.

All these lines are examined for their quality, strength and colour, because it is believed by palmists that their condition reflects the energy of whichever

The Fortune Teller *This 16th-century painting by Michelangelo Merisi da Caravaggio shows a gentleman having his palm read.*

aspect of life is ruled by that particular line. For instance, a feathery head line, lightly etched on the hand, indicates indecisiveness, while a thick, deeply marked heart line suggests intense emotions. In addition to the quality of the lines themselves, the positions where they begin and end on the hands are also held to be significant.

Breaks and interruptions to the lines, as well as other marks on the hands such as stars, squares and circles, are also taken into consideration when practising palmistry. These can all alter over time.

Foretelling the future

After looking at a person's hands to discover their character, a palmist usually examines the lines on the hands in order to predict the future. This is done by dividing each line into segments that indicate the different ages in life, and by looking for breaks or other markings that will be coming up in the near future. This is a relatively complex process and takes practice to perfect, but it can prove to be very accurate.

I CHING

If you are interested in the **I Ching**, you may also like to read about:
- **Uncovering the Unconscious**, pages 18–19
- **Confucianism**, pages 220–221

The *I Ching* is most often used as a form of divination, but this ancient text can also be read as a **philosophical work**. It has also attracted considerable interest from psychologists, notably **Carl Jung** in the first half of the 20th century. The *I Ching* consists of 64 **hexagrams**, each of which describes a different situation that someone might meet in life. Although the traditional way to **cast** the *I Ching* is with coins, it is now available in other forms too, including computer software programs. It is a simple matter to consult the *I Ching*, but what can pose more of a challenge to the contemporary reader is **interpreting** the text in its unmodernized form.

An ancient philosophical work

The *I Ching* originated in ancient China in approximately 2800 BCE. Four men are usually credited as being early authors of the work: Fu Hsi, Kin Wên, the Duke of Chou and Confucius (although some scholars are dubious about the extent of his involvement). However, the antiquity of the *I Ching* makes the exact details uncertain. The *I Ching* is also known as the Book of Changes, as a reminder that nothing stays the same.

Originally, the *I Ching* was cast with 50 yarrow stalks, but eventually that was considered to be impractical and the stalks were replaced by three coins, each with a heads and tails side. This is the method that is most commonly used today.

When it was first developed, the *I Ching* served two functions: it was a text intended to be read for contemplation and inner reflection, and it was also used for divination purposes. However, its function as a divination tool provoked dissent, and scholars abhorred that such an important philosophical text should, as they saw it, be misused.

The *I Ching* and Jung

Swiss psychologist Carl Jung was interested to see how the *I Ching* fitted his theory of synchronicity, which he described as a meaningful relationship between two events that take place simultaneously. He believed that this went beyond mere chance, and that even the most ordinary events will have the quality of a larger event when they occur at the same time. The *I Ching* gave him an opportunity to test this theory, as he described in his 1949 foreword to Richard Wilhelm's (1873–1930) German translation of an edition of the *I Ching* dating from the K'ang Hsi period of the 17th–18th centuries.

Casting the hexagrams

Three coins should be chosen, preferably of equal size and each with a clearly marked heads (obverse) and tails (reverse) side. Some paper and a pen or pencil are also required with which to draw the hexagram (six broken or unbroken lines) as it is created, plus a copy of the *I Ching*.

Begin by thinking of the question to ask the *I Ching*. As with other forms of divination, this works best if the question is kept simple so that it is easier

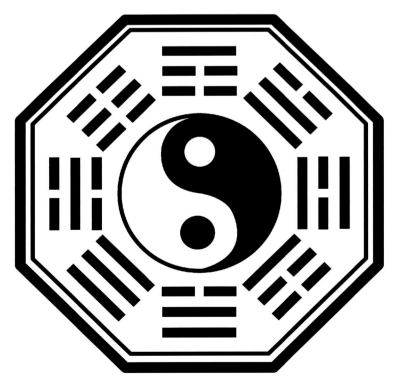

Hexagrams *This illustration shows the eight possible trigrams that can be thrown. The yin yang symbol is featured at its centre.*

to interpret the *I Ching*'s answer. The coins should be held in the hand and then tossed on to a flat surface, such as a table or floor. Note how they have fallen and count up their values. The heads, or obverse, side scores 2 and the tails, or reversed, side scores 3. There are four possible scores, with each one forming a different line in the hexagram: 6 gives an old yin line (broken and marked with 'X'); 7 gives a young yang line (unbroken); 8 gives a young yin line (broken); and 9 gives an old yang line (unbroken and designated with '0'). This first line forms the bottom line of the hexagram. Throw the coins five more times to create the rest of the hexagram, which is always created from the bottom upwards.

The meaning of the hexagram can then be looked up in the *I Ching*, using a special table of trigrams that gives the number of the hexagram that has been formed. If the hexagram contains any old lines (also known as moving lines), pay particular importance to their meaning when reading their interpretation. After reading about the hexagram, the moving lines should be converted into their opposites, so that a broken line becomes unbroken and vice versa. This will create a second hexagram, whose meaning is read as an adjunct to the first.

Interpreting the *I Ching*

Looking up the number of the hexagram in the *I Ching* is easy. What can be harder is to read that hexagram's narrative in the light of the question that has been asked, unless the text has been modernized. Traditional *I Ching* texts use particular phrases that can be difficult for contemporary readers to understand and interpret, referring as they do to maidens, sovereigns, the superior man, the mountain and so on. However, it helps to approach the *I Ching* in the spirit in which it was written, and to analyse its meaning carefully, rather than to expect it to provide ready-made answers. In this way, it regains the philosophy and spiritual wisdom that have made it such a valuable tool for contemplation for thousands of years.

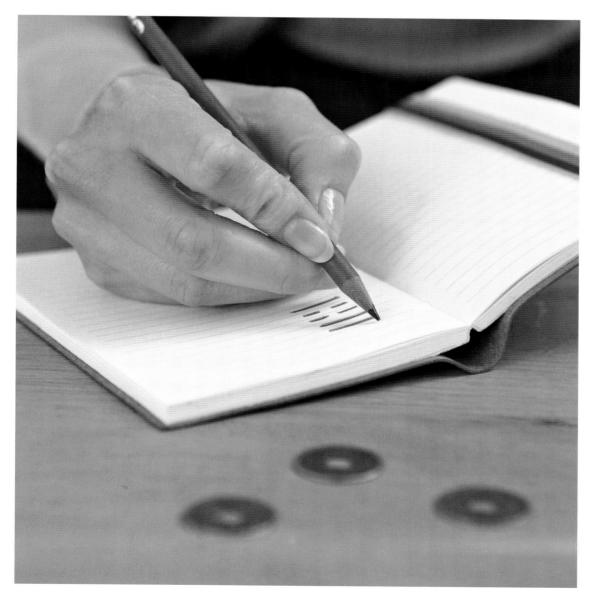

Throwing coins *In order to create a hexagram for the* I Ching, *three coins must be thrown on a flat surface six times. The different variations of the landing coins create the hexagram and lead the participant to a specific section of the* I Ching.

OTHER FORMS OF DIVINATION

If you are interested in **Other Forms of Divination**, you may also like to read about:
● **The Tarot**, pages 62–63
● **Numerology**, pages 66–67
● **I Ching**, pages 70–71

Divination can take many forms, which means that it offers plenty of scope in finding a technique for a specific purpose. When **dowsing**, a pendulum supplies straightforward answers to questions, while in **face reading**, a person's face is studied for information about their character. In addition, both **scrying** and **reading tea leaves** can provide considerable information about the future.

Pendulum dowsing

Dowsing is a traditional skill, often employing special rods to locate water, minerals or lost objects, but it can also be effective when used as a means of answering questions. Although you can use dowsing rods for this purpose, it is easier to use a ready-made pendulum – whether this is made from brass, crystal or wood – suspended from a length of cord. The cord is held so that the pendulum dangles beneath the hand, and questions are then put to the pendulum, to which it can reply 'yes' or 'no', according to the direction and shape of its swing. For instance, a circular swing may mean 'yes' and an elliptical swing may mean 'no', while an anticlockwise swing may indicate that the question should be rephrased.

It takes practice to become used to the pendulum and to train it to answer questions sensibly. The questions must also be simply phrased, one at a time. Another very important factor is that the questioner must distance him or herself emotionally from the answer, to avoid unconsciously influencing it in any way.

Scrying

This ancient form of divination involves gazing into a flat, shiny surface in order to see the future. Magicians from ancient Egypt scryed with bowls of water, ink or blood, while the Elizabethan magician John Dee (1527–1608) used a special black-backed mirror.

Crystal balls are often used for scrying, but these are expensive, so a small piece of polished crystal is another option. Alternatively, a bowl of water or a mirror can be used, but the scryer must make sure that they cannot see their own reflection in either of these, as that will act as a distraction and could diminish the results.

The results of scrying vary from person to person. Some people may see visions in the shiny surface, rather like watching a film. Others may see a single, symbolic image that needs to be interpreted, or they may see only clouds, which they also have to interpret according to their shapes and colours. Alternatively, the scryer may not see anything at all in a physical sense, but instead may work intuitively, as words or images come into their mind as they gaze at the surface.

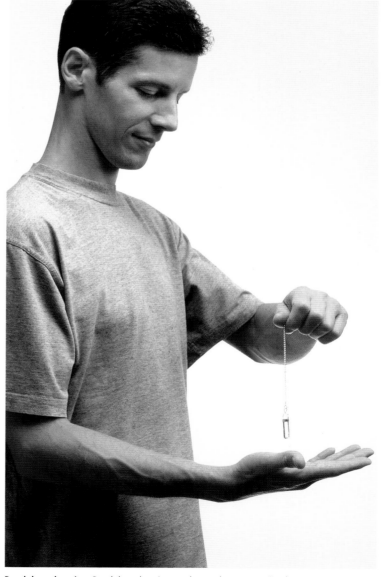

Pendulum dowsing *Pendulum dowsing can be used to answer simple yes or no questions and was traditionally used to predict the sex of an unborn baby.*

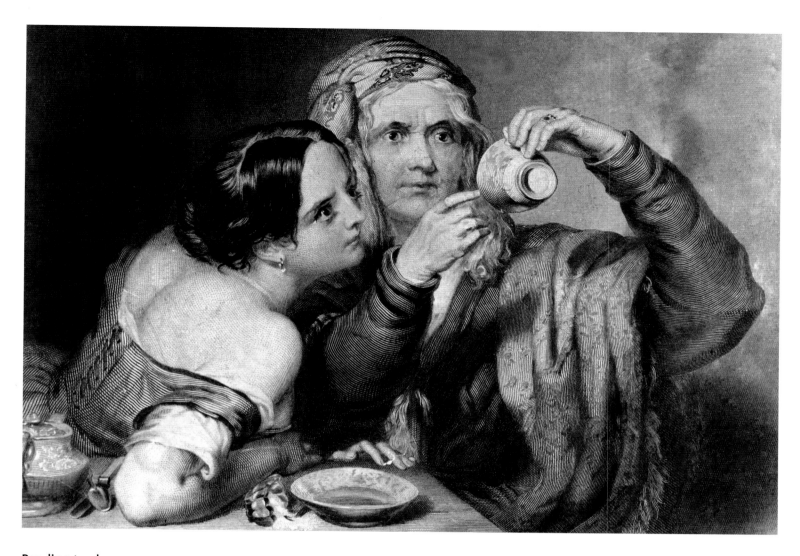

Reading tea leaves

Tasseomancy, the art of reading tea leaves, is one of the simplest forms of divination, but it can also be highly accurate. The tea leaves form patterns and shapes that provide information about a person's life and what the future holds for them.

One of the advantages of tasseomancy is that it requires very little equipment: all that is needed is a teapot, some loose tea leaves, a cup and saucer. The tea should be made in a teapot without an internal strainer so that the leaves can flow into the cup. The tea is then drunk while reflecting on the question to be asked. When there is only a very small amount of liquid left in the cup, turn it anticlockwise three times, cover it with the saucer and invert both cup and saucer so that the cup's rim is resting on the saucer. Leave the cup for a few seconds to allow all the tea to drain out, then pick the cup up and begin studying the shapes that the leaves have made. These are interpreted symbolically or literally, according to intuition and the circumstances of the person having a reading. The position of the leaves within the cup is also important, as it can indicate timing: leaves near the rim describe the near future, while those at the bottom of the cup indicate three or four weeks hence.

Tea-leaf reading *This 18th-century engraving depicts the art of tasseomancy, a form of divination that relies heavily on the instincts and skills of the reader.*

Face reading

Unlike the other forms of divination described here, face reading does not use any special equipment, nor does it describe the future in the same way. Instead, it interprets a person's facial features, based on the assumption that these describe the individual's character and therefore the path they will take through life.

Many cultures have practised face reading, but it has been particularly popular in China for thousands of years. In Chinese face reading, faces are divided into five different shapes, each named after one of the elements: water, wood, fire, earth and metal. Each facial feature has its own meaning. For example, the nose represents wealth, and the visibility of the nostrils is believed to describe a person's spending ability: open, flared nostrils indicate someone who enjoys spending money, while nostrils that are less visible belong to someone who knows how to hold on to their money. The ears are regarded as especially important because they indicate wisdom. Ears that are large and fleshy, with long lobes, indicate a long, healthy life.

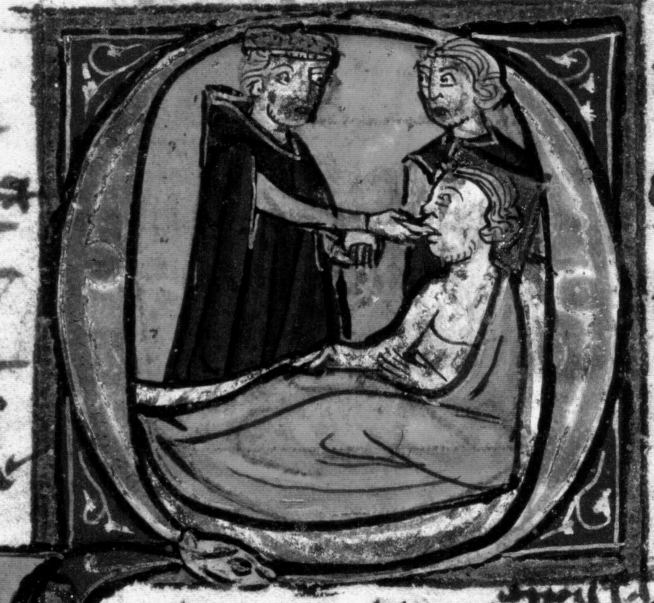

MIND
AND BODY

The 'mind–body problem', *psyche* versus *soma*, is one of the central and enduring mysteries of both science and philosophy. Can the mind directly affect the health of the body? Can we actually use the powers of our mind to prevent illness and to heal? Perhaps the single most important criticism of conventional medicine has been that it attempts to treat biology in isolation from psychology, insisting on a rigid dichotomy between mind and body. This section explores approaches and therapies that embrace a more holistic view.

Psyche versus soma

Although contemporary conventional Western medicine in general treats physiological and psychological ailments separately, other traditions have taken a very different view. The Indian ayurvedic system of health and traditional Chinese medicine has acknowledged the role of mind–body interactions since ancient times, but this was not just an Eastern approach. Hippocrates (c. 460–377 BCE), the father of Western medicine, emphasized the need to adopt a holistic approach: 'It is more important to know what sort of person has a disease than to know what sort of disease a person has.' Medieval European medicine deviated little from the Roman-era teachings of Galen (c. 130–200 CE), an influential Graeco-Roman physician, who propounded the theory of the four humours which made explicit the link between mind and body by explaining physical properties and characteristics, including disease, as the result of interaction between four types of bodily fluid, which were also held to determine personality, mood and other aspects of psychology. It was only during the Enlightenment in the late 17th and 18th centuries that the introduction of scientific method, with its need to isolate variables and remove from the equation capricious factors like personality, drove a wedge between mind and body.

Hippocrates *This book illumination from the 13th century shows Hippocrates treating the sick. Celebrated as the 'father of medicine', he advocated an empirical approach to the practice of medicine, but never lost sight of the importance of a holistic view of mind–body health.*

As allopathic medicine increasingly asserted authority over the practice of healthcare in the 19th and early 20th centuries, alternative and complementary systems such as homeopathy and chiropractic broke away to promote an alternative, holistic vision that included *psyche* and *soma*, mind–body and spirit.

The placebo effect

In the 1920s the neuroscientist Walter Cannon (1871–1945) described the 'fight or flight' response in animals, definitively linking psychological stimuli to hormonal and physiological responses, and conventional medicine began to recognize the link between mind and body. In the 1930s Hans Selye (1907–1982) developed the concept of stress as a major influence on health. And on the beaches of Anzio in the Second World War, Henry Beecher (1904–1976) uncovered the dramatic potential of the placebo effect; running short of morphine for wounded soldiers, he administered saline injections that proved to be almost as effective as the real thing.

The placebo effect is one of the powerful examples of the mind–body interaction. A placebo (from the Latin for 'I will please') is an inert substance given in place of a pharmacologically active agent (a drug). When patients are administered a placebo without knowing it, physicians often observe a 'placebo effect', whereby the patient's condition improves *as if* he or she had been given the real medication, apparently indicating that the patient's belief in the efficacy of treatment is what produces therapeutic effects.

Psychoneuroimmunology

Discoveries such as these launched a powerful new branch of science, psychoneuroimmunology (PNI). For conventional medicine, PNI is a route into a world already colonized by a profusion of complementary therapies that recognize the unity of mind and body, yet despite the mounting evidence for the efficacy and importance of PNI, conventional medicine continues to under-appreciate the centrality of the mind–body connection.

This section of the book explores a number of therapies that acknowledge the mind–body approach to holistic healing, illustrating Hippocrates' dictum that 'Natural forces within us are the true healers of disease.'

PSYCHONEUROIMMUNOLOGY

The study of the central nervous system and the immune system has revealed extensive **connections** between them. Psychological and social states, especially **stress**, can affect the functioning of the immune system and therefore health, and this offers a novel set of **interventions** for boosting/regulating the immune system, including stress-management programmes and laughter therapy.

If you are interested in **Psychoneuroimmunology**, you may also like to read about:
- Cognitive Behavioural Therapy and Mindfulness, pages 28–29
- Hypnotherapy, page 30
- Autogenic Training and the Endorphin Effect, page 80
- Meditation, pages 78–79
- Biofeedback, page 86

Mind–immune system connections

Until the 1960s conventional medicine refused to accept that the immune system might be affected by the central nervous system (CNS), and by extension by the mind and psychological states. This was despite a long history in medicine of recognizing and utilizing mind–body links, which stretches back to Hippocrates and beyond. Today psychoneuroimmunology (PNI) is an established and burgeoning discipline, thanks to a series of discoveries elucidating the three main pathways by which the CNS and the immune system can affect one another, as follows:

1. The CNS connects directly to parts of the immune system via the autonomic nervous system. This is the set of nerves that controls processes not under voluntary control, and includes nerve fibres that connect to the thymus, bone marrow and spleen – organs that are part of the lymphatic system, a vital component of the immune system. Meanwhile, the subdiaphragmmatic vagus nerve carries signals from the immune system to the CNS, so that communication goes both ways.

2. The endocrine system is made up of glands that secrete hormones – chemical messengers transmitted via the bloodstream. The endocrine system is partly controlled by the nervous system, while many immune cells carry surface receptors for hormones, such as cortisol, associated with stress. This allows CNS–immune system communication to be mediated by hormones; for instance, high levels of stress can lead to elevated cortisol levels in the bloodstream and this hormone can in turn bind to immune cells – up to a certain point this can stimulate cell function, but above a threshold it may instead suppress cell formation.

3. Cytokines are messenger molecules produced by immune cells; they help to direct and amplify the immune response. Proinflammatory cytokines, for instance, help to trigger inflammation in damaged or infected tissue. Cytokines can also affect brain function and nervous control of the endocrine system. Proinflammatory cytokines signal the CNS to increase body temperature as a way to retard bacterial growth, and also to shut down other body processes in order to preserve energy needed to fight illness. In other words, cytokines signal the brain to institute 'sickness behaviour', such as loss of appetite, drowsiness and the desire to rest.

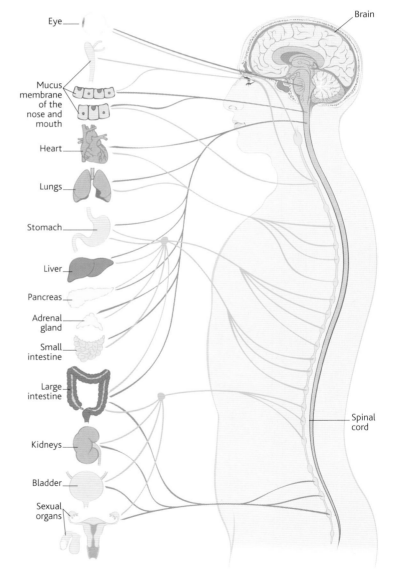

Autonomic nervous system *This diagram shows the major pathways of the autonomic nervous system, including the main organs that it controls.*

Labels: Eye, Brain, Mucus membrane of the nose and mouth, Heart, Lungs, Stomach, Liver, Pancreas, Adrenal gland, Small intestine, Large intestine, Spinal cord, Kidneys, Bladder, Sexual organs

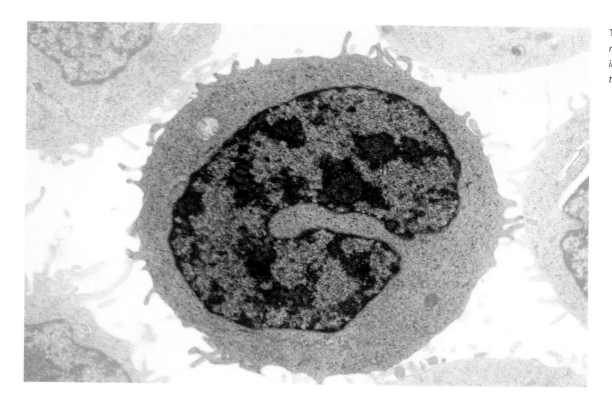

T **lymphocyte** *Research has shown that numbers of white blood cells can be increased and the immune system boosted through stress-management programmes.*

Stress

Extensive research has shown how acute and chronic stress can have positive and negative effects on the immune system. Acute (intense, short-lived) stress triggers the 'fight or flight' nervous and endocrine response, and this in turn mobilizes large numbers of immune cells, triggers release of antibodies and boosts production of cytokines. Chronic (long-lasting) stress, on the other hand, can suppress both immune cell function and antibody production, which may, for example, make a person vulnerable to infections and lengthen the time it takes to recover from illness. Stress can be broadly defined as anything that makes an individual feel threatened or anxious – for example, feeling lonely can be just as stressful as feeling put upon.

Psychological interventions to boost the immune system

If psychological and social states, such as loneliness, depression and chronic stress, can suppress the immune system, then interventions to alleviate these states should help to boost it. Patients with cancer and HIV have been particular targets of this research, because of the central role of the immune system in these diseases.

Stress-management programmes have been shown to boost immune function in some such patients, increasing the numbers and activity of some immune cells such as the all-important CD4+ T lymphocytes (white blood cells targeted by HIV); for instance, a study by Antoni et al., reported in the *American Journal of Psychiatry* in 2002, showed higher counts of CD4+ and other white blood cells after a ten-week stress-management intervention, while a July, 2008 study reported in the journal *Brain, Behaviour, and Immunity* found that 'mindfulness-meditation stress management training' was associated with higher CD4+ counts.

Disclosure of previously suppressed or undiscussed trauma through simple interventions, such as getting people to write or talk about traumatic events, has been shown to boost health and even improve response to vaccination, and may improve resistance to auto-immune diseases in the future. Relaxation is a powerful tool for improving psychological states, and there is some evidence that relaxation techniques and therapies, such as hypnosis and meditation, carried out regularly can boost antibody levels and increase numbers and activity of immune cells and therefore improve overall health. For example, research by K. G. Walton et al., reported in the *Annals of the New York Academy of Sciences*, 2004, revealed that long-term practitioners of transcendental meditation had significantly lower levels of the stress hormone cortisol than control subjects.

One of the most interesting applications of PNI is laughter therapy, which first secured mainstream medical attention with the publication of Norman Cousins' (1915–1990) book *Anatomy of an Illness*, published in 1964, in which he details his self-treatment of the painful and apparently incurable condition ankylosing spondylitis. When doctors appeared unable to do much for him, Cousins checked himself out of hospital and into a hotel room and watched comedy films and television programmes, such as the Marx Brothers and *Candid Camera*. He found that laughter alleviated his pain and allowed him to sleep. Other evidence suggests that laughter can indeed have direct positive effects on the immune system.

PNI may underlie much wider therapeutic benefits than these specific types of intervention. Some studies have suggested that a large proportion of drug treatments are effective because of the placebo effect, while others have suggested that placebos can be as effective as surgery or painkilling medication, underlining the importance of PNI.

MEDITATION

Achievement of tranquillity and spiritual discovery through a focusing of the mind have particularly strong roots in **Eastern spirituality**, but meditation in many different traditions shares **essential characteristics**. In the West, meditation, including the technique of **transcendental meditation** developed in the mid-20th century, has become important for its **therapeutic benefits**, with psychologists most recently concentrating on mindfulness-based stress reduction.

If you are interested in **Meditation**, you may also like to read about:
- Creative Visualization and Guided Imagery, page 33
- Mystical and Transcendent States, pages 34–35
- Yoga, pages 106–109
- Buddhism, pages 208–209
- Tibetan Buddhism, page 212
- Zen Buddhism, page 213
- Pilgrimage and Retreats, pages 298–299
- Breathwork, page 81

Meditation and Eastern spirituality

The practice of meditation involves clearing the mind of distracting thoughts and focusing consciousness. Form, purpose and content of meditation can vary widely, from simply focusing on breathing as an aid to relaxation, to repeating mantras (words or sounds), exploring the nature of reality, and seeking unity with the divine.

Meditation is important in Christianity, usually as a monastic practice involving prayer on scripture, and also features in Judaism (specifically Kabbalah) and Islam (especially in Sufism), but is usually associated with Eastern spirituality and religion. It is thought to have originated in Vedic Hinduism, and was an important feature of ancient yoga and of Taoism.

Whirling dervishes *Mevlevi Sufi dervishes demonstrate their meditative form of dance. The white robes represent shrouds and the conical hats tombstones, symbolizing earthly death and rebirth in mystical union with God.*

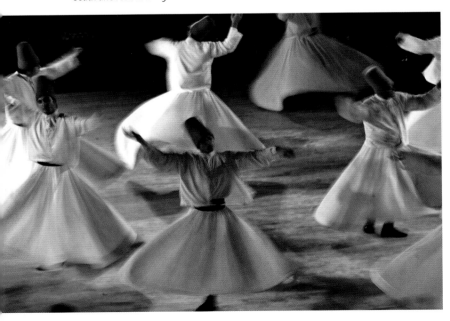

Meditation became one of the defining features of Buddhism, and Buddha is said to have achieved enlightenment specifically through meditation. In Buddhism a distinction is usually drawn between *shamatha*, sometimes translated as 'calm abiding', which involves focus on a single thought to achieve calmness and alertness, and *vipassana*, 'insight', the aim of which is to achieve wisdom about the true nature of reality. In Zen Buddhism meditation is elevated above all other routes to enlightenment as the key to discovery of self.

Essential characteristics of meditation

Most forms of meditation stress the need to quiet or still the mind and banish distracting, mundane thoughts. This allows achievement of a state of passive alertness, and focus on a single element. The nature of this element can vary widely. The process of breathing is a common focus. In transcendental meditation (see opposite) the focus is a personal mantra; in Tibetan Buddhism it is the mandala (a circular diagrammatic representation of the cosmos); in Christianity formulae such as the Lord's Prayer or the *Ave Maria* may be recited.

Meditation is often preceded by preparatory rituals for mind, body and place. A cross-legged, straight-backed posture is common, and is particularly important in belief systems featuring vital energy or life force, where it is believed to optimize the flow of energy. Meditation may be accompanied by chanting, props such as rosary beads, music, incense and even physical activity, as in t'ai chi or the dance of the whirling dervishes of Sufism.

Therapeutic benefits of meditation

Traditionally, meditation has been a route to tranquillity, physical and mental relaxation, inner knowledge, creative and spiritual development, psychic exploration, integration of consciousness, mystic and visionary experience, insight into the nature of reality and ultimate enlightenment. More recently in the West considerable attention has been paid to applications of meditation for therapeutic benefit.

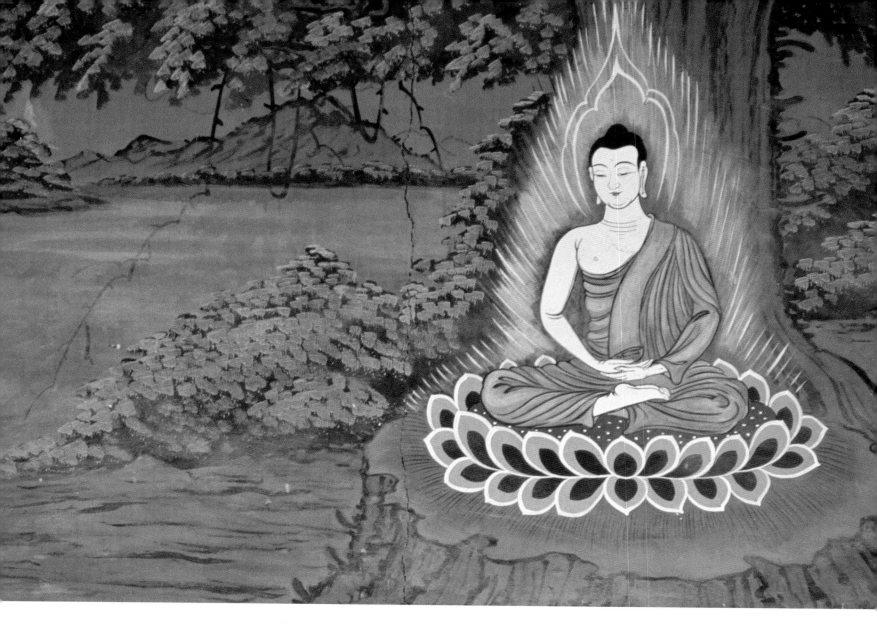

Relaxation is the primary therapeutic benefit explored. Meditation can help to relieve stress and anxiety, and induce calmness and tranquillity. It is recommended as part of a treatment programme for anxiety disorders and panic attacks, and also for conditions that may be stress-related, such as eczema, asthma, hypertension and irritable bowel syndrome. Research by Kabat-Zinn et al., reported in *Psychosomatic Medicine* in 1998 for example, indicated that meditation could improve stress-related psoriasis in a much shorter period of time than conventional techniques.

More generally, meditation can be an important tool for improving mental, emotional and social wellbeing. Increasingly, research is finding scientific evidence of meditation's ability to boost the immune system, balance/integrate mind and body, boost creativity, improve memory and aid learning and mental discipline. For example, research by Davidson et al. published in *Psychosomatic Medicine* in 2003 showed that mindfulness-based meditation (see page 29) boosted subjects' immune response to vaccination. The long-term practice of meditation also appears to have an effect on autonomic processes such as heart rate, blood pressure and metabolic rate.

Meditating Buddha *This painting of Buddha from the Temple of Yongju, Suwon, South Korea, shows a pose of meditation under a Bodhi tree, common in Eastern art.*

A 2004 study by Solberg et al. published in *Applied Psychophysiology and Biofeedback* showed that the heart rate of experienced meditators is significantly lower after a session of meditation than that of participants who only rested during the same period.

Transcendental meditation

In the 1950s Indian guru Maharishi Mahesh Yogi formulated an accessible version of ancient Vedic precepts for Western consumption, calling his system transcendental meditation (TM). TM is a meditation technique based on silent repetition of mantras for 20 minutes night and morning, which is said to lead to a heightened state of awareness known as cosmic consciousness, with benefits including improved mood, more energy and reduced stress. TM is said to lower the heart rate and blood pressure, reduce oxygen consumption and affect electroencephalograph (EEG) readings (see page 86).

AUTOGENIC TRAINING AND THE ENDORPHIN EFFECT

A system of **exercises and meditations** in body awareness and relaxation originally developed by German psychiatrist Johannes Schultz, autogenic training or therapy is believed to help relieve anxiety and many stress-related disorders. An associated programme of exercises known as the **Endorphin Effect** incorporates autogenic training.

If you are interested in **Autogenic Training and the Endorphin Effect**, you may also like to read about:
● **Psychoneuroimmunology**, pages 76–77
● **Cognitive Behavioural Therapy and Mindfulness**, pages 28–29
● **Body-Centred Therapies**, pages 82–83
● **Hypnotherapy**, page 30
● **Meditation**, pages 78–79
● **Buddhism**, pages 208–209

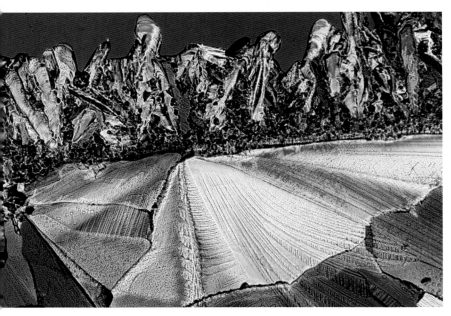

Beta-endorphin *This polarized light micrograph shows crystals of beta-endorphin, an opioid peptide that relieves pain.*

Autogenic exercises and meditations

Early 20th-century research in the mind–body field led Johannes Schultz (1884–1970) to develop a set of simple exercises that anyone could use to self-induce a trance state or state of hypnosis. 'Autogenic' means 'from within', and the key to Schultz's therapy was that the patient learned to carry out the hypnosis and subsequent healing on him or herself. Once learned, autogenic techniques form a valuable therapeutic tool that can be applied for self-management of conditions for life.

The key exercises are performed sitting, reclining or lying down in a comfortable position, and consist of repetition of simple formulae, allied with focus on different parts of the body. Schultz's aim was to counteract the 'fight or flight' autonomic response and induce a 'rest and digest' response, and the exercises/meditations follow from this. The formulae focus attention on bodily sensations associated with relaxation, including warmth and heaviness of the limbs, warmth in the abdomen, a cool brow, regular heartbeat and deep, slow breathing. The exerciser aims for a state of 'passive concentration', similar to the Buddhist technique of 'mindfulness', in which the conscious self becomes an alert but passive observer. Autogenic training takes place over about eight to ten weeks, including thrice-daily practice sessions.

Clinical research studies suggest that autogenic training may have promise as a treatment for circulatory problems (such as cold hands or feet), hyperventilation, gastrointestinal problems (such as constipation and diarrhoea), phantom limb pain, and fatigue and emotional problems in people with multiple sclerosis. Practitioners of autogenic training also claim that it can be used to treat high blood pressure, relieve stress and treat anxiety-related disorders such as insomnia, eczema, panic attacks and irritable bowel syndrome, and that regular practice of the techniques can increase concentration and focus, build self-confidence, combat jet lag and fatigue and boost creativity.

The Endorphin Effect

At the beginning of the 21st century, British holistic healer and author William Bloom explored the parallels between 'new' scientific discoveries in the field of psychoneuroimmunology (PNI) and the tenets and practices of many complementary and alternative therapies that emphasize the mind–body connection, with particular reference to endorphins, naturally occurring opiates that act as hormones and neurotransmitters, mediating positive sensations and emotions and relieving pain.

He developed a set of simple strategies and exercises for mind–body control aimed at allowing people to inhibit the production of adrenaline and cortisol – 'stress hormones' linked to the 'fight or flight' response – and boost endorphin production. These revolve around awareness and monitoring of bodily sensations and states, which Bloom explicitly links to the practices of focusing (see page 83). These 'Endorphin Effect' exercises include: focusing attention on inner sensations; sending positive thoughts to the body; cutting off the mind from external stimuli; and slowing down breathing to a relaxed, sleep-like rhythm.

BREATHWORK

Breathwork describes techniques for altering breathing as part of psychotherapy or meditation, based on the theory that breathing regulates vital energy and that psychological states can be expressed in the way we breathe. Perhaps the earliest form of breathwork is yogic **pranayama**; modern Western alternative therapies include Grof's **Holotropic Breathwork** and Orr's **Rebirthing-Breathwork**.

If you are interested in **Breathwork**, you may also like to read about:
- **Mystical and Transcendent States**, pages 34–35
- **Body-Centred Therapies**, pages 82–83
- **Yoga**, pages 106–109
- **Hinduism**, pages 204–205
- **Martial Arts**, pages 116–117
- **T'ai Chi**, pages 112–113
- **Energy**, pages 302–303
- **Chakras and the Aura**, pages 172–173

Pranayama

A Sanskrit word meaning 'lengthening of life force' (although *prana* can also be translated as 'breath'), pranayama can also mean 'breath control' or 'breath restraint'. It describes a set of yogic exercises involving breathing, aimed at stilling the mind and attaining higher states of awareness.

Yoga teachers view pranayama as just one aspect of an overall system, but in both India and the West it has become popular as an independent practice, and is said to have therapeutic benefits for stress relief, stress-related disorders, asthma, immune function and metabolism, and even to improve willpower and judgment and enhance perception.

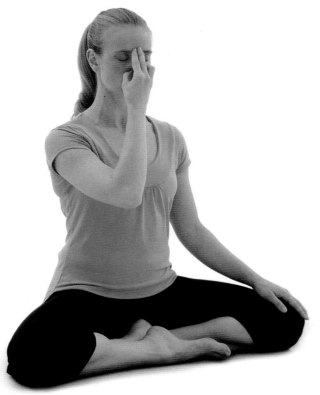

Nadi-sodhana pranayama *Alternate nostril breathing is a common breathing exercise used in yoga practice.*

Holotropic Breathwork

Developed by Stanislav Grof from his work on psychedelic psychotherapy, Holotropic Breathwork uses hyperventilation (referred to as intensive breathing) in conjunction with music, drumming, focused bodywork (massage and manipulation of areas of tension) and other adjuncts to access altered states of consciousness. Holotropic means 'moving towards wholeness', and Grof believes that intensive breathing can amplify natural psychic processes, induce self-healing and access visions and mystical experience.

Grof describes many types of experience accessible through his system, including hallucinations, heightened awareness, revisitation and resolution of trauma and repressed emotions, access to information beyond the normal boundaries of the self (such as out-of-body experiences, encounters with archetypes, reliving of significant past lives) and recollection and resolution of birth trauma (a point of similarity with Rebirthing-Breathwork).

Critics argue that hyperventilation is dangerous and that the technique can be damaging. Grof himself recognizes that the technique is unsuitable for some individuals and certain conditions, including epilepsy, pregnancy and psychiatric disorders.

Rebirthing-Breathwork

New Age guru Leonard Orr developed Rebirthing-Breathwork as a technique to resolve deep-seated psychological trauma caused by the process of human birth. The central technique is connected breathing, where there is no pause between inhalation and exhalation. It is claimed that this boosts oxygen levels in the blood to counteract supposedly chronically inadequate oxygenation of the blood, and to relieve the toxic levels of carbon dioxide believed to help maintain psychological and physical repression. In so doing, practitioners are believed to access and resolve perinatal trauma stored in their cellular memory, although the effectiveness of the practice is the subject of debate. Critics argue that there is insufficient evidence to support the concept of perinatal memories or cellular memory.

Caution: Breathwork therapies should only be undertaken under the guidance of a highly qualified therapist in the particular discipline involved.

BODY-CENTRED THERAPIES

Body-centred therapies is a term that describes a field of psychotherapy focused around core beliefs about how **energy**, thoughts, feelings and personality are **embodied**, based on the theories of psychoanalyst **Wilhelm Reich** and since developed into a **school** of therapeutic approaches, including Somatic Emotional Therapy, the Hakomi method, Integrative Body Psychotherapy, bioenergetics, Radix, Rubenfeld Synergy Method, focusing and many others.

If you are interested in **Body-Centred Therapies**, you may also like to read about:
- **Chiropractic and Osteopathy**, pages 132–135
- **Applied Kinesiology**, page 168
- **Yoga**, pages 106–109
- **Pilates**, pages 110–111
- **Alexander Technique**, pages 118–119
- **Shiatsu**, pages 124–125
- **Bowen Technique**, page 138
- **Rolfing**, page 139
- **Iridology**, page 140

Embodied psychology

Most body-centred psychotherapies share a set of core beliefs about the relationship between mind and body, the most fundamental of which is that there is no clear distinction between the two. All aspects of mind and psychology are embodied – that is, contained in and expressed through the physical substrate of the person: his or her body. Emotions, memories, thoughts and personality are not simply mental artefacts or constructs; they have real physical presence in the body, expressed through body structure, breathing, posture and movement, and the way the whole organism functions. Body-centred psychology is holistic.

In body-centred psychotherapy phrases such as 'pain in the neck', 'stiff upper lip' and 'feet on the ground' are more than just figures of speech; they communicate literal truths about how the body expresses its psychology. Most of the therapies stress the importance of breathing, and of expressive movement and posture modification as agents of change. Many stress the therapeutic benefits of touch, but only within boundaries agreed between client and therapist.

Body-centred psychotherapy, also known as body–mind therapy, is distinguished by its emphasis on taking therapy components from bodywork schools such as the Alexander technique, rolfing and the Feldenkrais method, which focus primarily on postural and structural body mechanics, although emotional and mental states are affected as a consequence.

Energy

Most body-centred psychotherapies develop a theory of bodily energy; terms used to describe this include vital force, chi, kundalini, bioenergy field and vibrations. The free and proper flow of energy in the body is understood to be essential to the functioning of the organism, and dysfunction and pathology are often linked to blocks or disturbances in this flow – for instance, as blockage of the chakras. Influential body-centred therapists like Keleman and Rosenberg describe normal function as a cycle in which energy or charge builds up until it is discharged. Interference with this cycle causes problems.

Wilhelm Reich's theories and practices

An Austrian psychoanalyst and protégé of Sigmund Freud, Wilhelm Reich (1897–1957) championed progressive ideas about sexuality and pioneered the holistic approach to mind–body interaction and therapy.

Reich insisted that the core of human psychology was a positive, life-affirming sexual energy. Specifically, he developed the concept of energy flow in the body, based on his experiences in analysis in which patients had reported 'streaming' sensations in their genitals when therapy was proceeding successfully. Both mental and physical problems, Reich argued, were the manifestations of blockages in energy flow, blockages that could be treated physically through 'bodywork' – repositioning and manipulating the body – rather than through talking.

In 1933 he laid out his theory that repression of the free flow and expression of sexual energy – the power of the orgasm – caused and was reflected by mind–body symptoms called 'character armour', in which 'rigidities' in a person's character were reflected in chronic muscular spasms. Later he claimed to have discovered a new fundamental force of nature to rank alongside electromagnetism. He called this new force 'orgone', believing that it generated sexual/life energy, and that all degenerative illnesses (or 'biopathies') were the result of blockages and deficiencies in the flow of orgone, which in turn were the result of emotional and social phenomena.

Eventually, Reich's controversial theories and practices provoked a hostile reaction from the authorities in the USA and he was sent to jail, where he died in 1957. His legacy, however, has influenced practically all subsequent body-centred therapies.

The body-centred psychotherapy school

There are over a dozen important body-centred psychotherapies:
- Bioenergetics was developed by Alexander Lowen, a student of Reich, and involves breathwork, yoga-style postures and stretching with the help of a 'breathing stool' – a padded bench across which the client can stretch to open the chest and spine.

Chakras *This diagram illustrates the position of the chakras, wheels of psychic energy that awaken kundalini energy.*

- Radix (from the Latin for 'root' or 'source') is another so-called 'neo-Reichian' therapy, developed by Charles Kelly and based in part on vision psychology and the Bates method. Radix therapists work through muscular tension in the face and head and then the rest of the body.
- Stanley Keleman was a student of Lowen who developed Somatic Emotional Therapy (somatic meaning 'of or concerning the body'), which teaches clients how to reorganize their muscular emotional patterns.
- The Hakomi method takes its name from a Hopi Indian word meaning 'who are you?' It was formulated by Ron Kurtz and uses mindfulness (see page 29), touch and gentle discussion and modification of body language.

- Integrative Body Psychotherapy, developed by Jack Rosenberg, uses awareness, breathwork, movement and self-release techniques to 'track' mind–body interruptions and develop 'somatic intelligence' to help better understand 'somatic experience'.
- Rubenfeld Synergy Method, a 'talk and touch' therapy developed by Ilana Rubenfeld, facilitates innate healing capacity to release mind–body 'holding patterns' and boost life energy, expressing and resolving repressed emotions.
- Focusing, developed by Eugene Gendlin, helps clients to tap into 'felt sense', a form of implicit, embodied knowledge or feeling. Awareness of this can help to 'unstick' clients and achieve a 'felt shift'.

NEUROBIOLOGY OF EMOTION

Emotion is a mind–body phenomenon, involving physical and psychological components. These are processed by brain structures such as the **limbic system** and the cortex, which interact according to an **information-processing model**. A controversial therapy known as **Eye Movement Desensitization and Reprocessing** (EMDR) claims to use this model to treat and cure trauma and other mental health problems.

If you are interested in **Neurobiology of Emotion**, you may also like to read about:
- **Cognitive Behavioural Therapy and Mindfulness**, pages 28–29
- **Psychoneuroimmunology**, pages 76–77
- **Autogenic Training and the Endorphin Effect**, page 80
- **Body-Centred Therapies**, pages 82–83
- **Breathwork**, page 81

Components of emotional response

According to the latest understanding of neuroscience, an emotion is a subjective experience derived from a combination of physiological and psychological factors. The physical side of an emotion is produced by a combination of neurology (the firing of nerve cells and activation of brain centres) and physiology (the action of hormones and neurotransmitters, and the effects they produce in the body). Physiological processes produce what

MRI scan *This magnetic resonance imaging scan shows a cross-section through the brain and skull. The MRI machine detects the magnetic field of hydrogen nuclei, which are more abundant in oxygenated blood, and so show areas of higher blood flow.*

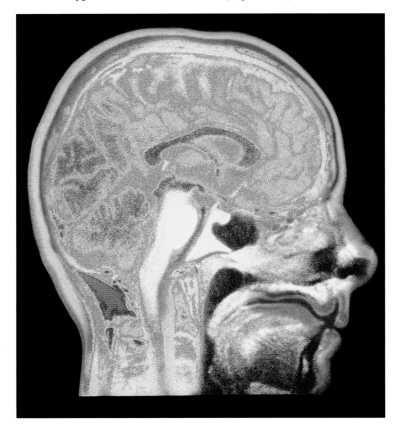

are known as the visceral sensations of emotion, such as a dry mouth, sweaty palms, racing heart, unsettled stomach and so on.

The psychological aspects of emotion include the effect of context and the input of 'higher' mental processes, such as learning, memory and knowledge. These influences are particularly important in more complex emotions, such as shame, guilt or wistfulness.

The limbic system

This is a set of structures that lies deep within the brain, which is heavily connected both to the cortex, the 'higher' brain where thinking, reason and analysis are located, and the brain stem, the part of the brain that produces visceral reactions. As well as emotions, the limbic system is central to other 'primitive' aspects of the mind – basic survival drives like sex and hunger – and to more sophisticated processes, such as memory and learning.

Two of the primary brain structures of the limbic system are the amygdala and the hippocampus. The job of the amygdala is to make initial assessments of information from the senses and trigger the relevant emotion – especially fear and other negative emotions. Depending on this assessment, the limbic system then activates glands in the brain and parts of the nervous system to produce a physiological response, readying the body for action. The hippocampus processes and directs the storage of memories, working in conjunction with the amygdala to attribute emotional content and intensity to memories.

The limbic system connects to the brain stem, which in turn triggers the visceral sensations of emotion. This 'embodied' component of emotion is important in complementary and alternative health systems such as mind–body therapies, breathwork, autogenic training and the Endorphin Effect. Connections to the cortex allow memory, knowledge and reason to modify emotion. Particularly important is the temporal lobe, where the subjective experience of emotion is primarily located.

Information-processing model

These components are typically understood to work together in an information-processing model, in which stimulus (information coming in

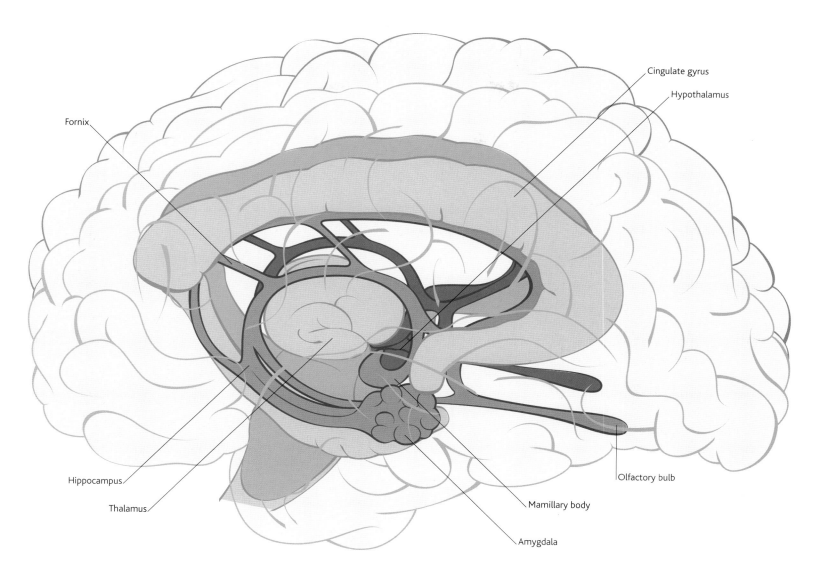

Fornix

Cingulate gyrus

Hypothalamus

Hippocampus

Thalamus

Mamillary body

Amygdala

Olfactory bulb

from the senses) arrives via the brain stem and is initially processed by the amygdala to assess the appropriate type and intensity of emotional response. At the same time the cortex is processing the stimulus and combining it with input from memory and knowledge, such as the context of the stimulus. The limbic system and cortex interact and combine to signal the temporal lobe and generate the subjective experience of emotion, while at the same time the limbic system is signalling the brain stem to trigger physiological responses. The limbic system and the cortex also work together to form and store a memory of the emotion.

When this model malfunctions, mental problems can result. An important example is post-traumatic stress disorder (PTSD), which is a disorder of memory and emotion where the two are dysfunctionally processed, labelled and stored, with distressing consequences.

Eye Movement Desensitization and Reprocessing

Francine Shapiro developed Eye Movement Desensitization and Reprocessing in 1987, but it remains a controversial and poorly understood treatment. She

Limbic system *This is a set of structures between the brain stem and the cerebral cortex that mediates and regulates emotion, memory and learning. Key structures include the hippocampus and the amygdala.*

found that getting PTSD sufferers to recall traumatic events while they tracked her finger movements with their eyes produced remarkable results: memories were stripped of their painful associations and clients were able to resolve problems and make dramatic improvements in their mental health. In addition to the eye movement there are extensive cognitive-behavioural components to the therapy to help identify 'Target Memories' (the traumatic ones to which the therapist wants to desensitise the patient).

There is evidence to suggest that EMDR is useful for treating PTSD and many other disorders, but there is also confusion over how it works. For instance, any kind of laterally alternating stimuli, such as sounds coming from one side and then the other, seem to produce comparable effects, and a form of EMDR has been used to treat blind patients. A related therapy, where the mechanism of action is even less clear, is energy psychology.

BIOFEEDBACK

If you are interested in **Biofeedback**, you may also like to read about:
- **Behaviourism and Attachment Theory**, page 26
- **Meditation**, pages 78–79
- **Body-Centred Therapies**, pages 82–83

Biofeedback is where a person is able to see in action physiological processes not normally available to the conscious mind – for instance by watching an EEG, the person can see a picture of their brain waves, and this in turn feeds back to those same brain waves. The individual is then able to carry out the procedure without the equipment.

The **applications of biofeedback** are wide-ranging and include the **HeartMath** system.

History of biofeedback

The concept that it is possible to exert conscious control over autonomic processes was controversial when it was first aired by American animal behaviourist Neal Miller (1909–2002) in the early 1950s. His experiments appeared to show that, using simple conditioning techniques, rats could be trained to perform feats such as lowering heart rate, dilating blood vessels in one ear at a time or controlling the rate of urine production in the kidneys. Miller was accused of scientific heresy, but in the late 1950s Russian psychologist Maya Ivanovna Lisina showed that humans could achieve similar feats. She hooked up test subjects to a polygraph displaying constriction or relaxation of the blood vessels, and found that if they were allowed to watch the polygraph readings they could learn to dilate their blood vessels by conscious effort of their will.

Applications of biofeedback

Biofeedback can be carried out with heart rate, skin conductivity, blood pressure, muscle function and many other processes that can be monitored and displayed. When using an electroencephalograph (EEG), biofeedback has proved to be a powerful tool for relaxation, relieving anxiety and boosting powers of visualization. An EEG displays brain-wave activity as lines on a graph or monitor and the subject watches the readout in real time. There is some evidence that EEG biofeedback therapy can boost immune function and increase both the numbers and activity of immune cells. Biofeedback therapy has also been applied to athletic performance, and practitioners claim that it may be an effective treatment for tension and migraine headaches, high blood pressure, incontinence, epilepsy, alcoholism, sleep disorders, irritable bowel syndrome, tinnitus, asthma, eczema and sexual dysfunction, although high-quality controlled studies confirming these claims are not as yet available.

HeartMath

One of the most popular and accessible applications of biofeedback therapy has been the HeartMath system. HeartMath is based on the theory that disordered or irregular heart rhythms, in which the heart rate fluctuates in a

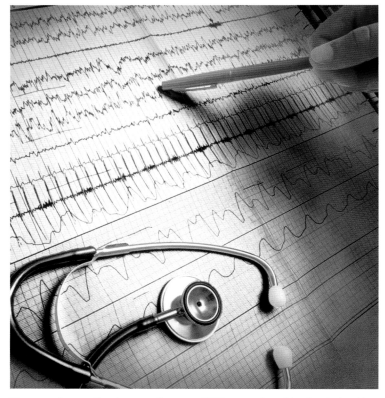

Electrocardiogram *The electrocardiogram or ECG is a recording of the electrical activity of the heart over a period of time, and is used to monitor heart function in a patient. If the patient is allowed to monitor the reading, an ECG can be used for biofeedback training.*

chaotic fashion, are responsible for a state of physiological 'incoherence', which in turn leads to illness and unhappiness. Proponents of HeartMath claim that by learning to regulate heart rhythm and bring about coherence, health and wellbeing can be enhanced.

One way to do this is to employ a biofeedback device marketed by the Institute of HeartMath, known as the emWave Personal Stress Reliever, which claims to monitor and display heart rhythms, so that with simple training the user can modulate and improve them.

ENERGY PSYCHOLOGY THERAPIES

If you are interested in **Energy Psychology Therapies**, you may also like to read about:

● **Acupuncture**, page 126
● **Acupressure**, page 127
● **Neurobiology of Emotion**, pages 84–85
● **Energy**, pages 302–303

Combining psychotherapeutic techniques with traditional Eastern acupressure techniques for manipulating **energy meridians**, energy psychology therapies include **Thought Field Therapy** and the **Emotional Freedom Technique**. They are similar in principle to Eye Movement Desensitization and Reprocessing (EDMR), but use pressure stimuli in place of auditory or visual ones.

Energy meridian regulation

Energy psychology borrows concepts about energy from traditional Chinese acupuncture, specifically the belief that proper functioning of mind and body depend on the free flow of energy through certain pathways in the body – energy meridians. Trauma, anxiety, unhappiness and ill health all result from disruption or blockage of these meridians. Simply talking about problems is not enough; energy psychology therapies treat them by using acupressure in conjunction with psychotherapeutic techniques (mainly cognitive behavioural ones). In essence, practitioners claim that tapping acupressure points while thinking about anxiety-triggering memories can restore balance to the body's energy flow.

An alternative explanation is that the tapping pressure stimulates mechanoreceptors – touch-sensitive nerve endings – and somehow mediates the release of chemical messengers (endorphins, for example); or that, as may be the case in EMDR, distraction/dual attention effects some sort of mental reprogramming.

Thought Field Therapy

Developed in the early 1980s, Thought Field Therapy (TFT; a.k.a. the Callahan technique) is a relatively complex technique for identifying appropriate acupressure points. The correct sequence – or algorithm – is determined using muscle testing, in similar fashion to kinesiology. Each problem or therapeutic target will have a unique algorithm. Roger Callahan, the founder, has claimed that TFT can cure phobias in as little as five minutes and malaria in just 15, and can also be used to treat addictions, anxiety disorders, depression and even cardiovascular diseases.

Emotional Freedom Technique

Gary Craig, who trained with Callahan, decided that complex algorithms were unnecessary, and that the sequence in which points were tapped was immaterial. He identified 15 specific acupressure points, and argued that although it is not necessary to tap all of them for every problem, there are few enough for more precise targeting to be unnecessary. He also incorporated elements of EDMR into his system. Craig describes his version of energy psychology as 'an emotional version of acupuncture, except needles aren't necessary'. Clients learn to tap themselves, while focusing on their problem and repeating simple cognitive behavioural therapy-style affirmations. Fast and effective, the system has shown benefits for phobias, asthma, migraine, high blood pressure, insomnia, diabetes and so on, and for emotional states such as loss of self-esteem. It does not replicate well under test conditions, since – as with so many subtle mind–body therapies – fear, insecurity and lack of trust are basic emotions that often interfere with the test procedure.

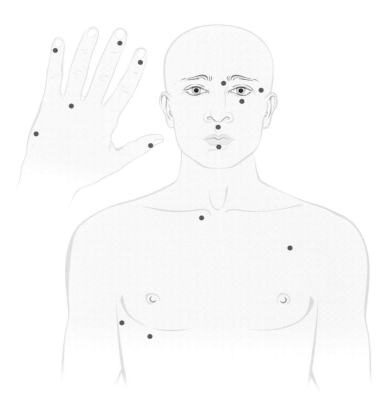

Tapping *The Emotional Freedom Technique uses acupressure points based on classical acupuncture meridians to help clients overcome a range of psychological problems.*

PART TWO
BODY

EASTERN APPROACHES 92

BODY WORK 104

NUTRITIONAL AND HERBAL APPROACHES 142

ENERGY THERAPIES 154

BODY AND SPIRIT 170

PART TWO
BODY

I qualified as a medical doctor in the early 1970s, feeling that my education had overlooked something. Knowing I had to find out what it was, I moved – like many a lad seeking his fortune – to London, where the counterculture was in full flower: East and West in slow collision. The Californian currents of Gestalt, transpersonal and encounter groups, along with the body-centred psychotherapies, were encouraging us to be more emotionally open; meanwhile, the traditions of yoga and meditation flowing in from Asia urged us to seek a higher self. Ecological, feminist and Afro-American movements stirred this turbulent mix, intensifying the feeling that social and individual transformation were just around the corner. A new awareness of human potential was breaking through: a sense that life and living are miraculously complex, that our bodies are wired for consciousness and potentially in synch with the living world where they evolved; an intuition that said if only we could tap the living forces of healing, nothing would be impossible. Faced with the 21st-century's many challenges, such a spirit of the time could still serve us well today.

These impulses for personal transformation and change continue to underpin the world of complementary therapies, and I am sure that this is part of the reason why people are attracted to them. But these approaches also speak about the body as a whole – something that Western medicine lost sight of as it reduced the body to component parts. Modern Western medicine's successes with infections, deficiency diseases, anaesthetics and surgery make a convincing case that when the parts need treating, medical science is very good at it.

But if medical science's role is to wage war on disease, then perhaps the older systems of medicine can help make peace in the body.

This is why I believe the two approaches truly *complement* one another. When I learned about homeopathy (and later osteopathy and acupuncture), many of Western medicine's missing pieces seemed to fall into place. These traditions became a place to seek wisdom that I could draw on for triggering self-healing, because they are founded on generations of observing people getting ill and recovering. So they have a lot to tell us about these processes, and how the mind and the body (which Western medicine kept separate) affect one another. Traditional systems often describe these processes in terms of how 'energy' flows or gets stuck: the same language that I encountered when I learned about body-centred psychotherapies. Though this way of speaking may not conform to strict scientific approaches, there is something very valuable in the way it expresses how being alive, and connected to other people and the living world, actually feels.

The big questions for 21st-century humankind are about wholes and wholeness: how mind, body, spirit and Gaia are one. Let the human genome project do its best to analyse life; the body as we actually *live it* is incalculably more than the sum of its parts.

David Peters

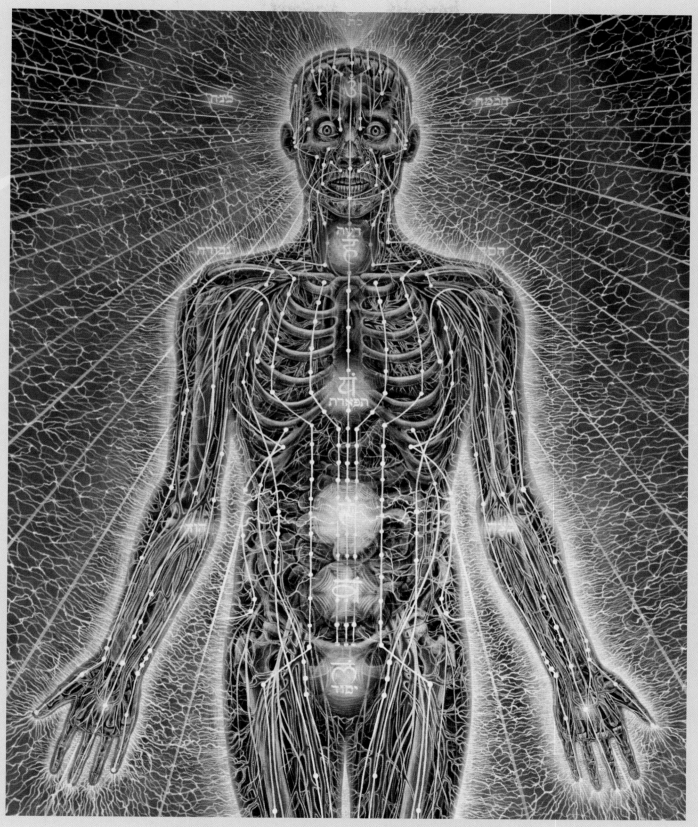

Body energy *Alex Grey's paintings often show the anatomical body as well as the 'energy bodies' as spiritual traditions imagined them. They remind us that the beautifully evolved physical body is profoundly connected to the 'mind-filled' universe that gives us life.*

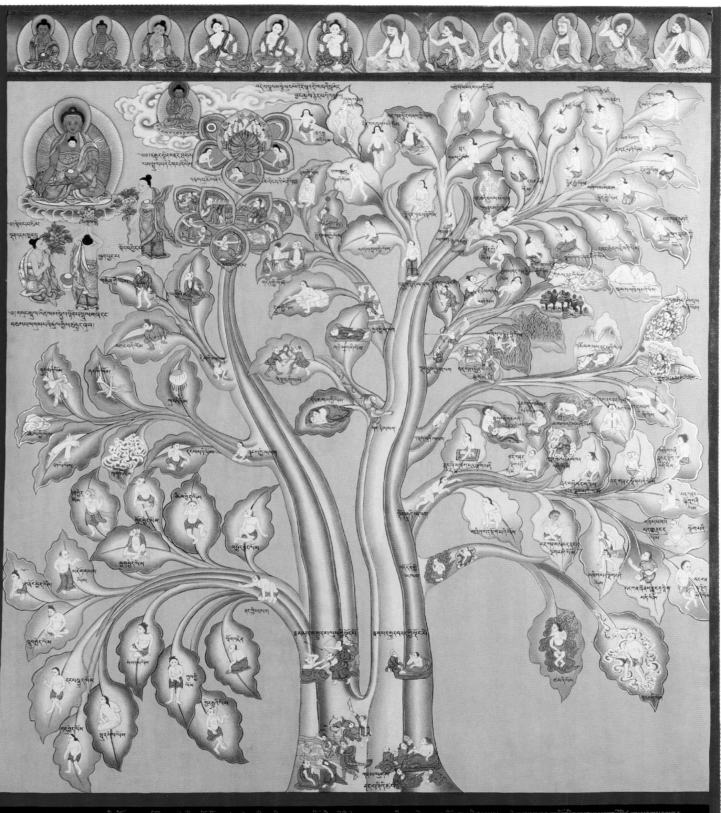

EASTERN APPROACHES

The modern Western approach to the body emphasizes matter over energy. The body is viewed as a sophisticated collection of systems and parts, with medical specialists becoming experts in treating one aspect only – for example, the heart, lungs or the endocrine system. When serious disease arises, usually a physician or general practitioner makes an initial diagnosis and then refers the patient to the correct specialist for further treatment.

The contrast between West and East

Western practitioners have traditionally considered the mind and emotions to be separate from the body, so that anger, grief or other powerful emotions are not thought to be integral to either the cause or the progress of illness. The Eastern approach to medicine offers a quite different perspective on the treatment of illness, one that considers the person as a whole – including the mind, spirit and emotions – and views him or her as a dynamic system.

If a serious or acute illness occurs, Western medicine may provide the heroic intervention needed to save a life. Western surgical techniques have achieved impressive results in the treatment of physical injuries, heart disease and cancer, and vaccination has safeguarded millions of people from infectious diseases. On the other hand, Eastern medicine, while capable of treating diseases (especially chronic illnesses), emphasizes prevention and the creation of wellbeing. Perhaps by integrating both Eastern and Western approaches, therefore, we can increase chances for recovery from illness and enhance overall quality of life.

Common principles

Ayurveda, Traditional Chinese Medicine and Tibetan medicine do not view their traditions as being in conflict with Western medicine. It is understood that Western medicine may have more to offer in an acute illness such as appendicitis or a heart attack.

Tree of health and disease *Used as a memory aid by students of Tibetan medicine, the tree of health and disease depicts the principles of disease prevention and cure.*

Unlike Western medicine, ayurveda, Traditional Chinese Medicine and Tibetan medicine are based on centuries of observation of how people stay well, become ill and recover, rather than on the science of biochemistry and pathology. From these observations the traditions have drawn conclusions about how the environment and the emotions affect the body. None subscribe to a 'one-size-fits-all' treatment. In all three modalities, the practitioner looks for configurations of signs (by examination of the pulses, face and tongue in particular) and symptoms (physical, emotional and mental changes) that constitute a recognizable pattern of underlying disturbance in the organs and energy flow. Consequently, each person's way of being unwell is individual and treatment is designed accordingly. In all three systems, when disease does occur, the goal is not only to treat the symptoms, but promote healing and bring the body into a better state of balance. Eastern medical modalities focus on the development of health, whereas Western allopathic medicine tends to focus on confronting disease and pathology.

Key concepts

A key principle of ayurveda is to balance the three *doshas*, or life forces, in a person in order to bring him or her in harmony with themselves and the universe, while the central aim of Traditional Chinese Medicine is to restore the movement of chi, or life energy, through the body so that all organs and symptoms function optimally. Tibetan medicine, an ancient blending of indigenous Tibetan, Traditional Chinese and ayurveda traditions, focuses on the mind as the major cause of illness, since it is believed that illness arises because a physical, mental and spiritual balance has been lost. Treatment entails balancing the three humours (similar to the three *doshas* in ayurveda), which may call for the application of Buddhist philosophy and spiritual practices as well as medications.

All three modalities – ayurveda, Traditional Chinese Medicine and Tibetan medicine – emphasize prevention, which in all three can include dietary changes. Prevention can include detoxification regimes such as *panchakarma* in ayurveda, meditation practices in Tibetan medicine, and movement practices such as t'ai chi in Traditional Chinese Medicine.

AYURVEDA

If you are interested in **Ayurveda**, you may also like to read about:
- **Yoga**, pages 106–109
- **Hinduism**, pages 204–205
- **Buddhism**, pages 208–209

Ayurveda is an **ancient Indian system of healthcare** and preventive medicine. Its **key concepts** are based on an integrative view of body, mind and spirit. It depends on the diagnosis of an individual's **constitution (*prakriti*)**, which is determined by the three **life forces (*doshas*)** and the effect of the *gunas* (mental attitude). Ayurvedic **treatment** focuses on rebalancing the *doshas*.

Ancient Indian system of healthcare

Ayurveda has been India's main healthcare system for at least 5,000 years. In earliest times, ayurvedic practices were handed down by word of mouth. This collective wisdom was committed to writing between 1500 and 400 BCE during the Vedic period. The sacred Sanskrit texts of ayurveda, the Caraka Samhita on internal medicine and the Sushruta Samhita on surgery, together explain the eight branches of ayurveda:

1. Internal medicine
2. Surgery
3. Head and neck diseases
4. Gynaecology, obstetrics and paediatrics
5. Toxicology
6. Psychiatry
7. Care of the elderly, longevity and rejuvenation
8. Sexual vitality.

Today as much as 80 per cent of India's population uses ayurveda, either exclusively or in combination with conventional medicine. An ayurvedic physician must learn anatomy, physiology, pathology, diagnostic systems and treatment strategies. This involves a post-graduate degree programme of comparable length to conventional medical training. Ayurveda is also practised in Bangladesh, Sri Lanka, Nepal and Pakistan, and, in the last decade, has expanded to become a recognized form of alternative medicine in Western Europe and the USA.

RESEARCH AND EVIDENCE

In a study performed in the Netherlands in 1989, a group of patients with chronic illnesses, including asthma, bronchitis, hypertension and diabetes, were treated with *panchakarma* and other ayurvedic remedies. Nearly 80 per cent improved and some chronic conditions were completely cured. Other studies have shown that *panchakarma* can lower cholesterol and improve digestive disorders. Diabetes, acne and allergies have been successfully treated with ayurvedic remedies, and many ayurvedic herbs have been proven effective in laboratory tests. Currently, the American National Institutes of Health is funding studies on the effectiveness of ayurvedic herbal therapies.

Key concepts

The word ayurveda is made up of the Sanskrit words *ayus*, meaning 'life', and *veda*, meaning science. Ayurveda aims to eliminate the causes of diseases, rather than just treating the symptoms. It also encourages personal responsibility for health and wellbeing. A daily regime may include self-monitoring of the body, special exercises, eating a diet appropriate for one's constitution and spiritual practices.

There are four main foundations in ayurvedic medicine:

1. All things, living and non-living, are interconnected. When diagnosing their patients' problems, ayurvedic practitioners consider the person's relationships with others, their relationship with the world (and possibly the stars) and their relationship with their own body and health.
2. All human beings are made up of the same elements found throughout the universe: earth, fire, water, air and space (ether). Inside the body the elements merge and flow, and their balance or imbalance determines health and disease.
3. If the mind, body and spirit are in harmony, the emotions are balanced and interaction with the universe and others is wholesome, then health will be good.
4. If a person is in a state of disharmony with him- or herself or the universe, then physical, emotional or spiritual disease may occur.

Constitution (*prakriti*)

According to ayurveda, a person's constitution, or *prakriti*, is determined by the unique combination of physical and psychological characteristics formed at the time of birth. This natal constitution remains unchanged throughout life. Determining the proper treatment depends on knowing a person's *prakriti*. Based on the individual's *prakriti*, the ayurvedic pratitioner gives guidance on diet and behaviour to help him or her heal disease or maintain health. The two types of *prakriti* are physical (*sareerika*) and mental (*mansika*). The physical or *sareerika prakriti* is based on the three life forces, or *doshas*, whose Sanskrit names are *vata*, *pitta* and *kapha*. The mental or *mansika prakriti* is based on the three tendencies of mind, or *gunas*: *sattva*, *rajas* and *tamas*.

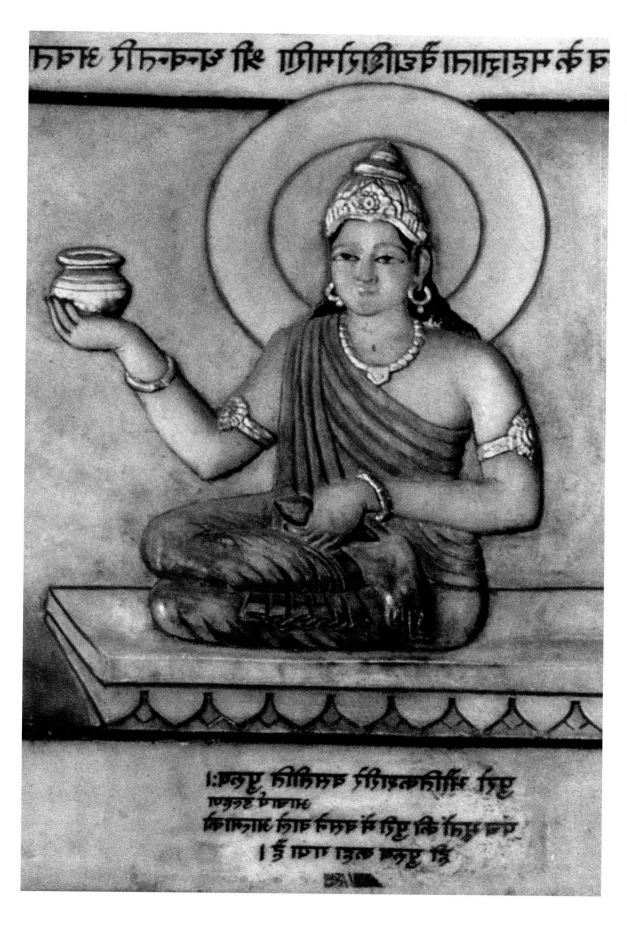

Dhanwantari *This relief shows Dhanwantari, known in the Vedas as the physician of the gods and the patron saint of ayurveda. In Hinduism, worshippers pray to Dhanwantari for good health.*

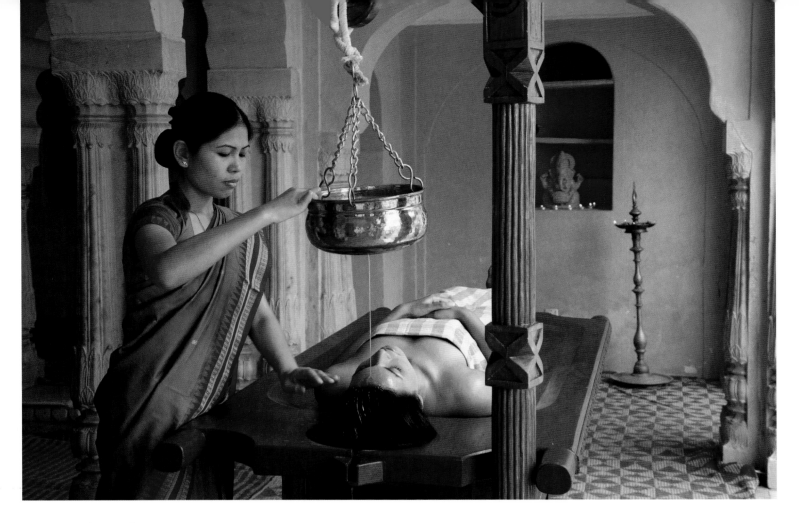

Life forces (*doshas*)

The way the three life forces are balanced affects health, in conjunction with the physical condition of the body, mental attitudes and lifestyle. *Doshas* have these elements in common:

- Each is made up of two of the five basic elements: earth, fire, water, air and space (ether).
- Each controls certain bodily functions – for example, *vata* controls the heart and breathing.
- Each person has a unique combination of the *doshas*, with one *dosha* usually more prominent than the other two. One can be a single *doshic*, *bi-doshic* or, more rarely, *tri-doshic*.
- Each *dosha* has its own physical and psychological characteristics.
- An imbalance of a *dosha* will produce symptoms that are related to that *dosha* – for instance, an imbalanced *vata dosha* causes fear and anxiety.

Vata dosha

Vata dosha combines the elements of space (ether) and air. It regulates major bodily functions such as blood circulation, breathing, heart rate, elimination and the mind. *Vatas* are lightweight with a thin build; they think and move quickly and have an aversion to cold, dry weather. *Vatas* have a tendency to worry and may suffer light, restless sleep. They find warm foods comforting. Physically, they are prone to having skin problems, neurological conditions, rheumatoid arthritis and heart disease. When unbalanced, they may suffer

Massage *Sirodhara, ayurvedic forehead oil-flow treatment, removes mental stress and anxieties and treats insomnia and headaches.*

from fear and anxiety and have physical tremors and tics. When balanced, they are highly creative.

Pitta dosha

Pitta dosha represents the elements of fire and water. *Pitta* controls hormones, metabolism and the digestive system. *Pittas* are of moderate build, with a strong appetite; they may have reddish complexions with moles and freckles, an aversion to hot weather and a preference for cold drinks and foods. *Pittas* can be perfectionists. A person with a *pitta* imbalance may experience negative emotions, such as anger, and become critical and judgmental. Digestion may be compromised by fatigue, too much sun or eating too many spicy or sour foods. *Pittas* are susceptible to hypertension, heart disease, infectious diseases and digestive problems such as Crohn's disease. A balanced *pitta dosha* builds qualities such as daring, courage and will.

Kapha dosha

Kapha dosha combines the elements of water and earth. *Kapha* helps to maintain strength and immunity and controls growth. *Kapha* lubricates and moisturizes body tissues, replaces old cells, heals wounds and balances *pitta* and *vata*. *Kaphas* usually have a solid and heavy body. They have great strength and endurance and are slow and methodical in whatever they do. Their skin is oily and smooth, their hair is lush, thick and dark and their sleep is sound and long. *Kapha* is unbalanced by greed, daytime sleep and eating too many sweet, starchy or salty foods. *Kaphas* are vulnerable to diabetes, cancer, obesity and respiratory illnesses. In balance, *kapha* gives vigour, strength and energy to the body, and calmness and steadiness to the mind.

The *gunas*

Gunas are natural tendencies of the mind and are major factors affecting one's mental state and health. The three *gunas* are *sattva*, the balanced, peaceful quality of being; *rajas*, the active mind; and *tamas*, the mind of darkness, inertia and ignorance. At any moment, the dominant *guna* affects how a person perceives the world. Ayurveda strives to increase *sattva*, through diet and other practices.

Sattva

Sattva, in Sanskrit, means balance, order or purity. A person who tends towards a *sattva* mental state is kind, calm, alert, thoughtful, lucid and serene. *Sattva* reduces *rajas* and *tamas*, encouraging health and spiritual realization. Ayurveda practitioners recommend eating *sattvic* foods and enjoying activities and environments that produce joy and positive thoughts. *Sattvic* foods include pesticide-free whole grains and legumes, fresh fruits and vegetables, nuts and some dairy products.

Rajas

A *rajastic* state of mind creates the desire for the possession of people and things, as well as the fear of losing them. *Rajas* are active, energetic, tense and wilful. To experience a *rajastic* mind is to experience suffering, craving and attachment. In order to reduce *rajas*, *rajastic* foods, overexercising, workaholism, loud music, too much TV or time spent on the internet, excess thinking and shopping should be avoided. *Rajasic* foods include fried foods, spicy foods, caffeine, salt and chocolate.

Tamas

Tamas means excessive, negativity, lethargy, dullness and sloth. It is often associated with delusions or ignorance. If a person embodies a *tamas* quality of mind, it means that they probably engage in self-destructive negative habits and inertia. *Tamasic* foods to avoid include heavy meats, cheeses, alcohol, tobacco, garlic, onions, fermented foods and overripe, stale, chemically treated and nutritionally deficient foods. By ingesting *tamasic* foods, a person becomes inert and greedy and is prevented from healing or accessing spiritual truths.

Diagnosis and treatment

An ayurvedic doctor performs a diagnosis by taking pulses and examining the tongue, face, lips, nails and eyes. Treatments focus on rebalancing the *doshas*. The most commonly prescribed treatments include:

- *Pranayama* – breathing exercises
- *Abhyanga* – massage or self-massage with herbal sesame oil to increase blood circulation and draw toxins out of the body
- *Rasayana* – meditation and mantra recitation
- Yoga – for improved circulation and digestion, the reduction of blood pressure and cholesterol levels, and for the reduction of anxiety and pain
- *Panchakarma* – the inducing of sweat, bowel movements and vomiting to cleanse the body of toxins
- Herbal medicines
- Dietary therapy.

Auyurveda hospital *A pharmacist at Siddalepa Auyurveda Hospital, Sri Lanka, prepares plant-based herbal formulas for patients.*

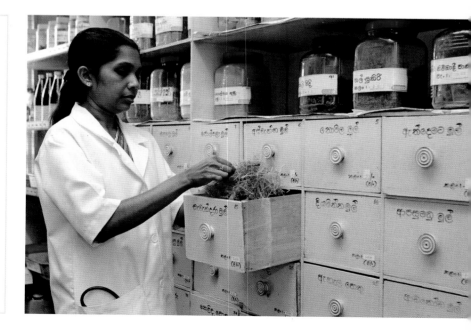

PRECAUTIONS

✖ *Panchakarma* Certain *panchakarma* methods are not appropriate for specific health problems. For example, *swedana*, a preparatory steam bath, is contraindicated for those with diabetes, and some procedures should not be performed on children, pregnant women and the elderly. Women should schedule *panchakarma* outside of their menstrual period. *Panchakarma* treatments should only be administered by qualified practitioners and are best experienced in a residential setting. During *panchakarma*, fatigue, malaise, headaches, congestion and an increase in symptoms may occur as toxins are released. *Panchakarma* can also cause mental and emotional disturbances, when old trauma is stirred up and released.

✖ **Herbal therapies** Ayurvedic medications may be toxic in large doses or in combination with other drugs. The National Center for Complementary and Alternative Medicine (NCCAM) in the USA funded a study published in 2004, which found that of 70 ayurvedic remedies manufactured in South Asia and purchased over the counter, 14 contained lead, mercury and/or arsenic at levels that could be harmful.

TRADITIONAL CHINESE MEDICINE

If you are interested in **Traditional Chinese Medicine**, you may also like to read about:
- T'ai Chi, pages 112–113
- Chi Kung, pages 114–115
- Martial Arts, pages 116–117
- Taoism, pages 216–217
- Confucianism, pages 220–221
- Acupuncture, page 126
- Acupressure, page 127
- Shiatsu, pages 124–125

Traditional Chinese Medicine (TCM) is a complex healing system that dates back over 5,000 years. The important theoretical elements of TCM include **chi**, **yin and yang**, the **Five Elements System** and the **12 meridians**. The symptoms and progress of disease are assessed by using the **Eight Principles**. The four diagnostic methods are: observe, hear and smell, ask, and touch. **Treatments** include herbal medicines, acupuncture, acupressure, massage, dietary therapy, chi kung and t'ai chi.

Chi

Traditional Chinese Medicine (TCM) is based on the concept of chi. The *I Ching* or the Book of Changes (c. 2800 BCE) describes chi as an all-encompassing invisible force that pervades and unifies the three energies in the universe – heaven, earth and human. In humans chi is said to flow through the 12 meridians, or energy channels, in the body. According to TCM, there are three sources of chi: from parents at conception; from ingesting food and liquids; and from breathing air.

Chi is said to circulate through the body's meridians in the same way that blood circulates in the arteries and veins. Its flow can manifest itself in one of three states: harmonious, deficient or stagnant.

Signs of harmonious chi include contentment, good stamina, restful sleep, creativity and productivity. Stagnant chi produces disharmony that results in aches, discomfort and pain. Deficient chi may lead to lethargy, low moods and persistent tiredness.

Yin and yang

According to Taoist theory, chi manifests itself through yin and yang. The interplay of yin and yang in the body, mind and spirit are fundamental to the TCM theory of health and disease.

Yin qualities are slow and gentle, insubstantial and diffuse, cold, dark, inward, damp and calm. Yang qualities are hard and fast, solid and dry, resolute, bright, outward, hot and confrontational.

The well-known black and white t'ai chi symbol expresses their complementary and never-ending interchange. The outside circle represents the great pregnant void or 'Tao' from which the two opposite energy principles of yin and yang emerge. Yin is symbolized by the black half and yang by the white. At the heart of each is a small circle of its opposite, symbolizing the dynamic nature of creation where nothing remains absolutely static: the yin becoming yang, and the yang becoming yin.

Some examples of yin and yang characteristics and phenomena include:

Yang	Yin
Active	Passive
Hot	Cold
Summer	Winter
Male	Female
Day	Night
Light	Dark
Sun	Moon
Creative	Receptive
Expansive	Contracting
Upward	Downward

The Eight Principles

A TCM doctor will use the Eight Principles, or four basic polarities, to assess a patient's symptoms and the progress of disease. The doctor will determine if the symptoms are:

- Excessive or deficient
- Hot or cold
- Yin or yang
- Internal or external.

Excess chi, or stagnant or congested chi, causes swelling and pain. If chi is deficient, it causes weakness, fatigue and a pale complexion. Heat symptoms manifest as fevers and a flushed complexion, and cold symptoms produce a runny nose, diarrhoea or a slow pulse. If the location of symptoms is deep in the body, relating to internal organs or blood, or if there is swelling, dampness or excess fluids, then the symptoms are considered yin. If the symptoms are associated with muscles, skin or with a scarcity of fluids, then they are yang in nature. If the origin of the symptoms is the weather, or exposure to germs, it is external. Most common illnesses, such as colds or flu, are considered external in nature. If symptoms are due to an imbalance between organs, or are caused by hormones, stress or emotions, they are considered internal. Symptoms can also manifest in combinations.

The Five Elements System

Whereas science in the Western world has been preoccupied with all that can be weighed and measured, that is *quantities*, in the East the study of *qualities* and their correspondences has predominated. In TCM, the Five Elements describe the distinct but related qualities of wood, fire, earth, metal and water, and, in the same way as they regulate growth and change in the natural world, they are said to encompass the phases of our physical, emotional and spiritual life. Each of the Five Elements has a unique quality and each person has a bias towards one or two in their make-up.

Each organ system and meridian is 'governed' by one of the Five Elements. As chi moves through the body's yin and yang organ systems and meridians, its quality of expression tends towards the associated element. The interdependence of the elements is defined by two sets of relationships, one generative, the other destructive or controlling. In the Generation Cycle (see diagram), wood feeds fire, fire creates earth (ash), earth bears metal (as when an ore melts), metal collects water (condensation on a metal bowl) and water nourishes wood. In the Destruction Cycle, water dissolves earth, earth absorbs water, water quenches fire, fire melts metal and metal cuts wood. When an element and its organ/meridian system are weak, the rest will suffer; when an element and its organs are strengthened, the others benefit.

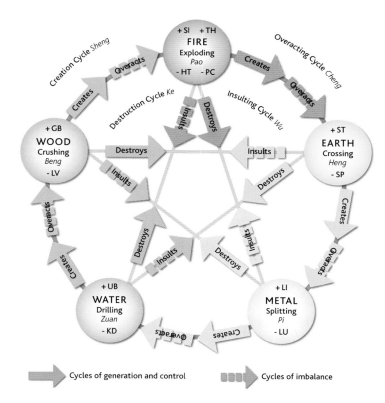

Cycles of generation and control

Cycles of imbalance

Cycles of generation and destruction *The Generation Cycle is also known as the* sheng, *creation or Mother–Son relationship. The Destruction or Control Cycle is also known as the* ke, ko *or Grandparent–Grandchild relationship.*

THE FIVE ELEMENTS SYSTEM

	Wood	Fire	Earth	Metal	Water
Season	Spring	Summer	Late summer	Autumn	Winter
Weather	Windy	Hot	Humid	Dry	Cold
Time of day	Morning	Midday	Afternoon	Evening	Night
Yin organs	Liver	Heart	Spleen	Lungs	Kidney
Yang organs	Gall bladder	Small intestine	Stomach	Large intestine	Bladder
Tissue	Muscles/tendons	Blood vessels	Flesh	Skin	Bones
Sensory organs	Eyes	Tongue	Mouth	Nose	Ears
Senses	Sight	Speech	Touch	Taste/smell	Hearing
Bodily fluids	Tears	Perspiration	Saliva/lymph	Mucus	Urine
Expression	Nails	Complexion	Lips	Body hair	Head hair
Colour	Green	Red	Yellow	White	Blue/black
Behaviour	Controlling	Crying	Worrying	Coughing	Shaking
Emotion	Anger	Joy	Compassion	Grief	Fear
Tone of voice	Loud/shouting	Laughing	Singing	Whining	Groaning
Spirit	Soul/vision	Consciousness	Intelligence	Instinct	Will to live
Mental activity	Planning/deciding	Integration	Reflection	Concentration	Meditation
Energy	Spiritual	Psychological	Physical	Vital	Ancestral
Dream	Forest/trees	Fire/laughter	Music/singing	Flying	Drowning

Meridians *These are energy channels that run through the body. They are part of the body's subtle-energy anatomy and cannot be imaged or found surgically. Various points along the meridians are accessed through acupuncture or acupressure massage to balance the body and restore it to health.*

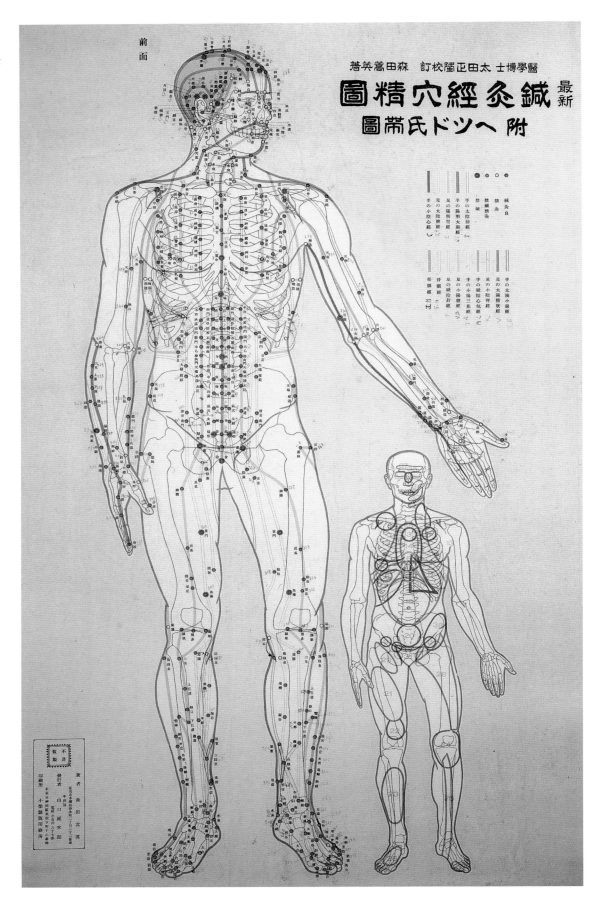

The 12 meridians

Chi flows through the meridians in a set order. Along the 12 major meridians, six yang and six yin, are a total of 365 specific points. These points are the gateways to chi, and are used both for diagnosing and treating the disruptions in chi flow. Through acupuncture or acupressure chi energy can be stimulated, if deficient, or sedated, if in excess, and so balanced. Herbal medicines and dietary changes may also be prescribed to treat imbalances.

Lung meridian (yin, metal) absorbs chi energy from the air through the breath. It controls the respiration and oxygen content in the body and has a close relationship with the heart and circulatory systems.

Large intestine meridian (yang, metal) supports the body's ability to remove waste and absorb water.

Stomach meridian (yang, earth) regulates the body's ability to take in food and fluid.

Spleen meridian (yin, earth) transforms food into energy and regulates and maintains the body's blood supply.

Heart meridian (yin, fire) regulates the spirit, blood vessels and the movement of blood.

Small intestine meridian (yang, fire) regulates the drawing out of nutrients and energy from food.

Bladder meridian (yang, water) oversees the urinary organs and the excretion of urine.

Kidney meridian (yin, water) oversees reproductive energy, the hormones and the bones.

Pericardium meridian (yin, fire) protects and controls circulation.

Triple warmer meridian (yang, fire) circulates heat and balances water in three parts of the torso: the upper associated with respiration, the middle with digestion and the lower with elimination.

Gall bladder meridian (yang, wood) regulates the creation of bile that helps transform food into chi energy.

Liver meridian (yin, wood) regulates the flow of chi throughout the body and maintains the body's blood supply.

Diagnosis and treatment

TCM treatments focus on rebalancing the chi energy in the body. A TCM doctor diagnoses a patient by taking pulses on each wrist and assessing the state of the meridians and associated organ systems. He or she would also examine the tongue and the appearance of the skin, and note the sound of the patient's voice.

Commonly prescribed treatments include:

- Acupuncture – stimulation of selected acupuncture points with needles
- Moxibustion – the burning of the herb mugwort at or near an acupuncture point to introduce heat
- *Tui na* – massage that stimulates acupressure points to correct imbalances of chi
- Herbal remedies
- Dietary therapy
- Chi kung and t'ai chi – health and energy-inducing practices.

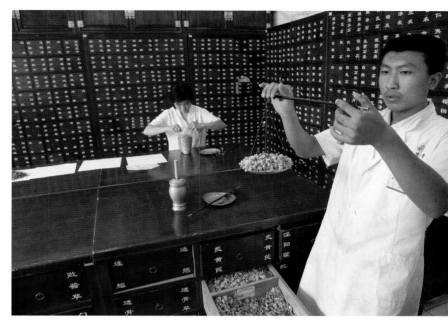

Pharmacy *A pharmacist preparing a herbal prescription weighs ingredients at a Traditional Chinese Medicine pharmacy.*

PRECAUTIONS

✖ **Acupuncture** Relatively few complications from acupuncture have been reported. When complications have occurred, it has been from inadequate sterilization of needles and from improper technique. It is crucial that practitioners use new disposable needles for each patient.

✖ **Herbal remedies** Some packaged Chinese herbal remedies have been found to contain heavy metals and bacteria. Look for the Good Manufacturing Practice (GMP) seal, which ensures that the product has been certified by the Department of Health, Republic of China. Some of the classical formulas include ingredients that we now know to be dangerous. These include cinnabar, lead, arsenic and magnetite. Modern herbalists use other ingredients in their place. Some preparations still include animal products such as bear's bile, the production of which involves cruelty. Consult a qualified TCM practitioner before taking any Chinese herbal formulas or supplements. The practitioner will aim to take into account all aspects of your current condition before prescribing a herbal formula specifically suited to you.

RESEARCH AND EVIDENCE

Acupuncture appears to be effective for a wide range of conditions. However, rigorous research is largely lacking. It is well established that acupuncture can reduce post-operative and chemotherapy-related nausea and vomiting and relieve dental pain. It can also be effective for osteoarthritic knee pain.

Chinese herbal therapy has been researched extensively in China, and reports generally conclude that it is effective for a wide range of health conditions. Research in the West has been less uniformly positive, but has found traditional Chinese herbal remedies to be effective in the treatment of irritable bowel syndrome, acne, psoriasis and polycystic ovary syndrome.

TIBETAN MEDICINE

Tibetan medicine is an ancient medical system that draws on many different healing traditions. Based on the beliefs of **Buddhism**, it places great emphasis on the mind and spirit in health and healing. **Treatment** is focused on the balance of the **three humours** and the **five elements**.

If you are interested in **Tibetan Medicine**, you may also like to read about:
- Ayurveda, pages 94–97
- Buddhism, pages 208–209
- Buddhist Sacred Texts, pages 210–211
- Tibetan Buddhism, page 212

Traditions and practice

The Tibetan medical system is thought to be a synthesis of many ancient medical traditions, including Indian, Persian, Greek and Chinese. But its main roots are in Tibet where traditionally people have lived in close relation to the natural world and have had to rely on their own resources to survive. Today Tibetan medicine's most important external influences are ayurveda and Traditional Chinese Medicine. Tibetan medicine continues to be practised in

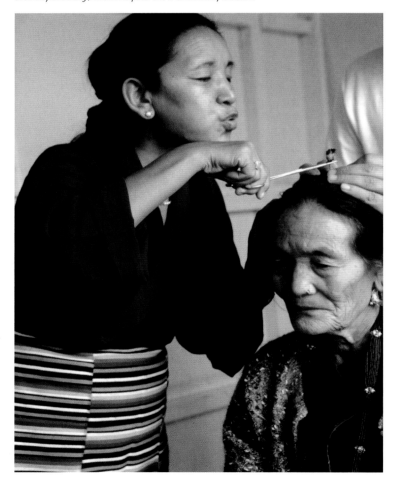

Moxabustion *A Tibetan doctor burning a herb, dried 'moxa' (Artemesia vulgaris), above the skin at an acupuncture point on top of the patient's head. The heat warms the chi and blood of the body, which helps in the treatment of disease.*

Tibet, India, Nepal, Bhutan, Ladakh, Siberia, China and Mongolia. More recently, versions of Tibetan medicine have become available in parts of Europe and North America.

The role of Buddhism

Tibetan medicine is based on the Buddhist belief that physical illness is linked to mental, social and spiritual illness. Illness ultimately results from the 'three poisons' of the mind: attachment, aversion and ignorance. Understandably, Tibetan medicine is reputed to have the oldest surviving written system of psychiatric diagnoses and treatments. Tibetan psychological medicine combines medical modalities with Buddhist theory and practice.

The classical Tibetan medical texts, the Four Medical Treatises, also called the Four Tantras and known collectively as the *Gyushi*, are said to be the discourses of Shakyamuni Buddha on healing, given in India during the 6th century BCE and reputed to have been committed to writing by the Indian sage Chandranandana in the 8th century CE. They form the basis of a famous set of 76 Tibetan medical paintings or *thangkas* called the Blue Beryl, which was created in the 17th century, containing more than 10,000 separate illustrations, each describing an aspect of Tibetan medicine. The *Gyushi* and the *thangkas* continue to be studied by doctors training in the Tibetan healing arts today.

The humours

Tibetan medicine declares that good health requires not only a balance in the body's three principal functions, or humours, but also a well-balanced mind. As in ayurveda, the mixture of humours determines a person's temperament and physical body type. The Tibetan humours (wind, bile and phlegm) are akin to the *doshas* in ayurveda: *vata*, *pitta* and *kapha*. In a similar way, the Tibetan humours are strongly influenced by environmental factors, such as the seasons, the weather and where one lives, as well as by internal factors such as diet, behaviour and mental state.

Diseases are generally thought to be caused by disturbances of one or more of the humours. Yet because this system is embedded in the Buddhist world-view, every disease is also said to be the result of negative emotions and spiritual ignorance – that is, the 'three poisons': attachment manifests in wind, anger in bile and ignorance in phlegm. These mental states together with other influences create the conditions that allow disease to occur.

BODY WORK

 Most systems of medicine, regardless of their origins or how their philosophies differ, see diet, massage and exercise as important ways of maintaining health and bringing about recovery. Ancient healers, observing the body in sickness and in health, recognized in-built healing processes at work, and early Chinese and Indian medical writings suggested that self-healing works effectively when the person is in a 'state of balance'.

Holistic approach

The therapeutic practices featured in this section illustrate some of the different bodywork approaches and methods available. Generally, their aim is to release the body's recuperative and restorative processes in order to alleviate pain, prevent ill health and optimize wellbeing. Although bodywork practitioners concentrate primarily on the physical body, their premise is that human beings are also mental, emotional and spiritual beings. All holistic practitioners view the body as a dynamic whole and believe that while restoring physical wellbeing, the work they do may also enhance other aspects of the person.

Balancing the flow of inner energy

Potentially self-healing we may be, but over the years the stresses and strains of everyday living can have a cumulative negative effect, particularly on the muscular and circulatory systems. Tensions and constrictions build up and effectively obstruct the normal self-regulating and healing systems of the body. In time, these 'blockages' can cause discomfort, and may predispose us to disease or emotional problems. If we approach bodywork in this light, its place alongside conventional medicine seems clear: while doctors battle with disease using drugs and surgery as weapons, bodyworkers strive to create peace in the body by dispelling, where possible, its tensions and conflicts.

The timeless power of touch to provide comfort is inherent in all 'manual therapies', and some bodyworkers emphasize this aspect more than others.

Acupuncture chart *This traditional Chinese medical chart shows some of the key acupoints along the stomach meridian.*

Some see what they do as purely a physical treatment; at the other extreme are practitioners who consider that they are dealing with the emotional, the energetic or even the spiritual body. The kinds of pressures used vary from the almost imperceptible touch of craniosacral therapy and the Bowen technique to the deeper manipulation of Swedish massage and rolfing.

Some traditional massage therapies, such as Thai massage and *kahuna* bodywork (Hawaiian massage or *lomi lomi*), bring a meditative element into massage. Acupuncture, shiatsu and chi kung (qigong) work towards balancing the flow of something they conceive of as an inner vital force, or energy, known as chi or qi (or ki in Japan; prana in India). Others, such as chiropractic and osteopathy, work more directly with the body's framework to detect and correct any imbalances between muscular tensions that may be impacting on health. Yet all these approaches have in common a concern to dissolve constriction and to create relaxation, space and flow in the body.

Mental and spiritual benefits

Some traditional therapies, such as yoga and the martial arts, originally developed as aspects of philosophies that shaped a whole way of life. Followers of these life-paths used physical exercise and breathing techniques not only for their health and wellbeing, but also as tools for spiritual development. While most people now practise body-oriented methods for health maintenance, others find that they can serve to enhance their awareness and sensitivity.

The Alexander technique, Pilates, the Feldenkrais method, Hellerwork and Tragerwork offer different methods of educating mind and body to recognize and unlearn the habitual responses that restrict the body's ability to move with ease and poise. The Bates method applies the same theory to eyesight.

Consulting a bodywork practitioner can be the start of a journey towards good health. Holistic practitioners believe in encouraging individuals to tune into their own bodies and become aware of their own tensions and tendencies. Once these traits are recognized, it may be possible to work with a practitioner to strengthen weak areas and unwind patterns of tension in the body. And, in the longer term, unexpected and yet powerful emotional and spiritual changes can also result.

YOGA

If you are interested in **Yoga**, you may also like to read about:
- Ayurveda, pages 94–97
- Hinduism, pages 204–205
- Hindu Sacred Texts, pages 206–207
- Chakras and the Aura, pages 172–173
- Meditation, pages 78–79

An ancient Indian healing practice, yoga was originally created as a path to **spiritual development**, but is better known today as a method of exercise and relaxation comprising *asanas* (postures) and **pranayama** (breath control). With regular **practice**, yoga can bring health **benefits**, including stress reduction and clarity of mind.

Spiritual development

The word yoga is derived from the Sanskrit word for 'union' – between mind, body and spirit. This holistic approach to life, which dates back some 5,000 years, is part of ayurveda, the ancient Indian medical system. Records show that it was originally practised by Hindu ascetics, or *yogis*, who regarded the purpose of yoga as a way of developing harmony between the physical, emotional, mental and spiritual aspects of life.

There are several branches of yoga including raja yoga (the 'royal path' or 'king of yogas'), which involves control of the mind and mastery of self in order to experience inner happiness and create positive change in society; bhakti yoga, of love and devotion; jnana yoga, of the intellect; karma yoga, of work and duty; and kriya yoga, of cleansing practices. The most popular practice in the West is hatha yoga, which means 'balance of body and mind' and was introduced by the Indian yogic sage Swatmarama and described in *Hatha Yoga Pradipika* in the 15th century.

The system of hatha yoga originated as a way of preparing the body for the meditation and spiritual practice of raja yoga, as defined by the Indian sage Patanjali in the Yoga Sutras (c. 200 BCE–500 CE), which includes the 'eight limbs', an eight-stage process or path towards spiritual growth. The first two limbs are the ethics of yoga, the vows and observances that should inform practice: *yama* (restraint, behaviour towards others) and *niyama* (self-discipline, behaviour towards oneself). Then come *asana* (posture); *pranayama* (breath control); *pratyahara* (sense withdrawal); *dharana* (concentration); *dhyana* (meditation); and *samadhi* (ecstasy, enlightenment).

Hatha yoga is concerned with creating balance by strengthening the body and calming the mind. There are several different approaches, including *iyengar*, a very rigorous form of yoga that pays attention to correct alignment of the body and concentrates on focusing the mind to perfect the detail of postures, as well as *satyananda*, *sivananda*, *ashtanga*, *bikram* and *dru*. Power yoga is a new form, developed in the USA, which offers a vigorous cardiovascular workout.

Asanas

A range of *asanas*, or physical postures, are practised to help stretch all areas of the body in a balanced way, working to strengthen weak muscles, stimulate nerve centres and internal organs and increase blood and lymph circulation, flexibility, stamina and body awareness. These postures may be dynamic or static. The latter are held for a length of time and then repeated. The traditional purpose of *asanas* is preparation for developing and exploring the more spiritual practices of yoga. The eventual aim is to develop sufficient strength, firmness and flexibility of mind and body to be able to sit quietly and comfortably for *dharana* (concentration) and *dhyana* (meditation) without distraction for extended periods of time.

Postures, which vary in difficulty and intensity, are mastered or worked towards in a gradual process without placing stress or strain on the body. These may include: Trikonasana (Triangle Pose); Talasana (Tree Pose); Svanasana (Downward Dog), Bhujangasana (Cobra Pose) and Padmasana (Lotus Position). The Sirsasana (Headstand) is considered the 'Father' of postures and the Sarvangasana (Shoulder Stand) the 'Mother' of postures.

Pranayama

Breath control is an essential feature of yoga practice and is said to develop the power of concentration and clarity of thought, as well as increasing mental and physical powers of endurance. Yoga is said to balance prana, 'the fundamental vibratory life force' that is apparent through awareness of the breath, and reduce any blockages that may diminish mental or physical health. According to yogic anatomy, prana flows through 72,000 channels called *nadi*, which distribute this vital energy to all parts of the body to ensure healthy function. A central *nadi* runs vertically along the midline of the body known as the *sushumna*, from which lead seven subtle-energy centres called chakras (see page 172).

Yoga breathing techniques, collectively known as pranayama, encourage slow, controlled breathing with the aim of expanding and making full use of the lungs, thus improving the intake and circulation of oxygen supplies to the organs and glands of the body. Coordination of the inhalation and exhalation of breath promotes mental focus and is an important preparation for and aid to *dharana* (concentration) and *dhyana* (meditation). Pranayama can also help calm an anxious mind by slowing, lengthening and deepening breathing.

Pranayama practice begins with an awareness of how the lungs function and the benefits of correct breathing. Simple techniques may subsequently be introduced, such as Bhramari (humming-bee breath), which can encourage relief from mental tension, and Nadi Shodhana (alternate nostril breathing) which restores, equalizes and balances the flow of prana.

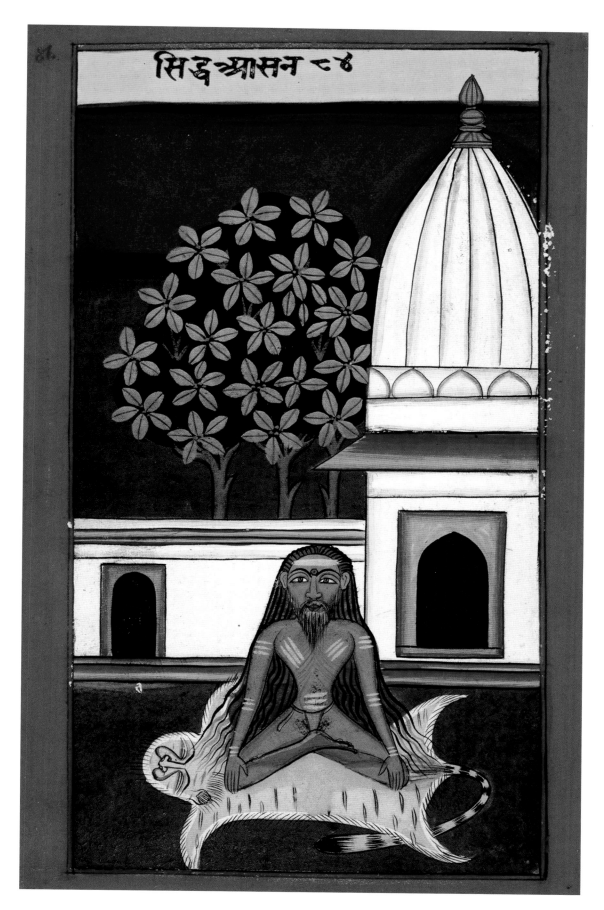

सिद्ध श्रासन ८४

Indian yogi *This 19th-century Indian illustration from* Asanas and Mudras *shows a* saiva yogi *in* siddha asana.

Practice and benefits

Yoga is taught in a class or one-to-one. Today there are a variety of classes tailored to suit people of all ages and abilities. They tend to be held weekly, last around 60–90 minutes and should always be supervised by a qualified teacher. Most yoga is practised on non-slip mats. Warm, comfortable clothing is recommended; shoes are not worn. Many yoga teachers advise students to begin by observing the breath, becoming aware of its movement and texture. This leads to warm-up stretches and a series of *asanas* and pranayama. The class finishes with complete physical and mental relaxation known as Sivasana (Corpse Pose). Some teachers include meditation or guided visualizations and also discuss the theory and philosophy of yoga.

Each individual is encouraged to work to their own level and to stop if any pain or discomfort is experienced. It is essential that yoga teachers carry out an initial assessment, discuss any medical conditions and offer advice on any variations of *asanas* to suit particular needs. *Asanas* are performed in many different positions, including standing and lying down, but can be adapted to suit individual needs. Yoga is taught in hospitals and hospices, even with exercises practised in beds, chairs and wheelchairs.

Once the postures have been mastered in a class, home practice of around 20–30 minutes daily is recommended.

Yoga can reduce stress and encourage relaxation, increase feelings of vitality and wellbeing, improve digestion, develop better posture and increase general muscle tone and strength. Yoga therapy involves the use of yoga to complement orthodox medicine by helping to treat and prevent a wide range of conditions, including back pain.

PRECAUTIONS

✖ Allow two to three hours after a meal before practising yoga postures or any movements or exercises involved in Pilates, t'ai chi, chi kung, martial arts and the Alexander technique (see pages 110–119).

✖ Discuss any health problems with your teacher. Some postures, movements or exercises may not be suitable if you have neck or back injuries, high blood pressure, heart problems or other disorders. Your teacher should be able to offer alternatives or variations.

✖ Be cautious if you are pregnant or menstruating – inform your teacher, who may suggest alternative postures, movements or exercises.

RESEARCH AND EVIDENCE

A systematic review of scientific evidence by the Natural Standard, an international research collaboration that produces scientifically based reviews of complementary and alternative-medicine topics, reveals that yoga may be a beneficial adjunct to conventional treatments for conditions including anxiety disorders or stress, asthma, high blood pressure and heart disease. There is some evidence to suggest that it may be useful in the treatment of epilepsy, some kinds of irritable bowel syndrome and in reducing cholesterol levels. A 2004 study published in the journal *Alternative Therapies in Health and Medicine* suggested that yoga may be helpful for treating depression in young adults.

Sun Salutation – *Surya Namaskar*

This has been practised, traditionally facing the rising sun, for hundreds of years. It can be used as an aerobic exercise, largely because of the two expansive movements: from standing upright with lifted arms down to the standing forward bend and back up again.

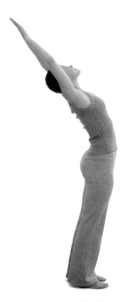

2 As you breathe in, lift your arms up in the air (next to your ears), arch backwards from your chest and stretch your arms and fingers upwards.

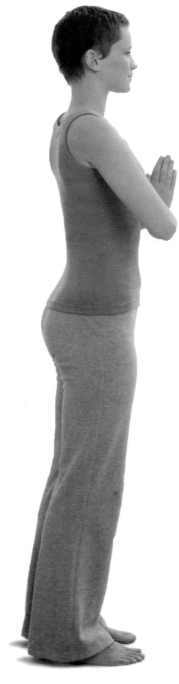

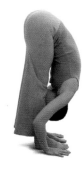

1 Exhale while you are standing with your feet together and palms together in front of your chest, fingers pointing upwards.

3 As you breathe out, bend forward and down until your head touches your knees. Bend your knees if necessary, then place your hands flat on the floor next to your feet. Only stretch as far as feels comfortable for you.

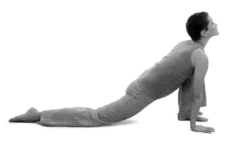

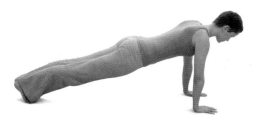

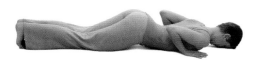

4 As you breathe in, place your right knee behind you on the floor, keeping your left knee bent between your arms, and look up.

5 Holding your breath, bring your left leg back into push-up position.

6 As you exhale, gradually bend your knees and lower your chest and forehead to the floor, but keep your hips off the floor.

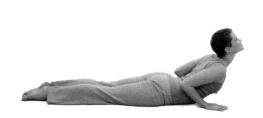

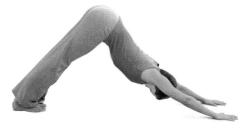

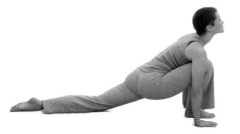

7 As you inhale, lie flat on the floor, stretch your toes so that the tops of your feet are on the floor, slowly lift your head and chest and look up. Keep your arms bent.

8 As you exhale, lift your hips up and push your heels as far as possible into the floor. Look towards your feet.

9 As you inhale, take a large step forward to bring your right foot between your hands, and lower your back knee to the floor so that the top of your back foot is on the mat. Look up.

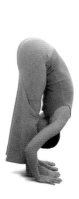

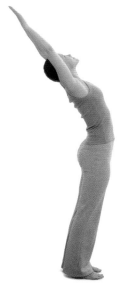

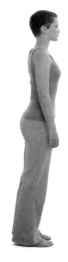

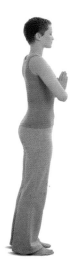

10 As you exhale, bring your left leg forward, straighten both legs as much as possible and bend down until your head touches your knees. Bend your knees if necessary, keeping your hands on the floor next to your feet.

11 As you inhale, stretch your arms forward and up, keeping your arms next to your ears. Arch back from your chest and stretch your arms and fingers.

12 As you exhale, return to a standing position, releasing your arms to hang by your sides.

13 Put your hands back in the prayer position as you exhale, and start again with Step 1. This time do movements 4 and 9 with your left leg first. Repeat the whole sequence 3–5 times in total.

PILATES

A complete exercise method, Pilates was developed by German born **Joseph Pilates** in the early 1900s. It is designed to improve physical and mental health by focusing on building the body's **core strength** and improving posture through precise, controlled **movements** and breathing.

If you are interested in **Pilates**, you may also like to read about:
- **Alexander Technique**, pages 118–119
- **T'ai Chi**, pages 112–113
- **Chi Kung**, pages 114–115
- **Yoga**, pages 106–109
- **Chiropractic and Osteopathy**, pages 132–135

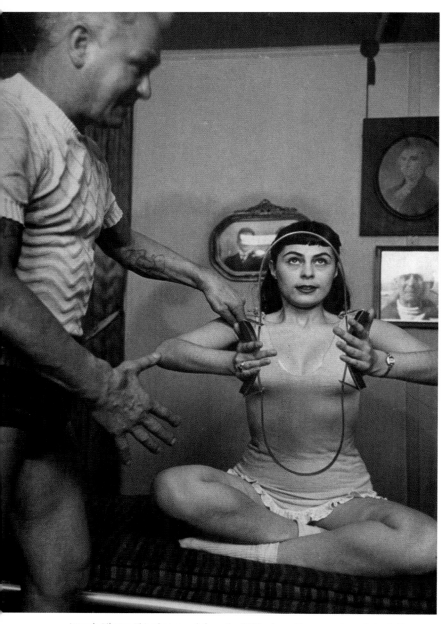

Joseph Pilates *This photograph from the 1950s shows the opera singer Roberta Peters squeezing an early form of the Pilates Resistance Ring, while training with Joseph Pilates.*

Joseph Pilates

The founder of Pilates, Joseph Pilates (1880–1967), suffered ill health as a child, leaving his body distorted and frail. Determined to overcome his disabilities, Pilates studied Eastern and Western approaches to exercise and devised a system that engaged both body and mind. In 1912 he moved to England to work as a circus performer, boxer and self-defence instructor.

While interned during the First World War, Pilates worked with fellow internees, many of whom were injured and bedridden, to perfect his system of body conditioning. His exercise group survived in reasonable health until the end of the war, despite suffering many illnesses that proved fatal to others living in similar cramped conditions.

In 1926 Pilates moved to the USA and opened his first exercise studio in New York. His regime of precise movements soon became popular with dancers, musicians, TV presenters and others who were attracted by the way that it appeared systematically to strengthen, stretch and tone the major muscles of the body in a uniform way, without adding muscle bulk or putting undue strain on the muscles and joints.

Pilates devised more than 500 different exercises at various levels of difficulty, and the movements are constantly being refined in the light of new research and knowledge. Pilates is recommended by many physiotherapists, osteopaths, chiropractors and medical practitioners for rehabilitation and prevention of injury and back pain, and is also used by athletes and dancers to complement their training.

Core strength

Pilates focuses on developing strength and stability in the centre of the body, or 'core', by working on the muscles of the pelvic floor, abdomen and back, all of which help maintain correct posture, balance and coordination. The starting point, known as 'neutral spine', is essential for performing each exercise effectively and safely. Once the body is well aligned with the core muscles held in tightly, individual muscle groups can be worked without putting strain on other areas. When performed correctly, Pilates exercise does not use excess energy or tension. Inhalation and exhalation coordinated with movement encourage the muscles to work more effectively and also help to maintain focus and control. Pilates is said to provide a complete body workout and to help promote harmony of mind and body.

Movements and instruction

The emphasis is on control and quality of movement; movements are minimal and extremely precise, and often only a few repetitions are required. It takes concentration to control each movement consciously, and this is thought to increase body awareness and enhance the ability to relax and release unwanted tension.

As precision of movement is paramount, it is important to have instruction from a qualified teacher with a sound knowledge of anatomy and physiology. Pilates teachers work on a one-to-one or group basis and can tailor the exercises to suit each individual. Classes, which usually last around an hour, include exercises in a standing position or lying on a mat on the floor, sometimes using resistance bands and exercise balls. Loose, comfortable clothing is worn. Shoes are not necessary. Advanced classes are held in studios fitted with specialist equipment such as 'the reformer', an exercise machine that adds extra intensity using the resistance of springs.

Pilates is suitable for all ages and levels of fitness. Some exercises are tailored to meet specific needs, such as chronic back problems or pregnancy.

Finding neutral spine

The starting point of Pilates exercise is finding the neutral position of your spine. This is a natural posture with the curves of the spine in correct alignment. Most people have habitual postures where the pelvis is either tucked or tilted. Neutral position is halfway between these two positions. Try this simple exercise to find your 'neutral spine' position. Stand with your feet hip-width apart parallel to each other. Relax your knees. Lengthen your spine and make a conscious effort to release any unwanted tension from your legs, shoulders and neck. Tilt your pelvis forwards and backwards. Be aware of these two positions. The neutral position is midway between the two extremes. Draw your navel and abdominal muscles back towards the spine and hold, without allowing your pelvis to tilt. Breathe normally. Try this exercise lying on your back, on all fours and lying on your side.

PRECAUTIONS

✖ See page 108.

RESEARCH AND EVIDENCE

Pilates has gained much attention over recent years, but despite anecdotal evidence, few scientific studies have been undertaken to establish the benefits as yet. A randomized controlled trial conducted in Canada, published in 2006, found that Pilates-based therapeutic exercises had a more beneficial effect on people with non-specific chronic lower back pain than conventional care, and this was maintained over a 12-month follow-up period.

Hip Rolls

This exercise strengthens the abdominal muscles, stretches out the hip flexors and lower back and releases tension in the upper spine.

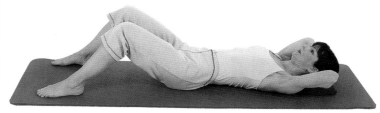

1 Lie on your back with your knees bent at a 90-degree angle and your feet slightly wider than hip-width apart. Your neck should be allowed to elongate and your spine to relax. Bend your arms and place both hands beneath your head, elbows wide. Inhale.

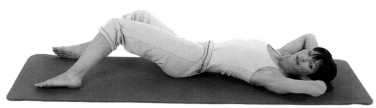

2 Exhale, drawing in the abdominals, as you roll your knees towards the floor. The soles of your feet will come off the mat. As you stretch, let your head roll in the opposite direction to your knees, so that you feel a stretch through your body. Inhale and rest in this position.

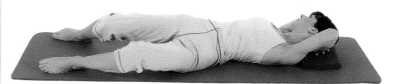

3 Exhale, drawing in the abdominals, to roll your knees all the way over to the other side. Let your head roll in the opposite direction. Imagine your lower abdominal muscles sinking down through your spine towards the floor. Inhale and rest in this position. Alternate smoothly from side to side. Repeat 10 times.

T'AI CHI

If you are interested in **T'ai Chi**, you may also like to read about:
- Chi Kung, pages 114–115
- Martial Arts, pages 116–117
- Traditional Chinese Medicine, pages 98–101
- Yoga, pages 106–109
- Pilates, pages 110–111
- Meditation, pages 78–79
- Taoism, pages 216–217

With **origins as a martial art**, t'ai chi is now better known for its health benefits and is becoming increasingly popular in the West. Flowing, controlled **movements** coordinated with breathing are said to facilitate the flow of 'chi' (intrinsic energy), through the body. Maximum **benefits** are achieved through everyday **practice**. Millions of people in China make t'ai chi part of their daily routine.

Origins as a martial art

According to legend, t'ai chi, or more properly t'ai chi chuan, is said to have been developed in the 13th century by a Taoist monk, Chang San-Feng, after he witnessed a fight between a crane and a snake. Legend has it that the monk was so inspired by the dynamic interaction between the forceful actions of the bird and the more subtle, graceful movements of the snake that he created a martial art based on the coordinated interplay of the complementary opposites yin (the soft, feminine principle) and yang (the hard, masculine principle). The name t'ai chi chuan can be translated as 'supreme ultimate fist'.

T'ai chi has since developed a worldwide following among people with little or no interest in martial arts, but who recognize its many benefits for general health and wellbeing. However, teachers stress the importance of understanding its original purpose and meaning as a martial art, where the intention is the full mobilization, proper coordination and direction of chi, the body's energy or life force. All movements should be performed with the mind and body in a state of conscious relaxation to enable internal energy to be focused in combat more effectively.

T'ai chi has been constantly evolved by practising Masters over many centuries, and the various styles bear the family names of the masters who developed them: Chen, Yang, Wu, Sun and Wu/Hao. The yang style is the most common type of t'ai chi practised in the West today.

Movements

T'ai chi is often called 'meditation in motion', because focusing the mind solely on performing the movements with grace and fluidity helps induce a state of mental calm, clarity and inner harmony. An expert can make the practice appear effortless, but it actually requires a great deal of concentration to maintain the correct postural alignment and coordinate the sequences in a calm, relaxed manner with natural breathing. All movements are slow and continuous, performed without strain or muscular tension. Each movement involves bringing energy up through the legs, hips, back and shoulders, and out through the arms and hands.

T'ai chi training involves learning solo routines (known as forms), two person self-defence routines (including pushing hands), as well as the martial applications of the postures. Standing in certain chi kung postures (see pages 114–115) for extended periods of time forms an integral part of most t'ai chi training.

Practice and benefits

Most people choose to learn t'ai chi in a class with others, although teachers also offer one-to-one lessons and residential courses. Loose, comfortable clothes and flat-soled shoes are worn. Classes tend to be held on a weekly basis, but daily practice and repetition are expected, because it is widely

T'ai chi master *This T'ai chi master practises in front of the old government palace in Kaifeng, Henan Province, China.*

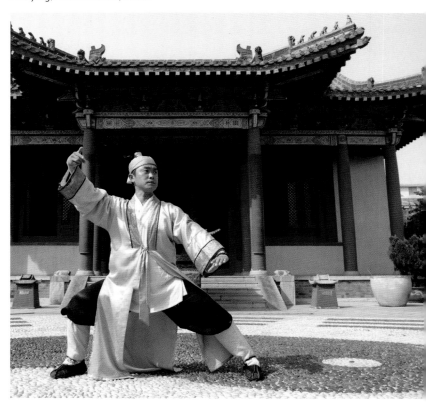

Cloud Hands

This simple exercise is an example of how t'ai chi can be used to relax the joints and associated muscles. This release of tension should relax your hands and fingers. Follow these instructions to work on the left side of the body, then come back to the start position and repeat the movements on the right side of the body.

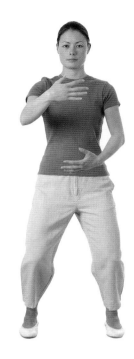 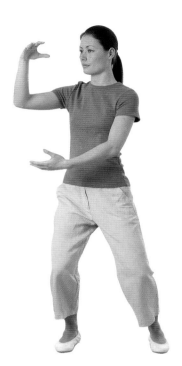 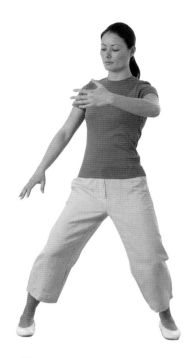

1 Assume a relaxed standing position with your feet facing forward, shoulder-width apart. Bend your knees slightly. Position your hands as shown, one above the other: your right palm at throat height, your left at stomach height.

2 Slowly turn your waist clockwise and, equally slowly, rotate your wrists to form a ball, with your right hand on top. Do not turn too far. Your bottom should remain tucked in and your knees retain plenty of space between them, remaining arch-like through the entire sequence.

3 Step to the left to a distance of one-and-a-half shoulder widths, then change hands so that the right drops to hip height while the left rises to throat height. Shift your weight onto your left side just before your right hand comes down.

---

recognized that dedication and patience are required to achieve the full benefits of t'ai chi.

T'ai chi can be practised anywhere where there is space to move around and the movements can be incorporated into everyday living. It is said that practising outside can help form a better connection with the earth, as well as getting you out into the fresh air. In China t'ai chi is widely practised daily in the parks, especially in the early morning.

As the movements involved in t'ai chi are so gentle, they can be effectively performed by all ages and abilities. Many older people have found that t'ai chi helps them to stay supple and flexible and experience less pain. The movements can even be adapted for people in wheelchairs or who are confined to beds.

According to Traditional Chinese Medicine, these gentle, rhythmic exercises combined with breathing can facilitate the free circulation of chi, which is said to support the body's own healing, thereby maintaining health and vitality and preventing disease. Regular practice can also help improve balance and posture, increase strength and range of movement, aid relaxation and help reduce and manage stress-related conditions.

PRECAUTIONS

✖ See page 108.

RESEARCH AND EVIDENCE

Research indicates that t'ai chi helps reduce mental and physical tension and improves coordination, balance and flexibility. A study at the Oregon Research Institute, published in 2008, showed that a regular t'ai chi programme benefited balance and reduced the number of falls among community-living older adults. Small-scale US studies report that regular t'ai chi sessions have helped lower blood pressure and improve cardiac health, reduce joint swelling and tenderness in osteo- and rheumatoid arthritis sufferers, and ease lower back pain.

CHI KUNG

Chi kung, or qigong, which can be translated as 'energy or breath work', involves the regulation of posture and breathing and the focusing of the mind in practice sessions. Most commonly known in the West for its health benefits, it can also be practised as a therapeutic intervention, martial art or as a meditative exercise.

If you are interested in **Chi Kung**, you may also like to read about:
- **T'ai Chi**, pages 112–113
- **Martial Arts**, pages 116–117
- **Taoism**, pages 216–217
- **Yoga**, pages 106–109
- **Pilates**, pages 110–111
- **Meditation**, pages 78–79

Energy or breath work

The term chi kung combines two ideas: *chi*, which means the breath of life or vital energy of the body, and *kung*, which means the skill and dedication of working towards self-discipline and the achievement of mastery of an art. The primary aim of chi kung is working with the breath in order to cultivate and balance the flow of chi through the body. Chi is said to release the body's potential for healing and provide the power and grace necessary for controlled movement.

It is believed that chi kung was first practised by Taoist and Buddhist monks over 2,000 years ago. Traditional Chinese martial arts such as t'ai chi incorporate the principles of chi kung. However, records show that it was not given its name until the mid-1950s. Although suppressed during the Cultural Revolution (1966–1969), there has been an awakening to chi kung over recent years in China and new 'sets' (movements) continue to be developed at the Peking University Institute for Health in Beijing.

Posture, breathing and the focused mind

Central to chi kung practice is awareness of being present in the moment. With a still mind and positive intention, it is believed that the flow of chi around the body can be directed, moved and balanced to help encourage healthy functioning of mind and body, increase energy and release tension. Master practitioners are said to build up a store of chi energy that can be directed towards promoting healing in others.

Moving or static postures are combined with breathing and the focused mind. The mental focus may be the breath itself or the *tan tien*, the area just beneath the navel, which is the centre of balance and gravity and a focal point for many meditative exercises. Some forms of chi kung include special methods of focusing on particular 'energy centres' in and around the body. Visualization and meditation may be used to concentrate and direct the mind.

Breathing should be natural and effortless, with emphasis on coordination with the postures. These usually start with connection to the earth through the feet, and to the heavens through the crown of the head, and include gentle, repeated movements, static postures, balance and walking techniques, tapping and shaking. An essential element of chi kung is feeling 'centred' and 'grounded'. Although not physically demanding, chi kung takes practice and dedication to perform well.

Practice sessions

Chi kung can be taught in a class situation or on a one-to-one basis. Although there are many different styles, sessions usually start with an invitation to free the mind and body from outside concerns and fully focus on the moment. This includes being aware of where tensions are being held, making subtle adjustments to posture and relaxing muscles in order to perform the sets in the correct way.

Many movements can be performed in a sitting or standing position and can be adapted for use in a wheelchair or bed. Clothing should be loose and comfortable and flat, soft shoes are worn. The basic postures are easy to learn and suitable for everyone, including children and elderly people. The best place to practise is in the open air surrounded by nature.

Health benefits

Positive effects tend to include relaxation and enhanced well being, which should be experienced within a few weeks of daily practice. Regular practice can help improve posture and balance, relieve stiffness and increase energy.

Chi kung is an integral part of Traditional Chinese Medicine and is even believed to help promote longevity. Medical chi kung has been integrated into many Chinese hospitals since 1989 and may be prescribed to help with a variety of complaints and for patients recovering from illness and/or surgery.

PRECAUTIONS

✖ See page 108.

RESEARCH AND EVIDENCE

Chinese research since the 1980s suggests that chi kung can bring many health benefits, including lowering blood pressure and improving immune function. A systemic review of randomized clinical trials into the efficacy of chi kung for pain conditions, published in the UK in 2007, suggested that Chi Kung can reduce chronic pain but concluded that further studies were warranted. A Swedish study, published in *Disability Rehabilitation* in 2007, suggested it could complement conventional treatment for reducing the symptoms of fibromyalgia.

Moving the Rainbow

This gentle exercise will stimulate chi flow along the meridians in your back.
It will help relieve lower back pain and correct poor posture in your upper back
and shoulders by gently stretching your muscles.

1 Begin by standing with your feet shoulder-width apart. Relax your knees and sink slightly as if you were about to sit. Inhale and slowly lift your arms in front of you to chest-height, parallel to the floor.

2 Move your left arm out to your left side, palm up, and lift your right arm above your head, with the palm of your hand slightly curving in. At the same time, shift your weight on to your right leg, keeping your left foot stationary on the ground, heel raised.

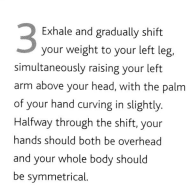

3 Exhale and gradually shift your weight to your left leg, simultaneously raising your left arm above your head, with the palm of your hand curving in slightly. Halfway through the shift, your hands should both be overhead and your whole body should be symmetrical.

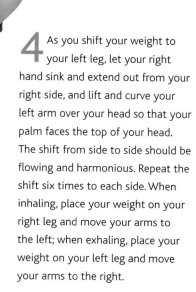

4 As you shift your weight to your left leg, let your right hand sink and extend out from your right side, and lift and curve your left arm over your head so that your palm faces the top of your head. The shift from side to side should be flowing and harmonious. Repeat the shift six times to each side. When inhaling, place your weight on your right leg and move your arms to the left; when exhaling, place your weight on your left leg and move your arms to the right.

MARTIAL ARTS

The term 'martial arts' encompasses a wide **variety of styles** of combat, with or without weapons. Mainly originating from ancient East Asian civilizations, and with a strong emphasis on discipline and practice, these self-defence methods all provide integrated approaches to **mental and physical training**.

If you are interested in **Martial Arts**, you may also like to read about:
- Chi Kung, pages 114–115
- T'ai Chi, pages 112–113
- Yoga, pages 106–109
- Meditation, pages 78–79
- Breathwork, page 81
- Taoism, pages 216–217

Variety of styles

Within the many different styles of martial arts there are divisions and subdivisions that have survived for centuries. Distinguished by methods of practice, movements and underlying philosophy, they all stress the importance of self-discipline and self-motivation, and that the skills and techniques must be used in a morally responsible manner.

There are two main categories of technique: percussive (striking) – blows with hands, feet and other permitted parts of the body; and grappling – throwing, joint locking, holds and wrestling moves designed to neutralize an attack and throw the opponent off balance. Some styles use weapons such as swords, staffs and spears made of wood or metal, but never firearms. Some teachers emphasize the spiritual benefits of regular practice of the discipline, while others focus more on self-defence and physical and mental exercise.

The following are some of the most popular forms of martial arts that are taught and performed in a variety of settings today:

Karate

Translated as 'empty hand', karate is a form of unarmed self-defence that employs techniques to strike, kick, punch and block the opponent primarily using a closed fist, although feet and other parts of the body may also be used. Originating on the island of Okinawa, it was modified and introduced to

Martial arts school *Students practise kung fu at a school near to the Shaolin Temple, China's most renowned home of this famous martial art.*

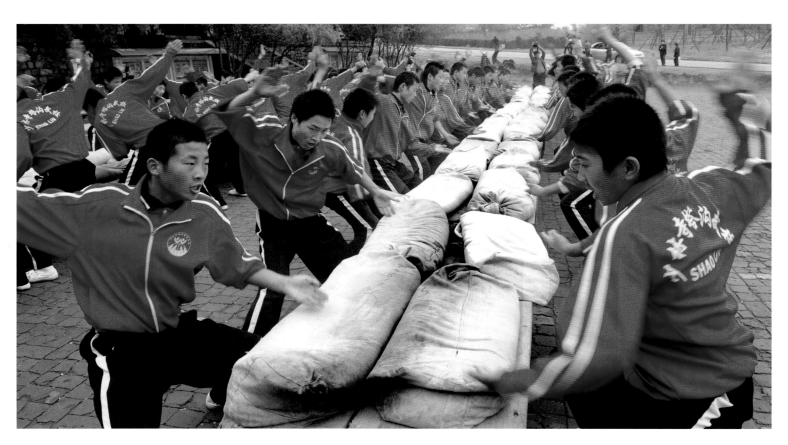

PRECAUTIONS

✖ See page 108.

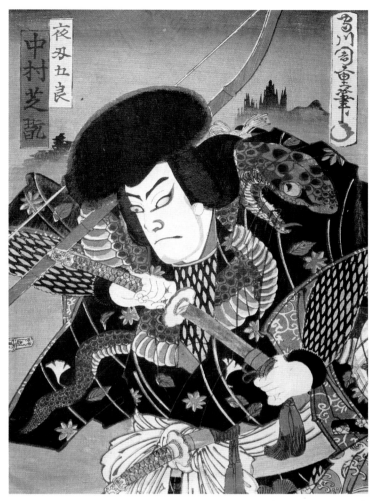

Samuri *This 19th-century Japanese woodcut depicts a samurai (also known as a ninja) initiated in* ninjutsu, *the martial art of invisibility.*

Japan in the early 1920s by Master Funakoshi (1868–1957), who emphasized the philosophical aspects and established karate-do (*do* meaning 'way or road') as a way of life. Students are encouraged to act with gentleness and humility towards others, both in training and in daily life.

Kung fu

Considered to be the oldest martial art, kung fu is reputed to have originated in China some 2,000 years ago. Kung fu, which can be translated as 'skill or knowledge of something physical', was made popular by the speed and coordination of the film star Bruce Lee in the early 1970s. There are many different styles, some teaching movements to turn an opponent's own force against him- or herself to unbalance them, some advocating a direct approach with strong kicks and strikes, while others use weapons such as swords, sticks and staffs.

Tae kwan do

Originating in Korea, where it is a national sport, tae kwan do can be translated as 'the way of foot and fist' and has absorbed many influences, including karate. It was founded in 1955 under the leadership of Korean General Choi Hong Hi (1918–2002), who required Korean soldiers to train in tae kwan do. Known for its kicking techniques, tae kwan do also uses the hands to strike an opponent or to block kicks and punches.

Ju-jitsu

Translated as the 'gentle art', ju-jitsu was originally developed in Japan as the primary unarmed combat method of the samurai warriors. It emphasizes using an attacker's strength against him- or herself to neutralize the attack. Techniques include joint locks, chokes, throws and strikes. Weapons such as swords, sticks and staffs may also be used.

Judo

Developing from ju-jitsu, judo, meaning 'gentle way', places emphasis on safety and physical conditioning. It uses skill and coordination rather than force or strength to overcome and unbalance the opponent. Techniques include throwing, control holds, arm locks, strikes and choking, without weapons. Judo became an Olympic sport in 1964.

Aikido

Also rooted in ju-jitsu, aikido can be translated as 'way of harmony' and focuses on working in harmony with the attacker's force to gain control. Techniques include throws and joint locks. Essentially non-combative, aikido is one of the more spiritual martial arts.

Mental and physical training

Traditionally, the practice of martial arts was directed towards self-improvement and self-mastery in the pursuit of inner development. Modern martial arts still advocate development of both mind and body, and students are expected to be committed to learning the skills in order to master the discipline. Benefits of regular practice include increased strength, stamina, flexibility and gracefulness, as well as improved wellbeing and confidence, fewer physical injuries and lower levels of anxiety. Many instructors consider martial arts to be a way of life and offer guidance on self-development.

Martial arts classes, clubs and competitions are now very popular. Most are suitable for people of all ages, including children, who might benefit from mental and physical discipline in a supportive group environment.

ALEXANDER TECHNIQUE

Developed by the Australian actor **Frederick Alexander** in the 1890s, the Alexander technique focuses on **re-educating mind and body** to achieve **natural posture**, ease of breathing and freedom of movement. The discipline, which is especially popular among those who practice the performing arts, can help bring about well-documented health benefits for people of all ages and walks of life.

If you are interested in the **Alexander Technique**, you may also like to read about:

- **Pilates**, pages 110–111
- **Yoga**, pages 106–109
- **Chiropractic and Osteopathy**, pages 132–135
- **Feldenkrais Method**, page 137
- **Rolfing**, page 139
- **Bowen Technique**, page 138
- **Martial Arts**, pages 116–117

Frederick Alexander

The Alexander technique was invented by Frederick Matthias Alexander (1869–1955) during his own search for a solution to his recurring hoarseness during theatrical performances. Careful and detailed self-observation in front of mirrors revealed that the underlying cause was apparently involuntary tension of his neck muscles in order to project his voice on stage. Although only a minor movement, this caused his head to be pulled back and down, constricting his throat and affected his breathing. Alexander subsequently learned how to correct his habit and as a result his voice improved, along with his general health and wellbeing.

Alexander concluded that ingrained postural habits and reactions, which tend to be especially prominent in demanding or stressful situations, not only impinge on performance, but can also affect the way the body functions and perhaps have a detrimental impact on general health and wellbeing. One of the early pioneers of the power of the mind–body connection, he believed that the most effective way of preventing long-held patterns of muscular tension and misuse was by learning the skills of calm and conscious self-awareness and direction of movement.

Alexander moved from Australia to the UK in the early 1900s, eventually setting up a school for teachers of the Alexander technique in London in 1931. Now widely used by musicians, actors and athletes to enhance their performance, the technique is popular in many countries and is recommended by some doctors as helpful in the management of pain, musculoskeletal problems and stress-related conditions.

Natural posture

One of the key principles of the Alexander technique is the achieving of a balanced relationship between the head, neck and back during all activities, whether running a marathon or answering the phone. Over the years, the natural and effortless poise and coordination we have as small children is hindered by the acquisition of bad postural habits, repetitive movements and accumulating stresses. Habitual tensing of muscles leads to misalignment of the head–neck–back relationship, resulting in problems such as rounded shoulders and an arched back.

As these habits become entrenched, poor posture can affect the way the whole body functions. Teachers of the Alexander technique believe that learning to recognize and correct poor use of body movements can help increase clarity of thought, improve muscle strength and stamina, ease backache and headaches, increase relaxation and result in a greater ability to cope positively with stress. Enthusiasts claim that applying the principles to daily life can also help make people feel taller and more graceful.

Re-educating mind and body

The technique which involves a course of practical one-to-one lessons with a teacher is suitable for all ages and levels of fitness. The first lesson usually includes assessment of posture, breathing, balance and coordination in everyday situations such as standing, sitting and walking. The teacher is trained to assess how habitual and subconscious patterns of muscle tension, acquired since childhood, are affecting ease and freedom of movement.

Students work with the teacher to learn to recognize and avoid these habits and to appreciate how it feels to move with minimum strain on the joints and muscles. To make the body work more efficiently teachers guide the pupil through a series of actions using their hands to direct, improve and modify posture and movement. Lessons take 30–45 minutes, often on a twice-weekly basis, and 20–30 are usually recommended, but dedication and homework are essential.

Long-standing habits can be hard to break, so it takes commitment and practice to learn the skills necessary to change these patterns. However, this new self-awareness of natural movement and posture eventually leads to a release of muscle tension and a natural realignment of the head, neck and back. This appears to help alleviate painful conditions and reduce the risk of further problems. The Alexander technique is now part of the curriculum in many schools of music, acting, circus and dance.

PRECAUTIONS

✖ See page 108.

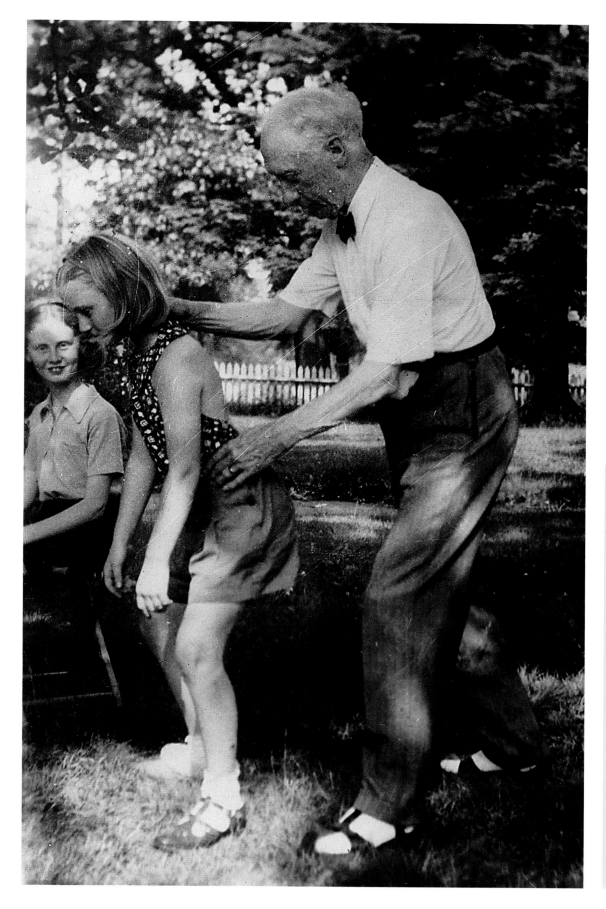

Frederick Alexander *This photograph shows Frederick Alexander teaching a student correct postural alignment.*

RESEARCH AND EVIDENCE

One of the first studies into the Alexander technique was conducted in 1956 by Dr Wilfred Barlow, one of Alexander's pupils, at the Royal College of Music in London. Photographs of students before and after lessons showed significant improvement in posture compared to those who undertook conventional postural exercises. Furthermore, this improvement enhanced singing performance. In the *British Journal of Therapy and Rehabilitation* in 1997, a review of further studies showed that the technique can be helpful in rehabilitating injured athletes and for increasing lung capacity and encouraging deeper, slower breathing. A 2008 UK-based clinical trial showed that Alexander technique lessons combined with exercise could have significant long-term benefits in improving quality of life for people with chronic and recurrent back pain.

SWEDISH MASSAGE

If you are interested in **Swedish Massage**,
you may also like to read about:
- Ayurveda, pages 94–97
- Reflexology, pages 128–131
- Aromatherapy, pages 156–157
- Bowen Technique, page 138
- Rolfing, page 139
- Indian Head Massage, page 123
- Thai Massage, page 122
- Shiatsu, pages 124–125

Massage, one of the most **ancient forms of healing therapy**, is a generic term for the systematic manipulation of the body's soft tissues (skin, muscles, tendons and ligaments) using the hands. Swedish massage, the most commonly practised method in the West, involves a practitioner applying a variety of **classic techniques** and degrees of pressure to attain **therapeutic benefits**.

Ancient form of healing therapy

Chinese texts dated as far back as c. 3000 BCE record massage being used to treat illness and injury, and pictograms in Egyptian tombs show people being massaged. Hindu texts include massage as an integral part of ayurvedic medicine, and its therapeutic benefits were also recognized by the ancient Greeks and Romans.

Swedish massage, or classical massage, evolved from a system of medical gymnastics and massage techniques devised by Swedish physiologist Per Henrick Ling (1776–1839). Ling's approach eventually gained official recognition from the Swedish government in 1813.

By the mid-19th century, Ling's methods were being adopted in many countries. In 1894 a group of nurses in England founded the Society of Trained Masseuses (which later became the Chartered Society of Physiotherapists), to develop and regulate the practice of physical treatments.

The technological advances of the 1940s and 1950s overshadowed manual methods of treatment, but interest has been rekindled in recent years by health professionals who offer holistic care alongside conventional medical approaches for a variety of conditions. Massage is now widely used in hospices, intensive-care units for premature babies, psychiatric institutions, health centres and pain clinics.

Therapeutic benefits

To reach out and touch is a natural, intuitive response to someone in distress. Touch can provide comfort, relaxation and pain relief. Perhaps because as babies we are aware of it before any other sense, touch 'tunes in' to some of our earliest experiences. Furthermore, certain sensory nerve endings in the skin may trigger the release of endorphins, which are natural painkillers that give a feeling of wellbeing.

The specific benefits of massage depend on the depth, speed and combination of various techniques tailored to individual needs. Massage can be soothing and calming, aiding relaxation and providing relief from stress-related conditions such as insomnia and irritable bowel syndrome. It can also be helpful for people with anxiety and depression. Firmer massage is used to help with muscle or joint problems or sports injuries. Massage is suitable for

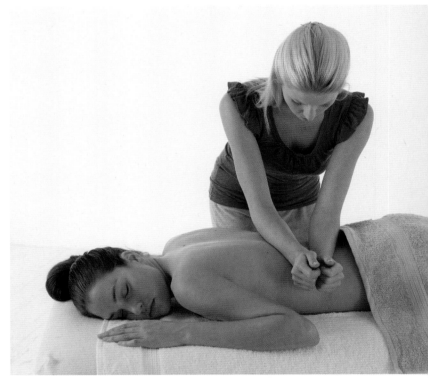

Swedish massage *Massage practitioners are trained to adapt their massage techniques to ensure the optimum benefits for each individual.*

all ages, including the elderly and very young, in which case only gentle pressures are applied.

Beforehand, the practitioner will ask questions about medical history, diet, lifestyle and general state of health. The client usually lies on a treatment couch. For a full body massage, all clothing, apart from underpants, is removed. Therapists maintain a high degree of privacy, using large towels for modesty. Massage oils and creams are used to ease the flow of hand movements. Massage should never cause pain. A practitioner will invite feedback on the level of pressure used to ensure optimum comfort throughout the massage.

Classic techniques

Swedish massage involves five classic techniques:

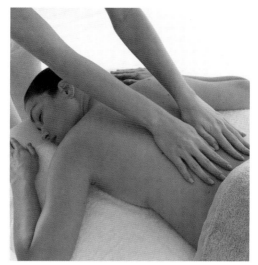

Effleurage A massage stroke applied with a light, medium or firm touch, which forms a major part of any massage routine, used at the beginning and end, and also to link movements.

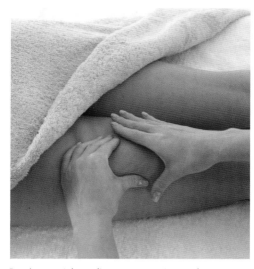

Petrissage A kneading, compression technique used to encourage the circulation of the blood and lymph through the muscle tissues and aid venous return.

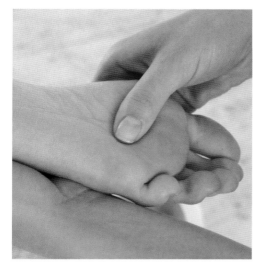

Friction A deep technique applied by concentrated pressure in a circular or cross-fibre motion on specific areas of muscle via the thumbs, fingers, heel of hand or elbow.

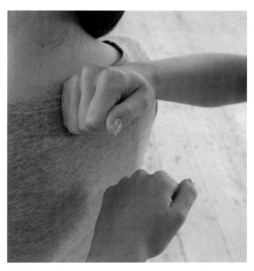

Tapotement A stimulating technique applied via a series of percussive movements that include hacking, cupping, pummelling and pounding.

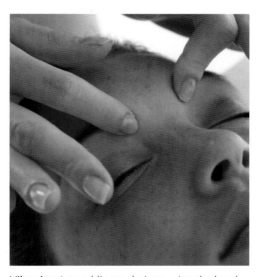

Vibration A trembling technique using the hands or fingers, which stimulates the nerve fibres and appears to have a relaxing effect.

PRECAUTIONS

✖ Consult your doctor if you have epilepsy, osteoporosis, cancer, diabetes, thyroid problems, thrombosis or any other serious health condition.

✖ Avoid vigorous massage in the first three months of pregnancy.

✖ Inform your practitioner if you are taking any prescribed or over-the-counter medication and if you are consulting another complementary or alternative-health practitioner.

✖ Avoid alcohol, large meals, hot baths and showers and strenuous exercise before and after treatment.

RESEARCH AND EVIDENCE

On-going research trials at the Touch Research Institute (TRI) in Miami, USA, show that massage can help with stress-related conditions such as insomnia, irritable bowel syndrome and chronic fatigue. Studies at TRI also show that massage can help premature babies achieve more rapid weight gain and development, and can improve body image and self-esteem among teenagers with eating disorders. In the *Journal of Pain Symptom Management*, a 1999 study showed that massage can be helpful for low back pain. The UK's National Institute of Clinical Excellence suggests that massage may be beneficial for people with multiple sclerosis. Evidence shows that massage is one of the most widely used therapies in supportive and palliative care and can have a significant impact on reducing anxiety, stress and pain in cancer sufferers.

THAI MASSAGE

If you are interested in **Thai Massage**, you may also like to read about:

- Yoga, pages 106–109
- Indian Head Massage, page 123
- Acupressure, page 127
- Shiatsu, pages 124–125
- Swedish Massage, pages 120–121
- Ayurveda, pages 94–97

The traditional healing massage of Thailand is regarded as a **meditative and spiritual practice**, bringing benefits to mind and body. It involves stretching techniques and pressure along the **sen** (energy channels or meridians), through which prana, or internal energy, is said to be transformed and redistributed through the body.

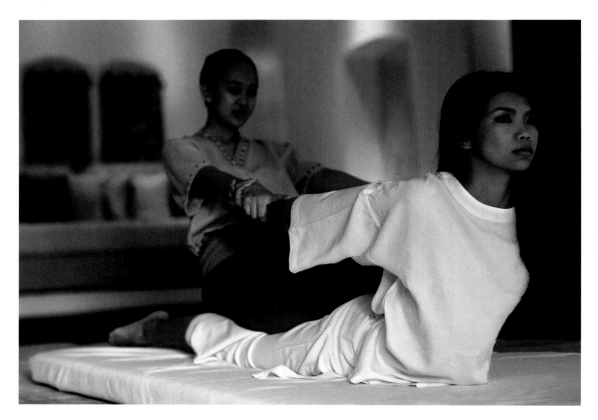

Thai massage *During a Thai massage, the client is passive and fully supported in all positions by a trained practitioner.*

PRECAUTIONS

✱ See page 121; if you are pregnant, inform your practitioner, as certain points should not be stimulated and some postures avoided.

RESEARCH AND EVIDENCE

While there is anecdotal evidence to support the claims of the beneficial effects of traditional Thai massage, including relief from mental and physical tension and increased energy levels, there has been little scientific research to date.

Meditative and spiritual practice

Thai massage reputedly developed during Buddha's lifetime over 2,500 years ago. As Buddhism spread from India to Thailand, so did massage for therapeutic purposes. Although strongly influenced by ayurveda, Thai massage has evolved its own principles and techniques.

Practitioners usually see Thai massage as part of a spiritual practice so it is normally carried out in silence to help facilitate meditation and mindfulness (concentrated awareness). Clients are encouraged to look within and give full attention to their physical and mental experiences.

Sen

The focus of Thai massage is the stimulation and rebalancing of the flow of prana, said to circulate through the 72,000 sen in the body. Practitioners structure their massage around the main ten energy lines, or sen, and use body weight to apply pressure with hands, feet, forearms, knees or elbows to specific points along the sen, accompanied by the stretching and mobilizing of muscles and joints and rhythmic rocking. Treatment may include being guided and supported in hatha yoga *asanas* (postures) that would otherwise be difficult to achieve.

Thai massage takes place on a mat or thin mattress on the floor. Loose, comfortable clothes are worn by both the practitioner and client. No oil is used. The session, which can take up to two hours, is intense, relaxing and supportive. Following a Thai massage, people often report feelings of wellbeing and relief from mental and physical tension. Other benefits are said to include pain relief, improved blood and lymph circulation, increased energy levels and better sleep.

INDIAN HEAD MASSAGE

If you are interested in **Indian Head Massage,** you may also like to read about:
- Craniosacral Therapy, page 136
- Aromatherapy, pages 156–157
- Bowen Technique, page 138
- Ayurveda, pages 94–97
- Thai Massage, page 122
- Shiatsu, pages 124–125

This seated massage therapy, developed from ayurveda, has its roots in traditional massage, as practised at home in **Indian families**. In order to aid relaxation and relieve stress, practitioners apply massage to the head, neck, upper back and face with the **optional use of oil** for additional benefits.

Family routines in India

Massage is an important part of the ancient ayurvedic medical system, and has long been part of everyday life in India. Traditionally, babies are massaged by their mothers from birth to aid healthy growth and development, and as young children are given regular head massage, while in adulthood head massage is incorporated into beauty and grooming routines.

Indian head massage was introduced to the UK in the 1970s and made popular by Narendra Mehta, a blind physiotherapist, who recognized its potential for relieving physical and mental stress among office workers. He extended the traditional massage to include the upper back, scalp, face and ears, combined with chakra (energy-centre) balancing, and launched the therapy as Champissage. In recent years, this therapy, now called Indian head massage, has been developed as a combination of Western and Indian massage techniques. It works to increase blood and lymph flow, relax taut muscles and, since it encourages deeper, calmer breathing, it could also have beneficial emotional and psychological effects. It is widely used in offices as a stress-relieving therapy, as well as in beauty and complementary therapy clinics. Some people experience almost immediate benefits, others need several sessions.

Optional use of oil

The massage usually takes place on a comfortable, upright chair. The therapist stands behind and uses a series of alternately soothing and invigorating movements, starting on the upper back and progressing to the neck and head, finishing with gentle strokes on the face. Each session lasts around 30–45 minutes, although it is often shortened for the workplace.

It can be practised without oils through light clothing. Alternatively, massage oils can be used to nourish the skin and hair; upper clothing is removed and a large towel offered for modesty. Oils used include sweet almond, coconut, olive, sunflower and sesame or traditional ayurvedic oils.

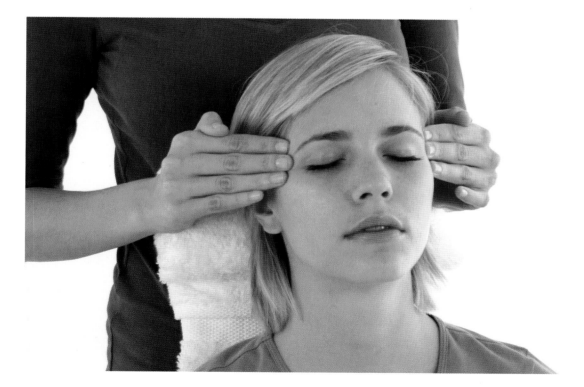

Indian head massage *Gentle massage to the face is extremely relaxing and can bring relief from a tension headache.*

PRECAUTIONS
✖ See page 121.

RESEARCH AND EVIDENCE

There has been little specific research into the benefits of Indian head massage to date. However, in the *Journal of Holistic Healthcare*, a 2007 descriptive study showed that it helped improve mood and reduce tension, and that it might therefore be a useful adjunct to conventional care for people with moderate mental health problems.

SHIATSU

A **traditional Japanese therapy**, shiatsu incorporates a variety of **hands-on techniques** which are used to detect and correct 'imbalances in the flow of ki', or vital energy, through the body. Shiatsu is a relaxing **therapeutic treatment** that is rapidly gaining in popularity in the West.

If you are interested in **Shiatsu**, you may also like to read about:
- Reflexology, pages 128–131
- Swedish Massage, pages 120–121
- Thai Massage, page 122
- Indian Head Massage, page 123
- Acupuncture, page 126
- Acupressure, page 127

Traditional Japanese therapy

Shiatsu, which literally means 'finger pressure', originates from an ancient form of Chinese massage called *anmo* or *tui na*, which involves applying pressure on certain points (*tsubos*) on the body with the aim of improving the flow of its vital energy, known as ki in Japan (chi in China), along channels known as meridians. This is said to enhance the body's innate ability to heal itself. In this way it is similar to acupuncture. When the principles of Traditional Chinese Medicine were introduced to Japan between 500 and 1500 CE by Buddhist monks, *anmo* gained popularity as a treatment practised mainly by blind therapists.

Shiatsu was developed in the early 20th century by Japanese practitioner Tamai Tempaku, who recognized the value of integrating gentle manipulation and stretching techniques from modern physiotherapy and chiropractic with diagnosis and treatment according to the principles of oriental medicine. Shiatsu was officially recognized as a clinical therapeutic practice by the Japanese Government in 1964, distinguishing it from the non-medical form of *anma* massage, which is also widespread in Japan.

Hands-on techniques

Early shiatsu practitioners developed their own styles and some founded schools that helped establish shiatsu as a recognized therapy. Today shiatsu practitioners work in different ways depending on their chosen approach, but all base their practice on Traditional Chinese Medicine principles. Some focus on specific *tsubos* on the meridians, as in acupressure, while others use massage along the meridians to assist the flow of ki. Some practitioners offer a more diagnostic approach to highlight problem areas. Most use a combination of dynamic, releasing manipulation techniques and stretches with gentle, nurturing moves and holds.

Although shiatsu helps reduce muscular tension, its primary intention is to harmonise the circulation of inner energies. It is thought that ki can stop

Passive rotation *A practitioner can use his or her body weight to increase the depth of a stretch. Rotating the legs in this way relaxes the lower back.*

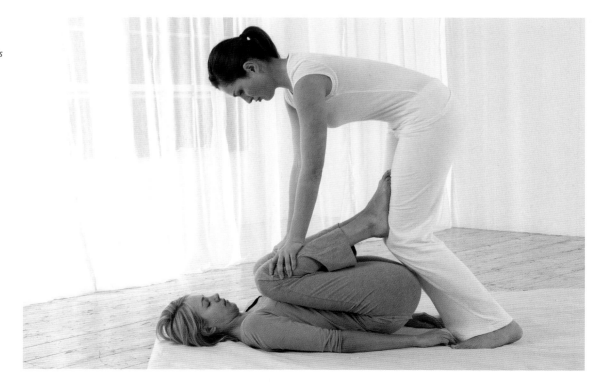

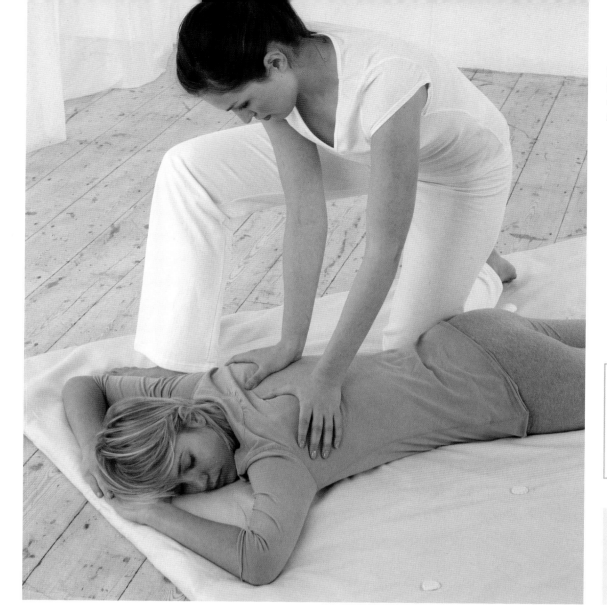

Palm pressure *Applied either side of the spine, palm pressure can be deeply relaxing and may help release tension held in the back and shoulders.*

PRECAUTIONS
✖ See page 121; if you are pregnant, inform your practitioner, as certain *tsubos* should not be stimulated.

RESEARCH AND EVIDENCE
At present there is little available research that relates specifically to shiatsu. See Acupressure, page 127.

flowing smoothly along the meridians for many different reasons, which results in imbalances which can manifest as physical symptoms or psychological disturbances. Specific techniques are chosen to help reduce excess ki where the flow is overactive or blocked (*jitsu*) or build it up in areas of weakness (*kyo*). Therefore a practitioner treating a neck problem will not only work on that area, but also on the flow of energy throughout the whole body to assist the body's powers of recovery.

Techniques include gentle holding and rocking, and pressing with palms, thumbs, fingers, elbows, knees and even feet on the meridians. If appropriate, the practitioner may work with rotations and stretching of the joints and limbs. The treatment is not painful, although minor discomfort may be felt when certain points are worked.

Therapeutic treatment

People generally report feelings of peace of mind and increased vitality after a shiatsu treatment. Some people feel that regular sessions help them maintain wellbeing and prevent the build-up of stress and tension. Shiatsu practitioners claim it can also help heal specific injuries and improve general health, back pain, headaches, joint pain and stiffness, depression, digestive problems and stress-related conditions.

Before treatment, the practitioner will ask the client about his or her current physical and emotional health, medical and family history, diet and lifestyle, and may also use traditional methods of pulse and tongue diagnosis. A feature of shiatsu is the use of gentle touch on the *hara* area (abdomen). Practitioners claim to be able to assess the health of the internal organs and to detect subtle imbalances in the flow of ki around the body from palpating the abdominal region.

Treatment usually lasts an hour and is given with the client resting on a special firm mattress, or futon, on the floor. However, it can easily be adapted to a chair or wheelchair. Shiatsu practitioners are trained to use controlled body weight to apply pressure without effort or strain. Treatment can be given fully clothed – loose, comfortable, warm attire is worn by both client and practitioner. No oil is used and there is minimal direct contact with the skin.

ACUPUNCTURE

If you are interested in **Acupuncture**, you may also like to read about:
- Reflexology, pages 128–131
- Acupressure, page 127
- Shiatsu, pages 124–125
- Craniosacral Therapy, page 136
- Traditional Chinese Medicine, pages 98–101

This ancient Chinese medical technique is now well established worldwide. The two main styles practised are **traditional Chinese acupuncture** and **Western medical acupuncture**. The **therapeutic treatment** involves the insertion of fine needles into the skin at specific points on the meridians to restore, promote and maintain good health.

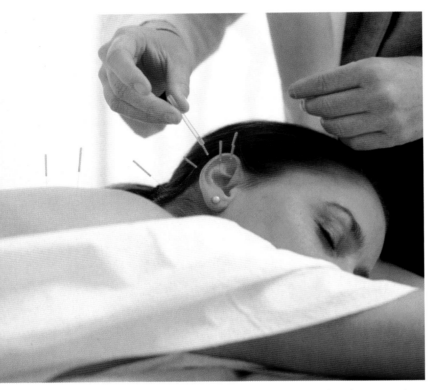

Acupuncture *During an acupuncture teatment, clients are invited to relax on a couch while needles are gently inserted into a specific combination of acupoints on the body.*

RESEARCH AND EVIDENCE

There have been many research reports on the effectiveness of acupuncture. In 1979 the World Health Organization listed some 40 diseases that could successfully be treated by acupuncture in a clinical setting, including breathing difficulties, digestive problems, disorders of the nervous system and painful menstruation. In 1989 *The Lancet* reported that acupuncture had a beneficial impact on people with alcohol addiction. In *Annals of Internal Medicine*, a 2004 study found that acupuncture significantly reduced pain in people with osteoarthritis of the knee. The *British Medical Journal* stated in 2006 that acupuncture for persistent lower back pain has been clinically researched more thoroughly than many orthodox treatments.

Traditional Chinese acupuncture

Traditional acupuncturists believe that health is dependent on the flow of chi, the body's informing energy, through channels (meridians), each linked to a vital organ, and that the flow of chi can be blocked for different reasons, including emotional disturbances, lifestyle, hereditary factors, infections and trauma. In order to plan individual treatment, traditional acupuncturists will take a full medical history, discuss lifestyle and assess the rhythm and strength of the meridian pulses and the appearance of the tongue for signs of imbalance. They will then insert very fine needles into the skin at chosen points thought to improve the flow and distribution of chi.

Western medical acupuncture

Since the 1970s many Western doctors, nurses and physiotherapists have trained in acupuncture and use dry needling to supplement conventional treatment. The insertion of needles is similar to traditional acupuncture, but diagnosis and treatment are based on conventional medical principles.

Therapeutic treatment

An acupuncture treatment usually lasts between 30 minutes and an hour and can be extremely relaxing. Acupuncture needles are very fine and do not cause any pain. Some people experience a tingling sensation. The number of treatments required depends on many factors, but some people report immediate benefits. Needles are left in place from a few seconds to 30 minutes. Acupuncture is used to treat all ages, including children. It is best known for its pain-relieving effects and is widely used in hospitals in China, especially during and following surgery. In the West it is gradually becoming more common in hospices, health centres and pain clinics. Traditional acupuncturists claim that it can help many other chronic and acute conditions, including addictions.

PRECAUTIONS

✖ See page 121; if you are pregnant, inform your practitioner, as certain points should not be stimulated. Also check that the practitioner is fully qualified and that disposable needles are used and hygiene is of a high standard.

ACUPRESSURE

If you are interested in **Acupressure**, you may also like to read about:
- **Acupuncture**, page 126
- **Shiatsu**, pages 124–125
- **Reflexology**, pages 128–131
- **Traditional Chinese Medicine**, pages 98–101

Working on the same principles as acupuncture but without needles, acupressure involves the **application of pressure**, usually with the finger and thumb. Widely practised in China as a **self-help treatment**, it is being introduced to workplaces in the West in the form of **seated acupressure**, a form of on-site massage.

Application of pressure

Pressure applied using the hands, fingers, thumbs or knuckles and occasionally the feet and knees in a 'press, hold, release' action on specific points on the body is said to 'balance the flow of the body's vital energy', chi. Pressure tends to be gentle but firm, and angled in the direction of the flow of chi along the channel (meridian).

Self-help treatment

Some acupuncturists use acupressure as part of their treatment and also offer advice on pressing specific points as a form of self-help for minor conditions. The points used are not always close to the part of the body where the problem is experienced.

Seated acupressure

This has become popular as a way of relaxing office workers, with therapists visiting the workplace to offer massage on-site. However, it is also used in other settings, including hospitals, hospices and complementary therapy clinics. Treatment is relatively quick and effective, lasting around 20 minutes or less, and the client remains fully clothed during the session. The client sits facing forward in an ergonomically designed massage chair and the therapist carries out a specific sequence of techniques and movements aimed at stimulating the acupressure points in the head, neck, shoulders and lower back. No oil is used. Benefits claimed include the relief of stress and muscular tension and improvements in backache and repetitive strain syndromes. Clients report feeling energized and refreshed afterwards.

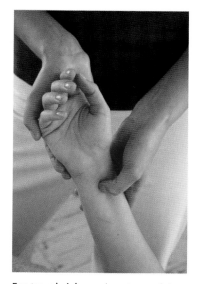

For stress and anxiety Locate a small hollow on the inner wrist in line with your little finger. Apply pressure with the tip of your thumb pointing towards your little finger. Hold for 20–30 seconds, release and repeat. Repeat on the other wrist.

For travel sickness Locate a point on the inside of your arm, about three finger-widths above the natural crease on your wrist. Support your outer wrist with your fingers and apply pressure with your thumb pad. Hold for as long as feels comfortable. Release. Repeat on the other arm.

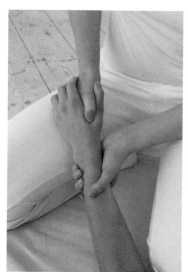

For constipation and indigestion Locate the point in the fleshy part between your thumb and forefinger. Place the forefinger of your other hand beneath and thumb on top. Gently squeeze and hold for 20–30 seconds. Release and repeat. **Do not use during pregnancy.**

PRECAUTIONS

✖ See page 121; if you are pregnant, inform your practitioner, as certain points should not be stimulated.

RESEARCH AND EVIDENCE

Forms of acupressure, including shiatsu (see page 124), have been suggested for many conditions, including nausea and vomiting. The Natural Standard (see page 108) reports that many studies support the use of wrist acupressure at point P6 for the treatment of nausea (see centre picture, left), especially when induced by motion, surgery, chemotherapy and pregnancy. Other trials suggest that acupressure may be helpful for improving sleep quality and for the relief of lower back pain and tension or migraine headache.

REFLEXOLOGY

If you are interested in **Reflexology**, you may also like to read about:

- **Traditional Chinese Medicine**, pages 98–101
- **Acupuncture**, page 126
- **Acupressure**, page 127
- **Shiatsu**, pages 124–125
- **Chakras and the Aura**, pages 172–173
- **Reiki**, pages 174–175

Developed from **zone therapy**, reflexology is based on the principle that **reflex points** on the feet and hands correspond to all parts of the body. This notion that the whole is represented in the part is a recurring theme in both bodywork and energy therapies. Applying pressure to these points with **reflexology techniques** is said to help release tensions and encourage the body's natural healing processes to restore and maintain **health** and wellbeing. There are also several **variants of reflexology** that have been developed in recent years.

Zone therapy

Foot massage has been practised for thousands of years and records show that it dates back to early Egyptian and Chinese civilizations. A pictogram in the Physician's Tomb at Saqqara in Egypt, dated c. 2300 BCE, depicts people giving and receiving hand and foot massage.

Reflexology in its current form was developed from zone therapy, which was introduced to the West in 1915 by Dr William Fitzgerald

(1872–1942), an American ear, nose and throat surgeon. He believed that applying pressure to one part of the body could have an anaesthetizing effect on another area. After further investigation, he claimed that the body is divided into ten equal zones, five on the left side and five on the right side,

Ancient origins *This Egyptian artwork depicting reflexology was found in the tomb of the ancient Egyptian physician Ankmahor at Saqqara, Egypt.*

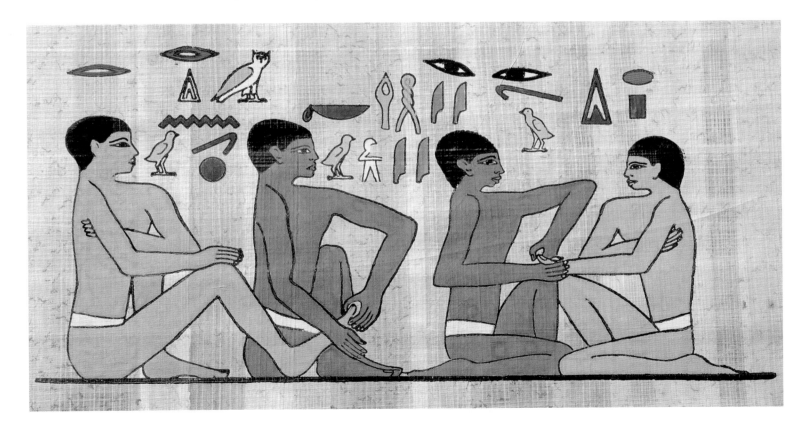

Plantar foot map

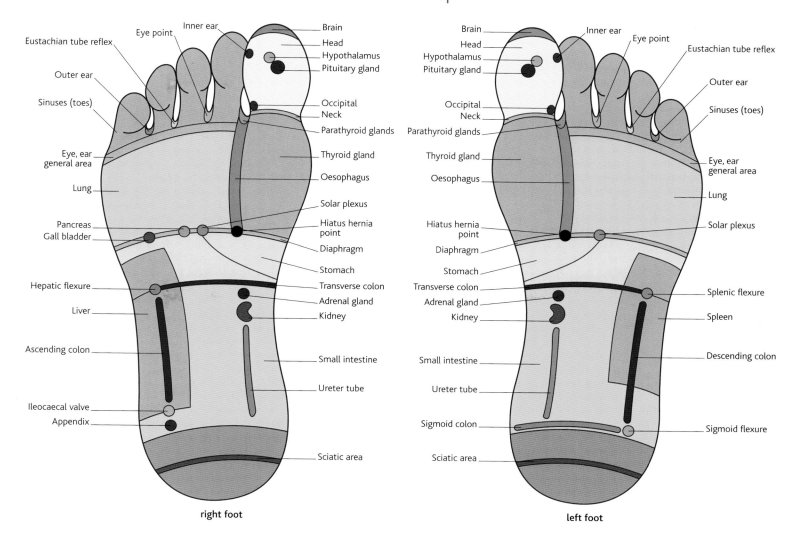

Plantar foot map *This map shows what reflexologists believe to be the reflex points on the sole or underside of the feet. The tops and sides of the feet also contain important reflex points.*

which run vertically through the body ending at the fingers and toes. He considered that pressure on one part of a zone affects all areas within the same zone, so it is possible to treat less accessible parts of the body by working in the same zone on the hands or feet. Dr Fitzgerald sometimes used clothes pegs and metal combs to exert pressure on the hands and fingers.

Despite much initial scepticism within the medical profession, the concept of zones remains a key principle of modern reflexology. Within each zone there is said to be a flow of vital energy which periods of illness, stress or injury, however minor, can interrupt, thus preventing the body from functioning properly. Working on points within each zone is said to help release blockages and restore the free flow of energy through the whole body. There is some similarity between the theory of zones and the meridians in Traditional Chinese Medicine. Both are based on a belief in a connection between various parts of the body, but unlike TCM's meridians the zones are of equal length and extend through the body from front to back.

Reflex points

Zone therapy was further developed in the 1930s by American physiotherapist Eunice Ingham (1899–1974), who introduced the Ingham Reflex Method of Compression Massage, later known as reflexology. She located and 'mapped' specific reflex areas on the feet relating to different organs, glands and parts of the body, and also developed pressing techniques for stimulating these areas. In the 1960s, one of her students, Doreen Bayly (1899–1979), introduced her ideas to the UK and other parts of Europe. Reflexology charts — based on experience of clinical effects rather than any basic scientific research — have been further developed over the years.

An important development was the introduction of transverse zones in the 1970s by German reflexologist Hanne Marquardt. She identified three horizontal lines across the feet, marked by the bones of the foot, which divide the foot into different areas and so enable more specific location of reflexes relating to different parts of the body.

Reflexology maps show points on the soles, sides and tops of the feet and hands. The right foot and hand correspond to the right side of the body and the left foot and hand to the left side. Some parts of the body are found on one side, the spleen for example, and so these are represented only on the appropriate foot or hand. Over recent years reflex points and areas have also been located and mapped on the ears and the face.

A full reflexology treatment involves working all the reflex points so that the whole body is treated. However, specific points can also be used for self-help and first-aid measures. Practitioners believe that crystalline deposits of waste products, usually calcium and uric acid, concentrate around the reflex points. Trained hands look for deposits or imbalances and work on a point to break down the crystals, encouraging elimination and stimulating the circulation. The big toe and thumb, for example, are said to correspond to the head and can be worked in a systematic way to help ease headaches.

Techniques

Practitioners are trained to use specific techniques to apply pressure to reflex points using finger and thumb techniques. Reflexologists claim that each foot contains 7,200 nerve endings and that relaxing the foot can have a soothing effect on the whole body. Therefore treatments usually include a variety of massage and relaxation techniques at the start and finish of each session. Among the more stimulating techniques is the 'caterpillar walk', which involves making small steps with a bent thumb or finger moving or 'creeping' like a caterpillar between reflex points.

The amount of pressure depends on individual preference, but reflexology should never be ticklish or painful. There may, however, be fleeting moments of discomfort, which are taken as an indication of congestion or imbalance in a corresponding part of the body. Extra attention may be given to areas of tenderness. Practitioners work with clients to assess which reflexes need more or less stimulation and provide a balanced and personalized treatment.

A treatment usually lasts around 45 minutes to an hour. The practitioner takes a case history, asking questions about symptoms, lifestyle and medical history to ensure that the treatment can be adapted to meet individual needs. Feet and hands may also be examined, as areas of hard skin or corns and discoloration and markings in the nails may provide information about the health of related parts of the body.

For foot reflexology, the client sits on a reclining chair or couch with feet raised, shoes and socks removed, with the practitioner seated so that both feet can be accessed comfortably. There is also a form of reflexology known as Vertical Reflex Therapy (VRT), which involves treating the client in a standing position. Originally developed in a nursing home to give reflexology to people sitting in a wheelchair, VRT is a brief but powerful treatment, working on the tops of the hands and feet in a weight-bearing position.

Health benefits

Initial responses to treatment can range from a sensation of wellbeing and relaxation to transitory feelings of tiredness, nausea or tearfulness after the first few sessions. A course of treatment varies in length depending on individual needs, but is usually between six and eight sessions. Many people have regular treatments to help maintain health and wellbeing.

Practised worldwide, reflexology is suitable for all ages, including babies and young children, and has been used to treat a wide range of acute and chronic conditions, including emotional problems. It is said to be particularly helpful for anxiety and stress-related conditions such as insomnia and constipation, and for pain relief. Many people report that reflexology has a positive impact on mind and body. It has become increasingly available in pain clinics, hospices, cancer centres and maternity units.

Variants of reflexology

Vacuflex reflexology, which was developed by a Danish reflexologist, Inge Dougans, combines traditional reflexology principles with acupuncture techniques. Vacuflex 'boots' are worn by the client to stimulate all reflex areas. When the boots are removed, practitioners look for temporary discolorations on the feet, which relate to corresponding reflexes and offer an indication of areas of the body that are out of balance. Treatment is then continued using suction cups on the surface meridian points on the client's hands, feet, arms and legs.

The Metamorphic technique, which was also developed from reflexology, involves a very light massage on spinal reflexes on the feet, hands and head. The practitioner gently works these points in a systematic way in order to help release 'energy blockages' said to have been developed during the nine months from conception to birth. Clients are encouraged to focus within and relax, so that their own energy can transform negative or unhelpful patterning established during the prenatal period.

RESEARCH AND EVIDENCE

There is much anecdotal evidence for the benefits of reflexology and an increasing number of clinical research trials are being completed. In *Obstetrics and Gynecology*, a 1993 US study indicated that reflexology may be effective in treating premenstrual symptoms. Several trials in the UK have found positive effects for reducing anxiety and improving the psychological wellbeing of people with cancer, and surveys reveal that reflexology is one of the most widely used therapies in cancer care. The UK's National Institute for Clinical Excellence suggests that reflexology may be beneficial for people with multiple sclerosis. However, there is no anatomical basis for the theories underpinning reflexology, or physiological explanation for its possible benefits.

PRECAUTIONS
✖ See page 121.

Foot reflex points

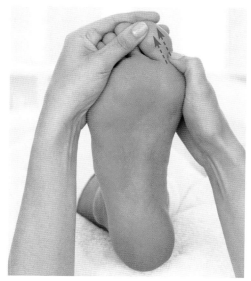

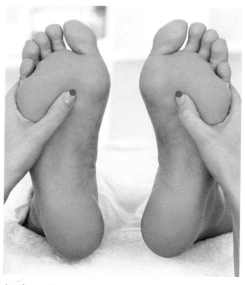

Sinus congestion Reflex points for the sinuses are located on the backs and sides of all five toes. The practitioner starts on the right foot, working each toe in turn, using fingers or thumbs to 'caterpillar walk', or squeeze, from the base upwards. Stimulation of these points is said to relieve sinus congestion and pain.

Anxiety Pressing on the solar-plexus reflex points may have a calming effect on the whole body and help ease anxiety. The practitioner uses the thumbs to press on solar-plexus reflex points on both feet. The client breathes in as pressure is applied and breathes out as pressure is released. This is repeated three times.

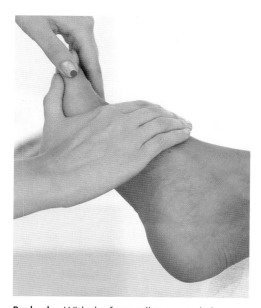

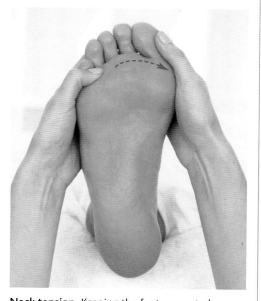

Backache With the foot well supported, the practitioner uses a thumb or finger to 'walk' along reflex points on the inside edge of the foot, starting at the big toe and following the natural curve of the foot, and back again. This is repeated on the left foot. Working these points is supposed to ease backache.

Neck tension Keeping the foot supported, the practitioner uses thumb- or finger-walking techniques to stimulate the reflex points that form a line along the base of the first three toes on the sole and top of the foot. The right foot is worked first, followed by the left. This is thought to ease tension in the muscles of the neck.

Hand reflex points

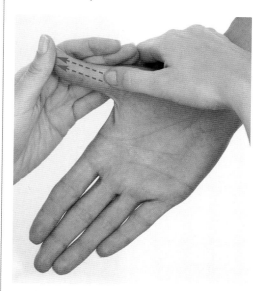

Headaches Use your thumb or finger to apply pressure with a 'walking' or pressing movement on the sides and top of the other thumb. Now press firmly on the tip of the thumb and each finger in turn. Repeat on the other hand.

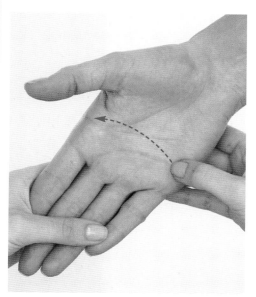

Constipation With 'walking', gliding or pressing movements, massage across the whole palm of each hand, working from the outer to the inner edge. Cover the whole of each palm with these movements.

CHIROPRACTIC AND OSTEOPATHY

If you are interested in **Chiropractic and Osteopathy**, you may also like to read about:

- Pilates, pages 110–111
- Yoga, pages 106–109
- Swedish Massage, pages 120–121
- Indian Head Massage, page 123
- Craniosacral Therapy, page 136
- Feldenkrais Method, page 137
- Bowen Technique, page 138
- Alexander Technique, pages 118–119
- Rolfing, page 139

Chiropractic and osteopathy both **developed** out of 19th-century North America's pluralist medical system, in which conventional medicine was only one approach among a range of 'alternative' healthcare options. Chiropractic and osteopathy are now well-established holistic approaches to diagnosis and treatment, whose practitioners focus on the link between the **structure and function** of the body and use a variety of **manual techniques** to encourage the body's healing response. Many different approaches and technique variations have evolved, and there are some specific **branches** of both methods.

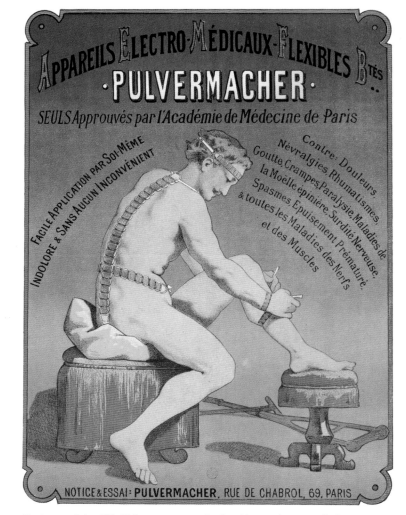

Electro-medicine *This 19th-century poster is advertising an electro-medical massage, which attracted a great deal of popular interest in the USA at the time.*

Origins and development

To understand the development of chiropractic and osteopathy, they need to be viewed in the context of 19th-century medicine and the industrialization of the USA. Colonial North America in the 17th and 18th centuries was even more riven with infectious disease than Europe, and yet medicine was even more basic. By the late 1700s new cities had built the first hospitals, but it was not until 1765 that the colonists founded a medical school in Philadelphia, Pennsylvania, at which time there were only a few dozen practitioners with an official medical degree. So, conventional medicine had only a precarious foothold in North America throughout the 19th century. Other approaches to healthcare competed for dominance, particularly on the frontiers furthest from the East Coast establishment. Physiomedicalists, Thompsonians, Eclectics, Grahamists, Hygienists and Hydropaths all claimed, in slightly different ways, that natural healing and lifestyle change were essential for good health.

As late as 1900, 15 per cent of the doctors in the USA practised homeopathy – treatment of disease using substances that cause similar effects to the symptoms that the disease would produce in a healthy person – rather than allopathy – the conventional treatment of disease with substances that have the opposite effects to the symptoms – and fewer than 10 per cent of American doctors were American Medical Association members. However, state licensing began to favour 'scientific medicine' and gradually the AMA's huge influence put an end to the country's pluralistic medical system.

During the 19th-century American industrial revolution, popular interest in electricity and magnetic fields – natural, artificial and even psychic – spread like wildfire and the popularity of electro-medicine and magnetic healing in all their diverse forms reached their height in newly industrializing Midwestern America.

Andrew Still (1828–1917), the founder of osteopathy, was practising regular medicine in Kansas at that time. He probably learned doctoring and

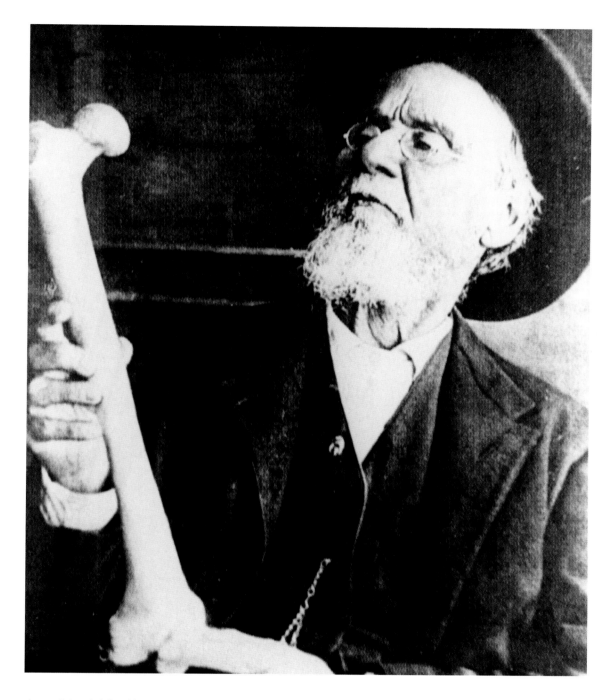

Andrew Still *The founder of osteopathy, Andrew Still, practised medicine from 1849 and served as a surgeon during the American Civil War. In 1892 he founded a medical school, and in 1894 a medical osteopathy journal.*

the traditional skills of bone-setting from his own father, who was a preacher and travelling lay healer. Impressed with magnetic healing and favouring natural hygiene approaches, Still rejected the use of allopathic medicine's alcohol-based drugs and began developing his ideas about the circulation of magnetic vital forces in the blood. His observations led him to link structure and function, and to apply massage and manipulation to realign the body's structure. In 1874 he unveiled his system of spinal manipulation, naming it osteopathy from the Greek words for 'bone' and 'suffering'. In 1892 Still opened the American School of Osteopathy in Kirksville, Missouri.

The founder of chiropractic, Daniel David Palmer (1845–1913), cited nerves rather than blood as the conductors of this magnetic vital force, which he called the 'Innate'. Palmer declared, perhaps even more than Still, his debt to the ideas and practice of magnetic healing and the laying-on of hands. Working in the magnetic healing tradition, Palmer saw the body as an integrated unit, and sought to develop precise spinal manipulations that would adjust the distorted nervous system and so release the healing flow of vital fluids. He named the treatment chiropractic from the Greek words for 'healing done with the hands', and in 1897 opened what became the Palmer College of Chiropractic in Davenport, Iowa.

Chiropractic and osteopathy are now practised worldwide. Chiropractors and osteopaths have been State Registered in the UK since 1994, and their value in treating musculoskeletal pain is widely accepted by the medical

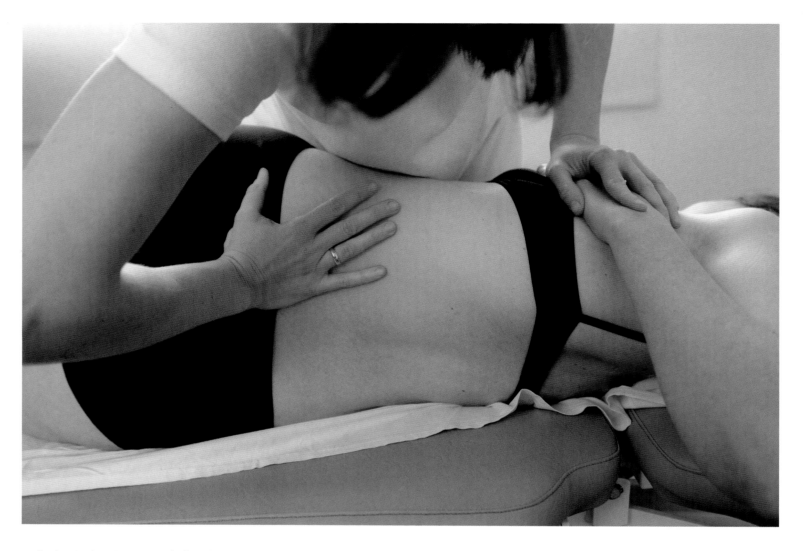

profession. In the USA osteopaths have been licensed as medical doctors since 1972. Both professions have international standards of education.

Structure and function

Still and Palmer both thought of the body as an intricate machine that could only function well and stay free of disease when the structure was properly 'adjusted'; the vital magnetic fluids depended on well-aligned structures. In the origins of chiropractic and osteopathy, we can see that the theory of flow (of fluids, energy or information) is central.

Chiropractic and osteopathy are both based on the principle that the body works as an integrated whole and that the musculoskeletal system of bones, joints, muscles, ligaments and connective tissue supports and protects the organs of the body. Both systems consider that mechanical faults and tensions can affect organs and systems anywhere in the body – leading, in varying degrees, to pain, altered breathing patterns, impaired nerve function and disorders of the circulatory, lymphatic and digestive systems. Originally, chiropractors and osteopaths treated every kind of health problem, but nowadays they specialize mainly in the diagnosis, treatment and overall management of problems with the joints, ligaments, tendons and nerves.

Osteopathic treatment *Practitioners use precise techniques to detect tension and improve the alignment of the spinal column.*

Practitioners say that injuries, anxiety, physical demands, ageing and postural strains can all disturb the musculoskeletal system, so contributing to long- or short-term health problems. Osteopaths believe that once the body's mechanical tension patterns are understood, then the problem can often be resolved. Back pain, for example, is commonly caused by tension around spinal joints, due to poor posture, joint dysfunction or an old muscle injury. Equally, recurring headaches may stem from stiffness and muscular tension in the neck.

Manual techniques and treatments

On a first visit, chiropractors and osteopaths will take a full medical history, including details of any accidents and injuries, and will assess the cause of the specific problem before discussing treatment options with the client. Assessment includes observation of movements while sitting and standing followed by use of a sensitive palpation for changes in tension and tenderness, temperature and flexibility. In these ways practitioners identify areas of weakness, tightness, stiffness or excess strain throughout the musculoskeletal system.

The approach is holistic and includes lifestyle advice, relaxation techniques and preventative exercises to practise at home to keep the problem at bay. If a practitioner thinks specialist investigation or treatment is needed, he or she will refer patients back to their doctor.

Practitioners use a range of manual techniques to relax muscles and joints, improve mobility and stimulate circulation. These may include stretching of soft tissues, massage and rhythmic movements. Gentle muscle energy techniques tend to be used on children and older people. In some instances, treatment may also include manipulation using short, quick movements called high-velocity thrusts to the spinal column and pelvic area. Although this is painless, it can result in an audible crack, which is thought to result from sudden pressure changes within the joints. Deep soft-tissue techniques working on sensitive tense muscles can be uncomfortable at first, but actual manipulative treatments should be gentle and painless, using a minimum of force on the joints. Stiffness and mild discomfort at the site of manipulation are common for a day or two following treatment, during which strenuous activity is not recommended.

Although chiropractors and osteopaths are best known for treating back and neck pain and stiffness, many people come for treatment of a wide range of other conditions, including arthritis, asthma and digestive disorders, migraine and painful periods. Treatment should be supported by advice on self-help measures, diet, lifestyle and exercise to help manage the condition and maintain general health and wellbeing.

Branches of chiropractic and osteopathy

A popular branch of chiropractic is McTimoney chiropractic, which was developed by British engineer and chiropractor John McTimoney (1914–1980) during the 1950s. Treatment uses very light force adjustment, not only of the spine, but also of the sacrum, pelvis and cranium (skull).

Many osteopaths practise cranial osteopathy. This treatment system, which involves very gentle manipulative techniques on the cranium, appears to be particularly effective for babies and young children. It is thought that childbirth, an accident or long-term tension can cause compression of the bones of the skull. This is said to impede the flow of fluid around the spinal cord, the spine and within the brain. Practitioners' hands gently influence the tension patterns round the cranium to help 'normalize the flow of cerebrospinal fluid'. Cranial osteopathy has been recommended to help ease conditions such as headaches and migraine, whiplash injury, glue ear, chronic sinusitis and recurrent infections in the head and neck area.

PRECAUTIONS

✖ Inform your practitioner before treatment if you are pregnant, have bone disease or disorders, or any serious medical condition, as it may be best to avoid certain techniques.

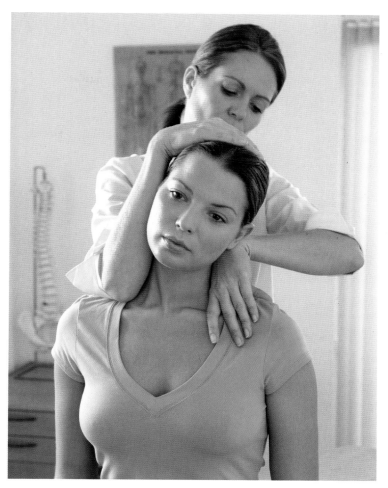

Chiropractic treatment *By using controlled techniques known as 'adjustments' to individual vertabrae, practitioners aim to encourage the body's own healing responses.*

RESEARCH AND EVIDENCE

Chiropractic There is a substantial body of evidence to support the use of chiropractic for lower back pain. Research is currently being conducted to investigate its effectiveness for other conditions, including neck pain, migraine and tension headaches, whiplash and repetitive strain injury. In the UK, a Medical Research Council clinical trial, reported in the *British Medical Journal* in 1990, found that chiropractic was more effective for back pain than hospital outpatient treatment. A follow-up trial in 1995 confirmed these results and showed that patients were generally more satisfied than those having conventional care. The Royal College of General Practitioners guidelines recommend manipulation for acute and sub-acute back pain.

Osteopathy Published in the international journal *Family Practice*, a 2003 trial showed some evidence that osteopathy may be helpful for low back pain and improvement in mobility. The UK's Royal College of General Practitioners recommends manipulation for acute and sub-acute back pain. There have been fewer studies of osteopathy techniques for neck pain, but there is some evidence that it may also provide some short-term benefits. The Natural Standard (see page 108) suggests that there is early evidence to show that osteopathy may also be beneficial for asthma, chronic obstructive pulmonary disease and emphysema, depression and menstrual pain.

CRANIOSACRAL THERAPY

If you are interested in **Craniosacral Therapy**, you may also like to read about:
- Chiropractic and Osteopathy, pages 132–135
- Swedish Massage, pages 120–121
- Thai Massage, page 122
- Indian Head Massage, page 123

This subtle touch therapy focuses on the **craniosacral system** to encourage the body's own natural self-healing processess to restore health. It involves the use of gentle 'listening' contact on the head and lower back in order to offer **diagnosis and treatment** for a range of acute and chronic conditions.

Craniosacral system

The focus of craniosacral therapy is on the membranes and cerebrospinal fluid that surround and protect the brain and spinal cord. The craniosacral system extends from the bones of the skull, face and mouth, down the spine to the sacrum and tailbone area. During the early 1900s, American osteopath Dr William Sutherland (1873–1954) found he could feel movements of the

bones in the skull and detect distinct, regular rhythms, which he believed were due to the pulsing of the cerebrospinal fluid (CSF). He thought that by influencing the flow of fluid he could help treat problems such as sinusitis and recurring infections in the head area. Another osteopath, Dr John Upledger, suggested in the 1970s that any imbalances in the flow of cerebrospinal fluid could reflect physical, mental, emotional or psychological tensions and injuries, not only in the local area, but anywhere in the body.

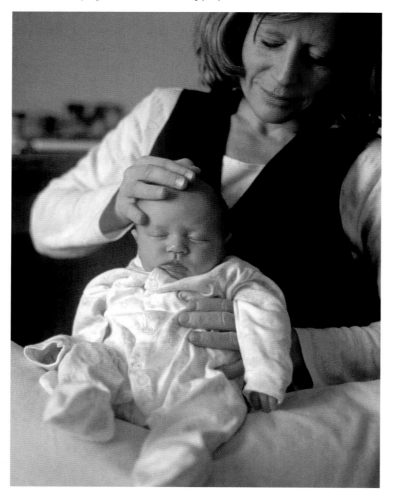

Craniosacral therapy *Treatment is so gentle and relaxing that it is suitable for young babies, children, pregnant women and elderly people.*

Diagnosis and treatment

Many people find that the light, almost imperceptible touch used brings about a deep sense of physical and mental relaxation. Treatment takes place fully clothed, usually lying on a therapy couch, but can be adapted for any relaxing position. The practitioner carefully rests hands on head (although palpation can take place anywhere on the body) in order to 'listen' to the rhythmic movement and sense any congestion or restrictions within the whole body, before using gentle touch to facilitate appropriate changes in these areas.

Therapists believe that by using the most subtle pressure they can restore even, rhythmic pulsing to the CSF. Some even suggest that a body may self-correct simply by the therapist being aware of the patient's craniosacral rhythm. Practitioners claim to help treat physical aches and pains, chronic disease and emotional disturbances, as well as improving wellbeing, health and vitality.

Before treatment, the practitioner takes a full medical history, including details of any medication. Treatment may last up to an hour. Children are said to respond very quickly, whereas an adult with a deep-seated condition may take longer. Generally, an initial four to six sessions are recommended.

PRECAUTIONS

✖ See page 121.

RESEARCH AND EVIDENCE

There is a growing body of anecdotal evidence to support the effectiveness of craniosacral therapy, but there have been no significant clinical trials to date, and scientific attempts to detect pulsaton in the CSF have been unsuccessful.

FELDENKRAIS METHOD

Named after its originator, Israeli **Moshe Feldenkrais**, this educational method offers a practical way of focusing on learning and movement to encourage wellbeing and achieve **health benefits**. There are two formats: **'awareness through movement'** (group classes) and **'functional integration'** (individual sessions).

If you are interested in the **Feldenkrais Method**, you may also like to read about:
- Alexander Technique, pages 118–119
- Pilates, pages 110–111
- Chiropractic and Osteopathy, pages 132–135
- Rolfing, page 139
- Bates Method, page 141

Moshe Feldenkrais

The Feldenkrais method was devised by Russian-born engineer and physicist Moshe Feldenkrais (1904–1984) as a way of healing a recurring knee injury. He drew on several sources, including martial arts, biomechanics and psychology, to develop a method aimed at relearning how to move with the maximum of efficiency using minimum effort. The method shares the objectives of, and similar benefits to, the Alexander technique, but uses a different approach. Originally taught in Israel and the USA, Feldenkrais group classes and individual sessions are now available worldwide.

Awareness through movement

During group classes the teacher gives verbal instructions to guide students through a series of gentle movements, with the focus on helping them to develop a heightened awareness of themselves and how they move. The intention is to reprogramme the nervous system, making it possible to identify habitual postures and movements and replace them with new patterns of behaviour.

Functional integration

One-to-one lessons are most useful for people with specific problems, including cerebral palsy and multiple sclerosis. The teacher uses touch and gentle manipulation to guide the student through specific movements and to encourage each individual to achieve their full potential.

PRECAUTIONS
✖ See page 108.

RESEARCH AND EVIDENCE

Small-scale studies and anecdotal evidence suggest that the Feldenkrais method may have a useful part to play in the treatment of musculoskeletal pain, anxiety and physical rehabilitation. However, the Natural Standard (see page 108) considers that further research is necessary. In the *American Journal of Pain Management*, a 1999 study into the effects of the Feldenkrais method on chronic pain showed positive results immediately after the course of treatment and in a one-year follow-up.

Health benefits

The Feldenkrais method is suitable for all ages. After the first session, most people are said to experience an immediate feeling of general wellbeing and greater freedom of movement. Longer-term benefits claimed include relief of tension and muscular pain, increased lung function, enhanced relaxation and greater ease in accomplishing everyday activities.

Feldenkrais treatment *During a Feldenkrais group class, students lie on the floor and are guided through many different sequences of movements.*

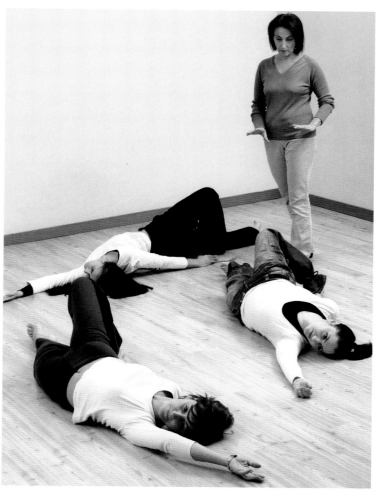

BOWEN TECHNIQUE

This gentle hands-on therapy, pioneered by **Tom Bowen** in Australia during the 1950s, is a remedial and holistic form of bodywork. The restorative **treatment**, which comprises sets of rolling-type moves interspaced with short breaks, has spread worldwide and is suitable for all ages. Claiming a range of **health benefits**, since the early 1980s it has flourished in many countries and has been taught in the UK since 1994.

If you are interested in the **Bowen Technique**, you may also like to read about:
- **Chiropractic and Osteopathy**, pages 132–135
- **Craniosacral Therapy**, page 136
- **Swedish Massage**, pages 120–121
- **Reflexology**, pages 128–131

Tom Bowen

A largely self-taught therapist, Tom Bowen (1916–1982) held a strong belief in the body's own power of healing. His special technique proved so popular that he set up his own clinic locally in Australia and is reputed to have helped thousands of people overcome or cope better with a wide range of injury, illness and disability. Bowen allowed six men to come on different days to watch him at work. One of these, an Australian osteopath called Oswald Rentsch, wrote down his observations on Bowen's methods and was the first to teach it after his death.

Treatment

The therapist uses thumbs and fingers on precise points of the body to perform Bowen's unique sets of rolling-type moves, which aim to stimulate the muscles, soft tissue and energy flow within the body. He or she may leave the treatment room for short periods to allow the client to rest while the body 'resets imbalances'. The treatment is gentle, subtle and relaxing. There is no manipulation and no force involved.

A treatment takes around 45 minutes and can mostly be performed through light clothing. It can be adapted to suit any situation, including beds and wheelchairs. It is claimed that four to five treatments at weekly intervals often achieve lasting relief.

PRECAUTIONS

✖ See page 108.

RESEARCH AND EVIDENCE

Despite anecdotal evidence there is limited scientific research into the efficacy of the Bowen technique. In *Complementary Therapies in Medicine*, a small 2002 study showed that it could help improve mobility and reduce pain in people with frozen shoulder. The Natural Standard (see page 108) reports that early evidence suggests that it may also offer benefits in the treatment of psychiatric disorders and job-related stress.

Health benefits

Practitioners claim that a wide range of complaints can be helped by Bowen technique, including back and neck pain, knee problems, repetitive strain injury, frozen shoulder, high blood pressure, headaches and infant colic. Some athletes and their physiotherapists recommend regular treatments to enhance performance, reduce the incidence of injury and speed up recovery. Other people use it for stress management and health maintenance.

Bowen technique treatment *This gentle therapy is usually carried out on a soft, low table with the client wearing loose clothing.*

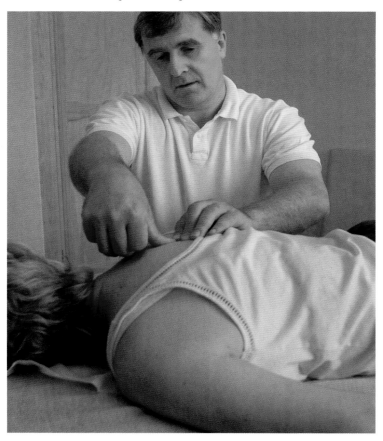

ROLFING

If you are interested in **Rolfing**, you may also like to read about:
- **Thai Massage**, page 122
- **Shiatsu**, pages 124–125
- **Chiropractic and Osteopathy**, pages 132–135
- **Craniosacral Therapy**, page 136
- **Feldenkrais Method**, page 137
- **Bowen Technique**, page 138
- **Alexander Technique**, pages 118–119

Named after American biochemist Dr Ida Rolf, who first developed the method in the 1950s, rolfing focuses on the body's **network of connective tissue** and involves a form of **deep-tissue massage and movement education** delivered over ten structured sessions. The aim is to balance tensions in the body and enable it to work more easily with gravity. Benefits are said to include enhanced physical and emotional wellbeing.

Network of connective tissue

Also known as structural integration, rolfing is concerned with the myofascial system – the muscles and fascia (the fine layer of tissue that runs between the muscles) – which holds the body together and initiates movement. Dr Ida Rolf (1896–1979) believed that emotional and physical stress affects the flexibility and health of connective tissue, leading to restricted movement of joints and muscles. Over time, limited movement in everyday activities sets up habitual patterns of bracing and tension, which have a detrimental impact on physical and emotional health.

Deep-tissue massage and movement education

Rolfers set out to remould and realign the body's myofascial system so that it can work *with* gravity, rather than against it, and to release the restrictions that limit movement. Rolfing comprises a series of ten sessions, each lasting around 70–90 minutes. Practitioners work with individual clients to develop body awareness and relaxed breathing. The treatments, usually around one to two weeks apart, are progressive, each one building on the achievements of the previous sessions. Each session involves a particular theme and area of the body and clients may be encouraged to carry out specific exercises at home. At the end of the ten sessions, clients are offered strategies for maintenance and ongoing improvement.

RESEARCH AND EVIDENCE

Rolfing has been suggested for many health problems, but there is limited scientific evidence as yet. The Natural Standard (see page 108) reports that small-scale studies indicate the need for further research into certain conditions, including anxiety, chronic fatigue syndrome and low back pain.

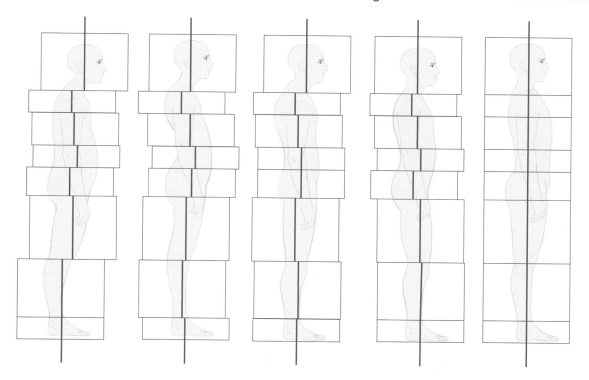

PRECAUTIONS
✖ See page 108.

Realignment *Clients and practitioners work together to free tensions and realign the body, so that it can work more efficiently with the downward force of gravity.*

IRIDOLOGY

If you are interested in **Iridology**, you may also like to read about:
- Bates Method, page 141
- Herbalism, pages 152–153
- Homeopathy, pages 160–161

Iridology is the **study of the iris** of the eye which practitioners claim may indicate overall physical and mental health. Detailed **examination of the eye** searches for signs of weaknesses in the efficiency of body systems and organs and the likely causes of illness. Practitioners usually advise natural therapies based on their **diagnosis**.

Study of the iris

The development of iridology in the 1880s is generally attributed to Hungarian doctor Ignatz von Peczely (1826–1911), who noticed a black line on the iris of an owl that had just broken its leg, which faded as he nursed it back to health. He recorded changes in patients' irises and drew up the first iridology chart. Many clinicians have since contributed to the development of the very detailed charts that iridologists work with today.

Iridologists work on the theory that because the iris contains thousands of exposed nerve endings, every part of the body is connected to the eye through the central nervous system. Digital technology and computer software are used to analyse irises and record and store data. Enlarged images of the iris are evaluated in the belief that they indicate the strengths and weaknesses of the body's organs and systems, levels of toxicity and even personality traits. This information is then used to suggest ways of preventing illness when there are only very early signs of it, before symptoms manifest.

Examination of the eye

Practitioners use a variety of equipment, from a torch and magnifying glass to a computer-imaging system, to assess the colour, texture and markings within each iris in a painless, non-invasive way. Iridologists estimate that there are around 200 differentiating signs on an average iris, making it unique to the individual. The outer rim, for example, is said to correspond to the skin and lymph zones. Yellow or orange marks on top of the base colour of blue, grey or brown are said to indicate metabolic disturbances. Sessions usually take around an hour.

Diagnosis

Iridology is a form of diagnosis rather than a treatment, so most practitioners are qualified in another therapy, often homeopathy, nutritional therapy or naturopathy. Following consultation and evaluation, the iridology findings inform recommendations that aim to enable the client to improve their overall health and wellbeing.

RESEARCH AND EVIDENCE

Despite positive anecdotal reports, scientific trials indicate that iridology has failed to detect disease even when it is present. These include a study published in the *British Medical Journal* in 1988, which concluded that iridology was not a useful diagnostic aid for suspected gallstones. There is a need for further trials to substantiate the effectiveness of this diagnostic approach.

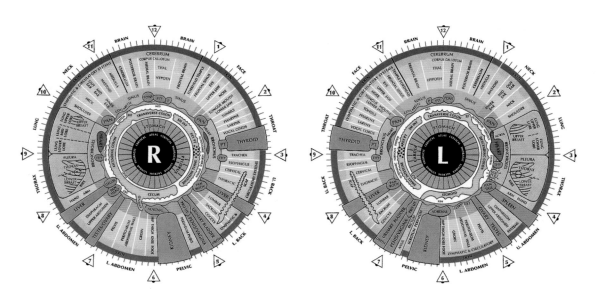

Iridology charts *The right iris is said to represent the right side of the body, and the left iris is said to represent the left side of the body.*

BATES METHOD

If you are interested in the **Bates Method**, you may also like to read about:

● **Iridology**, page 140
● **Breathwork**, page 81
● **Meditation**, pages 78–79

Developed from the **research findings** of American medical ophthalmologist Dr William Bates, the Bates method aims to improve eyesight naturally without the use of lenses or surgery. An integral part of the method is incorporating **basic techniques** into daily life to re-educate the eyes and aid vision problems.

Research findings

Dr William Bates (1860–1931) began developing his theories after realizing that his patients' vision was extremely variable from day to day. Through his research he found that: normal sight is inherently variable; defective sight can get better as well as worse; poor sight and eye disease seemed to be related; and that eyesight may be an important indicator of mental, emotional and physical health. He concluded that most people predominantly see the world around them with the mind and only partially with their eyes.

Basic techniques

The emphasis of the Bates method is on improving the use of the eyes in everyday life, and learning to use the eyes and the mind in a relaxed and natural way. This is achieved through practising techniques based on three principles: relaxation, awareness and movement. These techniques are suitable for anyone, including children and older people, who wishes to maintain or improve their sight.

Practitioners suggest that in mature years people's vision problems, including eye conditions, are often due to acquired habits of straining the eyes, and can therefore be both prevented and reversed in many cases. The method claims other benefits, such as increased energy, better balance, improved concentration and faster reading.

Palming

Sit in an upright chair. Cover your closed eyes with the cupped palms of your hands, without pressing on the sockets. Allow your eyes to rest in the warmth and darkness. Turn your attention to a visualization or relaxing music for ten minutes. Do this two to three times a day for relaxed vision.

Swinging

With your eyes focused on a point in the distance, sway your body to the left while blinking your left eye, then to the right, blinking your right eye. Do this 100 times. This helps to lubricate the eyes and reduce eye strain.

Splashing

Every morning splash warm and then cold water over the eyes 20 times to stimulate circulation to the eyes; repeat in the evening using cold water first.

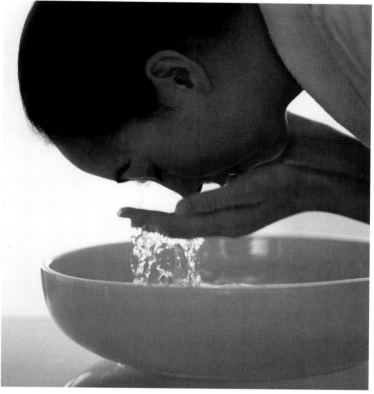

Splashing *Practitioners believe that, as with any educational process, those who learn to integrate the basic skills into their daily life will gain the most benefit.*

PRECAUTIONS

✖ Consult your doctor and a trained Bates method teacher before doing the above exercises if you have any eye disorder, including glaucoma or cataracts.

RESEARCH AND EVIDENCE

The Bates method relies on anecdotal evidence and small studies to support its claims. There have been no significant clinical research trials as yet.

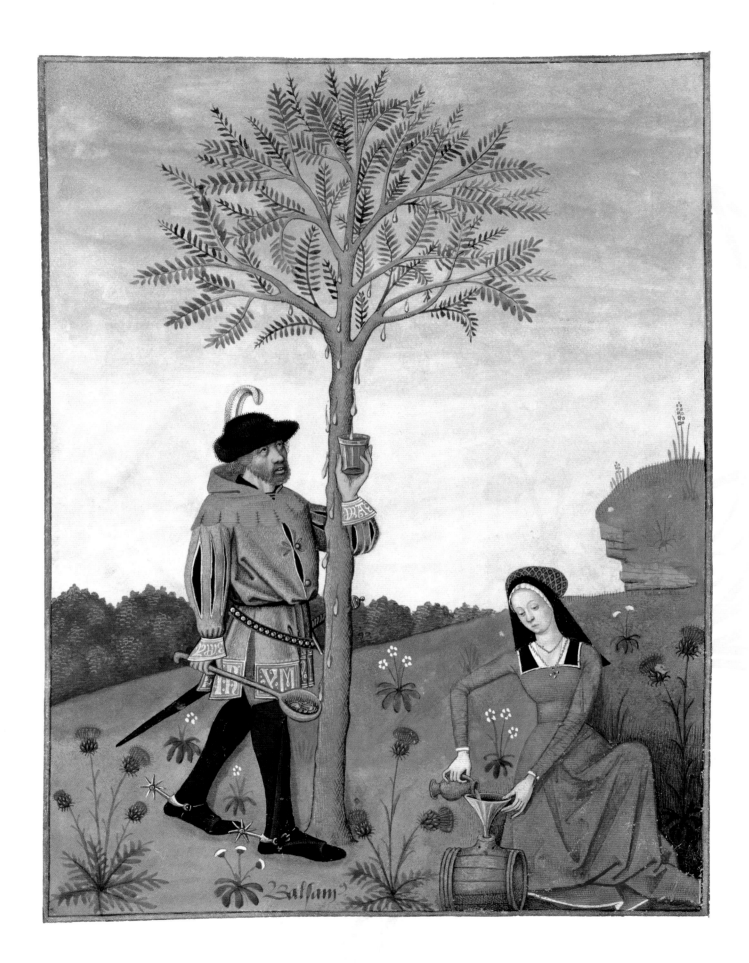

Balsam

NUTRITIONAL AND HERBAL APPROACHES

Today the fact that fitness and health depend greatly on a healthy diet seems obvious, yet this view has been contested in the past, and it runs counter to the idea that health depends on doctors and medical science. Nutritional therapies use vitamins, minerals and other non-herbal nutritional supplements to address various health conditions. When appropriate, dietary changes may be prescribed, such as low-sugar or low-salt diets, diets that eliminate certain foods or medically supervised fasting. Naturopaths recommend lifestyle changes in addition to dietary and herbal supplements.

The nutrition–health connection

Public-health reformers in 19th-century England realized that poor diet undermined health, but it was not until the late 20th century that the link between diet and chronic disease was fully accepted. The late 19th-century Nature Cure movement in Europe and the Dietary Reform movement in the USA proclaimed a radical rejection of synthetic drugs and doctors' dominion over healthcare.

Despite these assertions by healthcare radicals for more than 200 years, those who saw connections between nutrition and disease were ridiculed until relatively recently. Most doctors derided American health expert Victor Lindlahr's book *You Are What You Eat – How to Win and Keep Health with Diet* when it came out in 1940, and yet nowadays the phrase he launched, which the 1960s' counter-culture took as the slogan for the wholefood-organic food movement, has become a cliché. Doctors now know for certain that better diet and physical activity can help prevent most long-term diseases, including obesity, diabetes, cardiovascular disease, many kinds of cancer, dental disease and osteoporosis. Lindlahr and his predecessors may have been ahead of their time, but their theories have stood the test of time to become widely accepted today.

Herbalism *This 15th-century illustration from the* Book of Simple Medicines *by Mattheaus Platearius shows sap being drawn from a tree for its recognized medical and health benefits.*

Nutritional therapy and naturopathy

Nutritional therapy evolved from naturopathy, a holistic approach to health that includes food medicine and herbalism. The basic idea behind nutritional therapy is that eating healthy, high-quality food is an effective way of creating health and wellbeing: the wrong foods harm us, and the right ones help to heal us. Nutritional therapists also take a great interest in the body's ability to digest and deal with the toxic products of digestion.

Nutritional therapy attempts to combine findings from biochemical and nutritional research with the practical principles of drug-free medicine. It aims to optimize resilience by correcting significant vitamin or mineral deficiencies, by improving digestive function (because eating well is one thing, but being able to absorb nutrients from food effectively is another) and by eliminating 'toxins'.

Nutritional therapists and naturopaths assess a person's nutritional status and level of functioning, recognizing that they are shaped by inherited and other influences, including diet, lifestyle and environment. Positive vitality, so they believe, requires good digestion, absorption and detoxification. Consequently, nutritional interventions include dietary change, food supplements, herbal nutrients and 'functional foods' such as probiotic yogurt. Dietary supplements may be advised as a complement rather than a substitute for a healthy, well-balanced diet. Assessments sometimes involve blood, urine and stool tests. In addition, some nutritional therapists and naturopaths use a broad range of treatments to address non-nutritional risk factors. These might include massage and manipulative therapy, exercise, hydrotherapy, acupuncture, detoxification and stress-management methods such as meditation and imagery and relaxation techniques. Personal spiritual development may also be encouraged as an important part of an overall health programme. Because naturopaths manage to combine so many therapies successfully, it can be difficult to single out specific illnesses for which naturopathy is recommended. Naturopaths treat a range of both acute and chronic conditions, from arthritis to asthma and from congestive heart failure to infertility. Above all the naturopath aims to treat the whole person, rather than just treating a disease or its symptoms, striving to maintain a balanced state of good health in their patients.

NATUROPATHY

Naturopathic medicine first developed in the early 19th century in Europe, evolving from the **Nature Cure movement**. Its **key principles** emphasized the body's own ability to heal and a holistic approach to wellbeing, and the **practice of naturopathy** today focuses on a range of therapies, including **nutrition**, physical therapy and psychotherapy.

If you are interested in **Naturopathy**, you may also like to read about:
- **Healing Water**, pages 164–165
- **Herbalism**, pages 152–153
- **Fasting and Detoxing**, pages 150–151
- **Macrobiotics**, page 149
- **Food Combining**, page 148

The Nature Cure movement

Pioneers of this movement included Vincent Priessnitz (1799–1851), born in what is now the Czech Republic, who developed a reputation as a healer after treating himself and his neighbours with water therapy. His fame grew to the point where he established his own sanatorium and was invited, in 1826, to Vienna to heal the Emperor's brother, Anton Victor. Johann Schroth (1798–1856) was a native of the same region as Priessnitz and founded a health spa at Bad Lindewiese. In addition to hydrotherapy, Schroth employed clinical nutrition and developed the Schrothkur regime, which featured cold wraps, the use of steam and an austere dietary regime still observed by many people throughout central Europe. Sebastian Kneipp (1821–1897), a Bavarian priest,

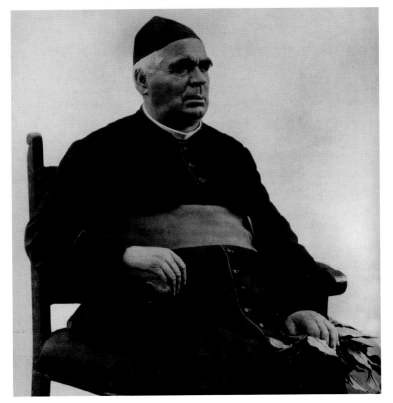

Sebastian Kneipp *Bavarian priest Sebastian Kneipp advocated a naturopathic approach to healthcare based on five key principles.*

is considered one of the founding fathers of naturopathy. He advocated five key approaches to health: hydrotherapy, herbalism, exercise, nutrition and spirituality. Kneipp lived in the spa town of Bad Wörishofen in Bavaria for over 40 years, and his water cure is still available there today.

Emigration from Germany to North America led to the spread of naturopathy's central principles to the New World. American Bernarr MacFadden (1868–1955) was a strong advocate of the relationship of physical exercise to health and also promoted fasting as a path to well-being. Dr Henry Lindlahr (1862–1924) brought all the various aspects of naturopathy together, founding the Lindlahr Sanatorium in Chicago and writing the seminal works *Nature Cure* (1913) and *Philosophy of Natural Therapeutics* (1922). Lindlahr trained in Europe before opening his first practice in Chicago in 1902. His 'Nature Cure' included a vegetarian diet, sun baths, air baths, exercise, hydrotherapy and manipulation. His son, Victor Landlahr, was the author of the highly influential book *You Are What You Eat*, published in 1940.

Key principles of naturopathy

Naturopathy typifies some key principles that are rooted in a timeless understanding of human needs and wellbeing, and which have become characteristic of 21st-century integrated healthcare, as follows:
- First, do no harm; opt for effective healthcare with the least risk.
- Promote the self-healing power of nature.
- Remove the causes of illness, rather than merely eliminating symptoms.
- Educate and encourage self-care.
- Whole-person care of the individual should take into account all aspects of mental, physical and spiritual wellbeing.
- Individual wellbeing also depends on healthy relationships, communities and biosphere.

The practice of naturopathy today

The core aspects of naturopathy as it is practised today include:
- Clinical dietetics, applied nutrition and detoxification techniques
- Hydrotherapy
- Physical therapy, such as osteopathy and chiropractic
- Psychotherapy.

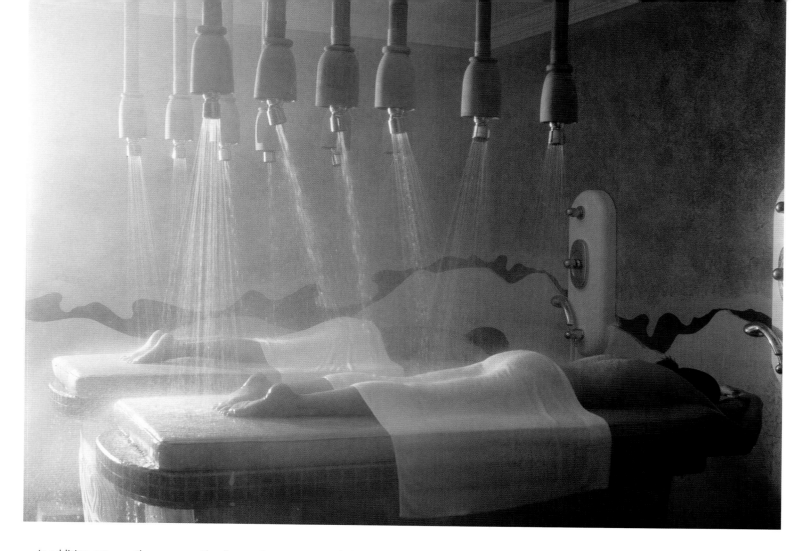

In addition naturopaths may use other forms of treatment in which they have appropriate qualifications, such as medical herbalism and acupuncture. A naturopath would begin by taking the patient's medical case history and assessing their lifestyle. He or she may perform a clinical examination of the patient, which could include iridology (examination of the patient's pupil) and tongue or nail diagnosis, and may also use diagnostic tests such as blood tests and imaging. Naturopaths believe that there can be a wide range of factors responsible for ill health. A course of treatment, therefore, would generally involve attention to many different aspects of the patient's lifestyle, including emotional health and the environment in which the patient lives.

Naturopathic nutrition

Nutrition is an integral part of naturopathy. Practitioners recommend the use of whole and organic foods and also recognize the benefits of oriental medicine and its approach to food. Naturopaths are familiar with a wide range of dietary approaches, including vegan, vegetarian, raw foods, macrobiotic and food combining, and may recommend specific diets to address a patient's health issues. In particular they study nutritional approaches to the treatment of a wide range of ailments, such as musculoskeletal disorders, cardiovascular disease, respiratory disorders and skin problems.

Hydrotherapy *The massaging effects of water jets on the body can be used to relax muscles, release tension and stimulate the circulation.*

PH balance

Naturopathic nutrition also focuses on acid–alkali balance. Practitioners believe that an excess of acid-forming foods such as high-fat foods, red meats, sugary and processed foods can cause fatigue and poor health. Naturopaths also say that many healthy foods such as vegetables, legumes, oily fish and whole grains, though alkaline by nature, may become acid-forming as a result of the manufacturing processes. Their general rule is to balance each meal with 75 per cent alkaline to 25 per cent acidic foods.

RESEARCH AND EVIDENCE

Most claims for the effectiveness of naturopathy are based on individual cases, medical records and summaries of practitioners' clinical experiences. Virtually no controlled studies on naturopathy have been published.

PRECAUTIONS

✖ See pages 146, 148, 149, 151, 152 and 164.

VITAMINS AND MINERALS

If you are interested in **Vitamins and Minerals**, you may also like to read about:
- Food Combining, page 148
- Fasting and Detoxing, pages 150–151

A surprisingly recent **discovery**, vitamins are organic substances that cannot be produced or synthesized by the body in sufficient amounts and must be obtained from the diet. We also need trace minerals, such as magnesium, because without them crucial enzyme systems in the body are disabled. A balanced **daily intake** of nutrients is essential.

The discovery of vitamins

Polish biochemist Casimir Funk (1884–1967) first conceived of 'vital amines' in 1912 when he identified the first B vitamin, but their existence had long been suspected; in the mid-1700s British naval doctor James Lind (1716–1794) realized he could prevent scurvy – a common disease among sailors – by giving limes to his crew. However, it was not until 1932 that Hungarian physiologist Albert Szent-Györgyi (1893–1986) unravelled the chemical structure of vitamin C.

Daily intake

The Recommended Daily Allowance (RDA) is the average minimum amount of a nutrient needed to stave off a deficiency disease, though nutritional therapists claim that people often require rather more because of the nutrient-depleting pollution, tobacco and stress of modern-day life. The best way to ingest vitamins and minerals and ensure good health is a diet rich in whole grains, fresh fruits and vegetables, legumes, nuts, seeds and oily fish, and low in nutrient-poor fast foods, refined foods, sugar, salt, processed meats and other foods containing additives, preservatives and toxins. However, the nutritional content of fresh food may be depleted, through age or damage or through modern agricultural and production processes. Although not an adequate substitute for a balanced, varied diet, a quality multivitamin and mineral supplement may help guard against vitamin and mineral deficiencies.

YEAR OF DISCOVERY	VITAMIN	SOURCE
1909	Vitamin A (retinol)	Cod-liver oil
1912	Vitamin B1 (thiamine)	Rice bran
1912	Vitamin C (ascorbic acid)	Lemons
1918	Vitamin D (calciferol)	Cod-liver oil
1920	Vitamin B2 (riboflavin)	Eggs
1922	Vitamin E (tocopherol)	Wheat-germ oil
1926	Vitamin B12 (cyanocobalamin)	Liver
1929	Vitamin K (phylloquinone)	Alfalfa
1931	Vitamin B5 (pantothenic acid)	Liver
1931	Vitamin B7 (biotin)	Liver
1934	Vitamin B6 (pyridoxine)	Rice bran
1936	Vitamin B3 (niacin)	Liver
1941	Vitamin B9 (folic acid)	Liver

RESEARCH AND EVIDENCE

The medical and scientific communities are accumulating powerful evidence concerning the role of nutritional supplements in health promotion, disease prevention and treatment of a wide range of conditions ranging from fatigue and PMS to infertility and high blood pressure.

PRECAUTIONS

✖ We only require small amounts of vitamins and minerals. Water-soluble vitamins (B vitamins and vitamin C) are not stored in the body, but high doses of fat-soluble vitamins A and D can build up. This is particularly dangerous in pregnancy, as large amounts of vitamin A can be harmful to the developing foetus.

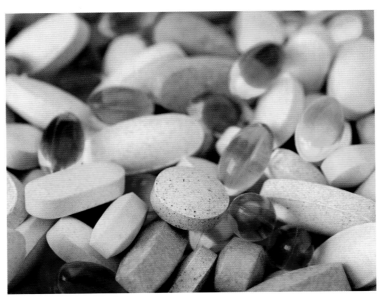

Vitamins *The best source of vitamins is a healthy diet, but vitamin supplements can help to support the immune system if the diet is deficient in some way.*

SUPERFOODS

If you are interested in **Superfoods**, you may also like to read about:
- **Vitamins and Minerals**, page 146
- **Food Combining**, page 148
- **Fasting and Detoxing**, pages 150–151

'Superfood' is a relatively new term that entered the language sometime in the late 1990s. It refers to foods rich in essential vitamins and minerals and in complex compounds that are not often combined in such density in other foods that we eat regularly. **Spinach and apples** are among many **well-known examples**.

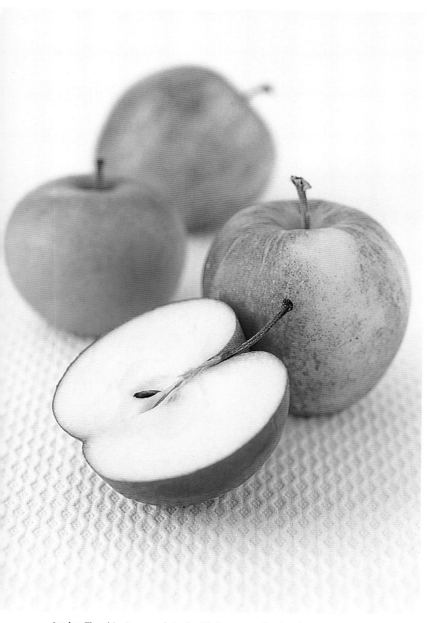

Apples *The ubiquitous apple is classified as a superfood and contains a quarter of the daily Recommended Daily Allowance of vitamin C.*

Spinach and apples

Perhaps the best example of a superfood is spinach. It is not only a rich source of energy-boosting folate and manganese, but also of potentially health-protecting flavonoids (see Research and Evidence).

Apples are high in immune-boosting, anti-ageing antioxidants, especially vitamin C for healthy skin and gums. One apple provides around a quarter of the daily Recommended Daily Allowance (RDA) of vitamin C. Apples also contain a form of soluble fibre called pectin that can help to lower blood cholesterol levels and maintain the healthy function of the digestive system. The sugar in an apple carbohydrate has a low glycaemic index (GI). Low-GI foods are digested slowly and are only gradually absorbed into the bloodstream, and therefore do not cause a sudden rise in blood sugar levels. Low-GI foods may help with weight control, and will tend to support diabetics' long-term control of blood sugar levels.

Other well-known examples

Among the most well-known superfoods are oily fish (such as salmon, mackerel and tuna) for omega-3 fatty acids, blueberries (fresh or frozen) for vitamin C, Brazil nuts for selenium, carrots for beta-carotene, tomatoes (fresh and canned) for lycopene, olive oil for the anti-inflammatory compound oleocanthal, red wine for resveratrol and garlic for allicin, considered to be the most powerful antioxidant. Other everyday superfoods include beans (in their dried form they help lower cholesterol), tea (green or black), walnuts and oats.

RESEARCH AND EVIDENCE

There is a growing body of research and clinical studies supporting the healing power of superfoods. According to work published by Japanese researcher I. Kuriyama in 2005, flavonoids, contained in spinach for example, may help reduce the risk of developing cancer. In 1997 M. P. Longnecker from the National Institute of Environmental Health Sciences observed the association between the intake of fruits and vegetables, such as carrots and spinach, and vitamin A and a lower risk of breast cancer. Other research has suggested that foods such as blueberries and spinach can prevent and/or reverse age-related declines in motor learning, memory and neurodegenerative diseases. For example, in 1998 the US Department of Agriculture reported that a six-month supplementation of spinach was linked to a reduction in age effects on neurodegenerative diseases in rats.

FOOD COMBINING

Food combining is an approach to eating that stresses the importance of **combining** different types of foods and **timing their consumption**. According to advocates, **'miscombining'** food can cause some people to develop health problems, digestive upsets, low energy levels, poor concentration and depression.

If you are interested in **Food Combining**, you may also like to read about:
- **Vitamins and Minerals**, page 146
- **Superfoods**, page 147
- **Herbalism**, pages 152–153
- **Fasting and Detoxing**, pages 150–151

Combining and timing food consumption

New York physician William Howard Hay (1866–1940) devised an acid–alkali balancing diet in the 1920s, and Herbert M. Shelton (1895–1985) subsequently published *Food Combining Made Easy* in 1940. According to their theories, it is difficult to digest certain combinations of foods because the different food types require different digestive enzymes.

One of the most important 'rules' of food combining is to avoid mixing carbohydrates and proteins at the same meal. Carbohydrate-rich foods such as bread, potatoes and rice require carbohydrate-splitting enzymes, whereas protein-rich foods such as meat, milk, eggs, beans, nuts and seeds require protein-splitting enzymes. While most people can secrete different types of

Citrus fruit *According to the principles of food combining, citrus fruits such as lemons should not be eaten alongside carbohdrates.*

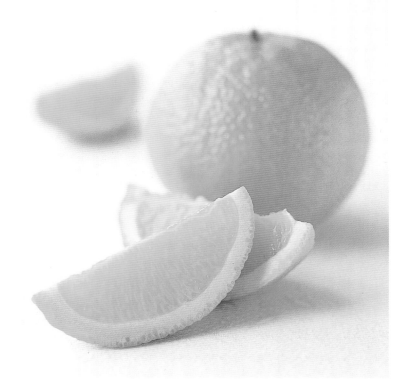

enzymes effectively, clinical experience suggests there are some who find that protein–carbohydrate combinations cause them digestive problems.

Another rule is always to eat fruit alone and wait at least 20 minutes before eating other food. According to food combining, we should:

- Avoid eating carbohydrates and citrus fruits together because the enzyme that digests carbohydrates can only function in an alkaline environment and citrus fruits create an acidic environment.
- Avoid eating proteins and fats at the same meal because fat takes a relatively long time to digest. Some foods, especially nuts, are over 50 per cent fat, therefore requiring several hours for digestion.
- Avoid eating proteins and acid foods (meat and citrus fruits) together because the acids of acid foods inhibit the secretion of the digestive acids required for protein digestion. Advocates believe that undigested proteins putrefy in bacterial decomposition and produce toxins.
- Avoid rich desserts because, eaten on top of meals, they may remain longer in the intestines and thus relatively undigested, fermenting into alcohols and acids.

Miscombining food

Supporters of food combining believe that 'miscombining' food can lead to irritability and ailments such as irritable bowel syndrome and acne. They claim that feeling tired after eating is usually a sign of miscombining.

RESEARCH AND EVIDENCE

Research studies do not support the assumptions used to justify food combining and there are as yet no clinical trials suggesting that it is beneficial. However, there are many testimonials from people who claim not only that food combining made them feel more energized, but that it also improved common digestion-related conditions, including acid reflux, bloating and stomach ache.

PRECAUTIONS

- ✖ Consult a dietician or your doctor before trying food combining, as it can lead to nutritional deficiencies.
- ✖ Food-combining diets are not recommended for children.

MACROBIOTICS

If you are interested in **Macrobiotics**, you may also like to read about:
- **Vitamins and Minerals**, page 146
- **Superfoods**, page 147
- **Herbalism**, pages 152–153
- **Fasting and Detoxing**, pages 150–151
- **Traditional Chinese Medicine**, pages 98–101

Macrobiotics, **originating** from Japan, is a dietary regime that stresses the importance of eating **whole foods** and of paying close attention to the optimal balance between food types. It is **holistic in approach**, and proponents suggest that there is a strong link between the food we eat and our physical and emotional health and wellbeing.

Origins

Japanese philosopher George Ohsawa (1893–1966) drew on oriental and Japanese folk medicine to create his own version of the Taoist philosophy of health in the 1950s. His teachings on these 'macrobiotic' ideas about eating, living and healing spread to the USA and Europe, where they remain influential today.

In Greek, *macro* means 'big or great' and *biotic* means 'concerning life', and the word may have been coined to indicate that macrobiotics takes a broad view of life and the significance of diet, or that the diet can prolong life. According to some proponents, the underlying principles of macrobiotics are reflected in many long-lived traditional cultures, such as the Incas and the Chinese in the Han Dynasty (206 BCE–220 CE).

Whole foods

The macrobiotic diet is typically low in fat and high in complex carbohydrates and fibre. It advocates the consumption of seasonal whole foods that have been grown locally. The staple food of the macrobiotic diet is grain — rice, barley, wheat, rye, oats or millet — which makes up at least 70 per cent. Pulses and lentils are also important, as are seaweeds and local fruits and vegetables. Foods considered to be extreme yin foods, such as sugar, and those viewed as extreme yang foods, such as salt and meat, are to be entirely avoided.

Macrobiotics also addresses *how* one eats, recommending against overeating, eating under pressure and not chewing thoroughly.

A holistic approach

Followers of the macrobiotic approach believe that food and food quality powerfully affect health, wellbeing and happiness. The guiding principle used in macrobiotics is yin and yang, the notion that complementary opposites are present in all things, and when balance is achieved in the diet, a powerful sense of health and wellbeing should result. Other guiding principles are: whole grains are the main staple food; food is best if it is whole, natural and unrefined; food is best if it is locally grown and eaten in season. Living the macrobiotic lifestyle also means regular exercise and experiencing the positive effects that result from the guiding principles that emphasize respect for the world, the natural environment and all forms of life.

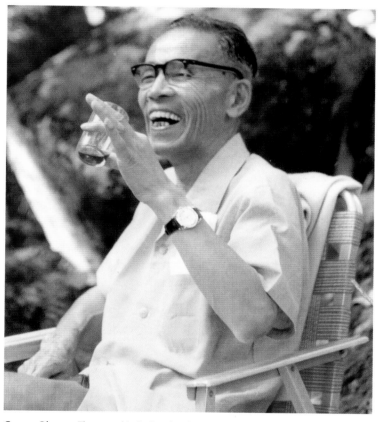

George Ohsawa *The macrobiotic diet, developed by George Ohsawa in the 1950s, has become easier to follow today with the increasing number of health-food stores.*

RESEARCH AND EVIDENCE

There is evidence that the macrobiotic diet, with its emphasis on whole grains and vegetables and being low in saturated fat, red meat and preserved meat products, can help prevent cancer, according to a study at the Tulane University, New Orleans, USA, published in 1993.

PRECAUTIONS

✖ Consult a dietician or your doctor before embarking on a macrobiotic diet, as it may lead to nutritional deficiencies.

FASTING AND DETOXING

If you are interested in **Fasting and Detoxing**, you may also like to read about:
- **Naturopathy**, pages 144–145
- **Herbalism**, pages 152–153
- **Macrobiotics**, page 149
- **Vitamins and Minerals**, page 146
- **Superfoods**, page 147
- **Pilgrimage and Retreats**, pages 298–299

The benefits of fasting can be to rest the digestive system and to flush out unhealthy 'toxins', which are thought to accumulate when we eat too much or unhealthily. Other detoxification methods include a **liver or kidney cleanse** and **colonics**. There are numerous anecdotes about the **benefits of colonics** but research is limited and scientists have yet to confirm its benefical effects.

The benefits of fasting

The rationale behind fasting for spiritual reasons is to deny the needs of the flesh. Many religions, including Christianity, Judaism and Eastern religions used and still use fasting for spiritual purification and to signify a turning away from physical concerns and towards the divine. Prolonged fasting may also encourage altered mental states which some traditions view as conducive to prayer, meditation or visions.

According to practitioners of alternative medicine, over time toxins build up in our bodies as the result of the pollutants that we breathe and the chemicals in the food and water that we consume. Periodically, our bodies release these toxins into the bloodstream, causing the body to experience a 'low' cycle when we may suffer headaches or depression. Fasting is said by its proponents to be a safe way to help the body move through this low cycle more quickly and with less discomfort. Those who fast regularly claim that it can rest the digestive system and speed up the elimination of toxins, which in turn boosts circulation, immunity and stamina. Some people undertake solely liquid fasts, consuming only water, broth or juices. Others undergo specific or 'mono' fasts, such as short-term fruit fasts, when they eat only fruits and juices, or brown-rice fasts. The most common fast is abstinence from all food and liquid except water.

Naturopaths believe that an excess of acid-forming foods, such as high-fat foods, red meats, sugary foods and processed foods, can cause fatigue and poor health. Therefore many fasts avoid these particular foods.

Liver and kidney cleanse

After digestion has broken down the food we eat, it is absorbed into the blood flowing in the vessels around the intestines. This blood then passes through the liver, where the products of digestion are broken down into safer substances that can be removed from the body through the gut and kidneys.

Nutritionally oriented practitioners believe that poor diet, stress and overconsumption of alcohol put added strain on the liver, causing it difficulty in dealing with the products of digestion, which results in toxins circulating in the blood. This, say practitioners, can cause fatigue, depression, poor health and possibly weight gain (the liver is also involved in the metabolism of fat).

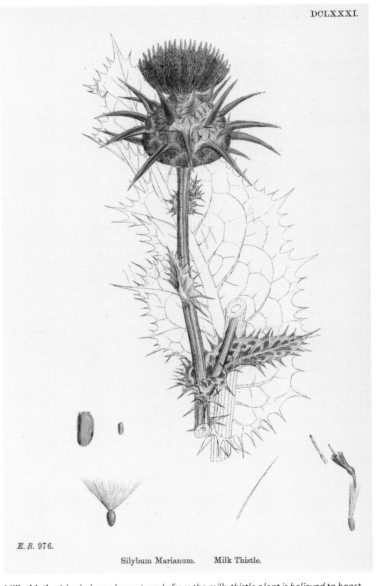

DCLXXXI.

E. B. 976.

Silybum Marianum.   Milk Thistle.

Milk thistle *A herbal supplement made from the milk-thistle plant is believed to boost the functioning of liver cells.*

While the first step to a healthy liver is a healthy diet, some nutritional therapists recommend a liver cleanse. This entails abstaining from high-protein foods for a few days; red meat is avoided and only moderate amounts of healthy protein are allowed, such as oily fish, nuts and seeds two or three times a day. Plenty of liver-boosting vitamin C- and E-rich foods, such as oranges, berries, kiwi fruit, peppers, dark-green vegetables, green tea and wheat germ, may also be recommended, as well as milk thistle, a herbal supplement thought to stimulate liver function.

The kidneys also filter out toxins, waste products and excess sodium from the blood into the urine. Some nutritional practitioners believe that a high-salt diet strains the kidneys and therefore recommend a kidney cleanse. This involves reducing salt intake, drinking plenty of water, eating naturally diuretic foods such as watermelon and reducing foods that are likely to irritate the kidneys, such as red meat and chocolate. Ginkgo biloba is a herbal supplement said to improve blood flow to the kidneys.

Colonics

Some people have several bowel movements a day; others can have none for several days with no harmful effects. In fact it is the hardness of stools rather than their frequency that defines constipation. Constipation can usually be dealt with by eating more fibre, drinking more water and taking regular exercise. 'Autointoxication' is the theory that stagnation in the large intestine (colon) allows toxins to form and be absorbed, and that this undermines wellbeing and can cause fatigue and chronic ill health. Although this theory is totally unproven, colonics are designed to encourage the excretion of toxins from the body. A colonic involves flushing the colon using a rubber tube inserted as far as 76 cm (30 inches) into the rectum. Warm water is pumped in and out through the tube, a few litres at a time. Some practitioners add probiotic herbs, coffee or other material to the water.

The benefits of colonics

Colonic irrigation may have been used as early as ancient times in Egypt, China, India and Greece. This practice gained some popularity in 19th-century European spas, and it has been used in modern times for general wellbeing and a variety of conditions.

Proponents of colonic irrigation believe that it can improve mental outlook, modulate the immune system and eliminate toxic substances. The theory is that intestinal flora (bacteria that normally live in the intestine) or waste products can affect the immune system and may therefore trigger diseases outside of the gastrointestinal tract. It is said that washing away these waste products can have beneficial effects.

RESEARCH AND EVIDENCE

For many methods of detoxification there is little or no evidence from clinical trials to support their use.

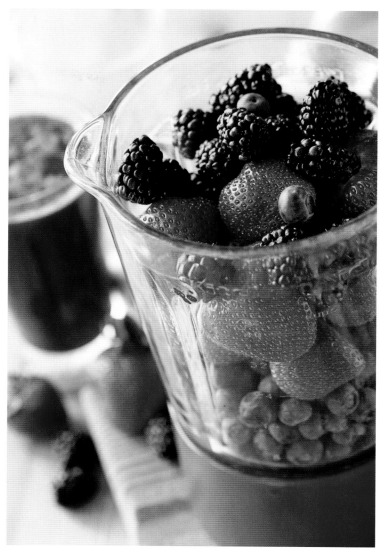

Juices *Fruit juices and smoothies are a good way of obtaining vitamin C and may be taken as part of a short-term fruit fast.*

PRECAUTIONS

✖ **Fasting** Mono fasts should not be prolonged for more than a few days or without advice and approval from your doctor. This is especially important if you are on medication, have a pre-existing medical condition or are pregnant. Prolonged fasting can be fatal.

✖ **Colonics** Colonics can be expensive, sometimes uncomfortable and, if the equipment is not properly sterilized, dangerous. Outbreaks of serious infections have been reported, as well as a few cases of fatal bowel perforation and heart failure from excess fluid absorption and electrolyte imbalance. Anyone who is pregnant or suffering from an inflammatory bowel disease or haemorrhoids should avoid colonics. If you are unsure about whether or not a colonic is safe for you, consult your doctor. Most doctors do not recommend colonics for any medical condition, although enemas to cleanse the lower colon may be appropriate in certain situations.

HERBALISM

Herbalism is the treatment of various ailments using natural sources found in plants, and has incorporated many **ancient traditions**. Herbs contain potent mixtures of chemical compounds that have physiological effects on the body. Although many pharmaceutical drugs are derived from herbs, drug companies isolate the **'active ingredient'** of the herb as the basis for the drug, whereas herbalists believe using the **whole plant** can deliver a range of **health benefits**.

If you are interested in **Herbalism**, you may also like to read about:
- **Ayurveda**, pages 94–97
- **Traditional Chinese Medicine**, pages 98–101
- **Vitamins and Minerals**, page 146
- **Superfoods**, page 147

Ancient traditions

Although the different traditions of herbalism have borrowed from one another over hundreds of years, three main branches can be distinguished: the Western herbal tradition based on Greek, Roman and medieval sources, including Arabic medicine; the ayurvedic and *unani* traditions from the Indian subcontinent; and Traditional Chinese Medicine, in which practitioners still largely adhere to the ancient traditional principles of how herbs work. Western herbalists generally prescribe herbs for the ingredients they contain and for their known physiological effects, in a similar way to conventional medicine. The traditional herbalists of the East, however, follow an entirely different approach, based on the concept that ill health is an imbalance in the flow of 'vital energy', which the appropriate herbs can harmonize.

PRECAUTIONS

✱ Check with your healthcare practitioner before using any herbal product, especially if you are taking prescription drugs, but also non-prescription medications and vitamins. Many herbal remedies can interact with other drugs. Also make sure that your healthcare practitioner is aware of your medical history, including allergies.

✱ Contact your healthcare practitioner without delay if you experience abdominal cramping, abnormal bleeding or bruising, changes in your pulse or heart rhythm, vision changes, dizziness or fainting, hair loss, hallucinations, inability to concentrate or other mental changes, hives, itching, rash or other allergic symptoms, appetite loss or dramatic weight loss.

✱ Discontinue herbal remedies at least two weeks before surgery, as they can interfere with anaesthesia and cause heart and blood-vessel problems.

✱ Avoid herbal preparations if you are pregnant or breast-feeding. If you are a woman of childbearing age, check that your birth control will not be affected before taking a herbal remedy.

✱ Do not use herbal remedies for children or adolescents unless under responsible medical supervision.

✱ Herbal remedies should not be used for serious or potentially serious medical conditions, such as heart disease or bleeding disorders.

Active ingredient versus the whole plant

Perhaps a quarter of modern medicines have plant origins; aspirin, quinine, morphine and digitalis are old examples, but even some recently formulated cancer drugs were initially extracted from plants, such as the Madagascar rosy periwinkle, from which vincristine is produced. However, although many drugs come from herbs, modern drug companies use only the 'active ingredient' of the plant or herb in a pure form as the basis for the drug. Herbalists, by contrast, use the whole plant.

A significant benefit of using the whole plant is that side effects are absent or minimal. For instance, the foxglove plant (*Digitalis purpurea*) has been used for centuries by herbalists for heart problems. Today scientists extract the main ingredient of the foxglove (digoxin), but by doing so they create a drug with a risk of toxicity. If, however, the whole plant is used, any toxicity should build up slowly enough so that it can be detected before it becomes dangerous.

Potential for herb–drug interactions is considerable, but as yet too little researched. For example, ginseng is relatively harmless, but it can increase the anticoagulant effect of the prescription drug warfarin, causing spontaneous bruising and bleeding.

RESEARCH AND EVIDENCE

Herbal remedies are prescribed for a wide range of conditions and there is a growing body of scientific evidence to suggest that some herbal remedies may be effective and beneficial for a number of health conditions, including depression, infertility, memory loss, hormonal imbalance, stress and anxiety; for example, St John's wort for moderate depression, ginkgo biloba for dementia, saw palmetto as a symptomatic treatment for benign prostate hyperplasia, and horse-chestnut seed extracts for chronic venous insufficiency. However, in the UK and the USA herbs are not yet regulated as medicines and there are currently unacceptable disparities in their quality in relation to cultivation and manufacture.

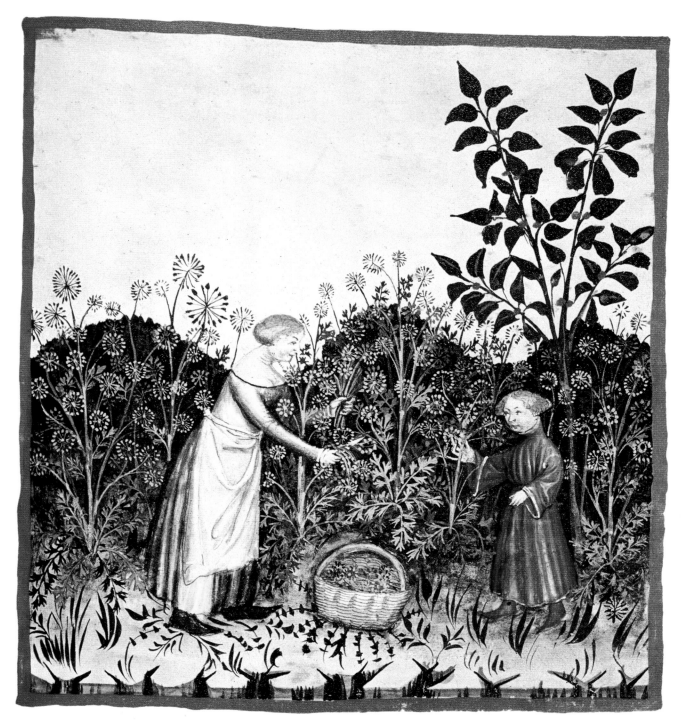

Health benefits

Herbalism aims to stimulate a return to health by strengthening the body's organ systems. Herbal medicines are available fresh or dried, or in tablet or liquid (tincture or juice) form. They can be taken by mouth, as an inhalation or applied to the skin.

Like any medicine, herbal remedies work better for some health conditions than others. According to herbalists, those conditions that respond well include colds, digestive disorders, headaches, fatigue, depression, rheumatism, arthritis, skin problems, anaemia and many hormonal,

Herbal medicine *This 14th-century illumination from* Tacunium sanitatis in medicina *(a Latin version of an Arabic science-of-health book) shows a medieval woman and child collecting herbs to create remedies.*

menstrual, menopausal and fertility problems. Herbalists also maintain that herbal medicine can provide preventative medicines.

As well as having healing properties, some herbal medicines, such as garlic and asparagus, are foods that provide vitamins and minerals as part of a healthy diet.

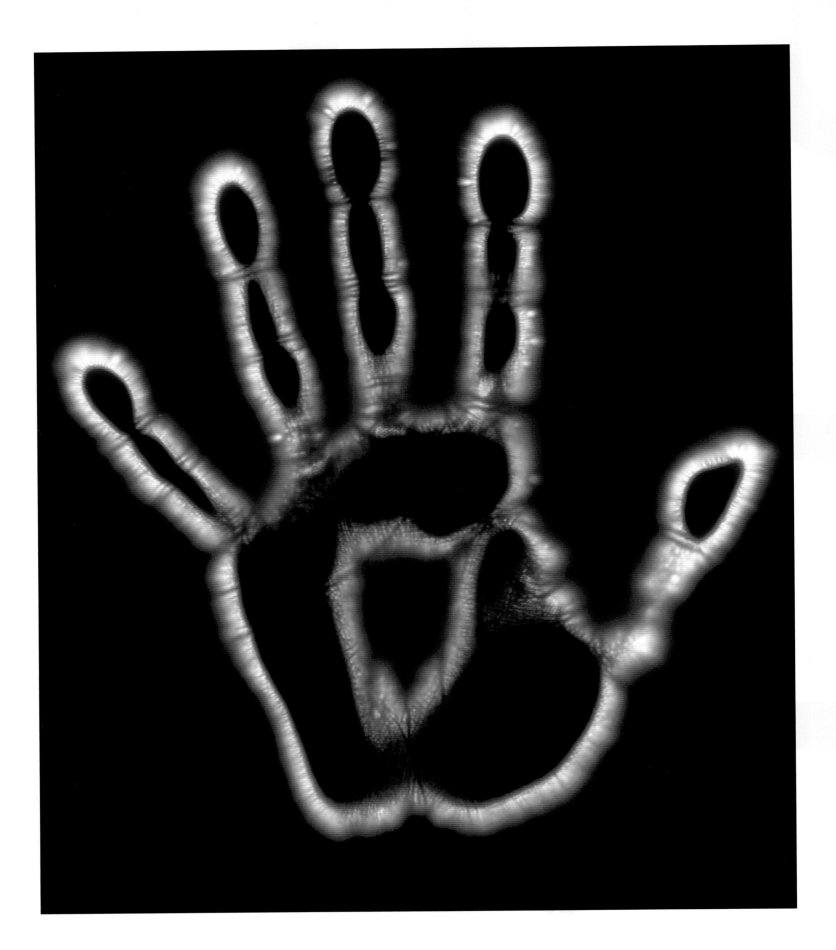

ENERGY THERAPIES

All matter is made up of atoms and molecules vibrating in particular ways, and in the electromagnetic energy spectrum it is the various rates of vibration that differentiate between light, radio waves and X-rays. Although these are scientific facts, if anything they only make matter and energy more mysterious. Yet the ideas behind energy therapies are stranger still. Therapists working in this way believe that energy is not confined to the physical world. Their view is that thoughts and feelings produce vibratory patterns in the physical body, and thus create non-material emotional, mental and spiritual 'energy bodies'. The various energies, so they tell us, pass freely between these 'bodies', the energy of one body affecting the state of the others. What should we make of these ideas, which seem to describe a flowing of information between body, mind and spirit?

At one time science studied the body and the mind as separate entities. Nowadays we have the technology to tune into their two-way conversation, and there is now a mass of scientific evidence for mind–body interaction: how stress undermines immunity; how emotions begin in the body and how they affect the brain; even how meditation boosts brain centres linked with positive emotions. Yet long before science confirmed these connections, people sensed the interconnectedness of body, mind, emotion and spirit.

The life force

The notion of a vital force or 'animating energy' is common to most complementary therapies. The different disciplines have various names for this force – chi, ki or prana – but the central idea is the same: that the living organism contains a special kind of 'energy' that vitalizes the physical body, linking the body and the mind and animating our emotions, thinking and creativity. Chi in Traditional Chinese Medicine is conceived of as a part of a wider flow of information whose workings can be seen throughout nature. So, chi is not unique to living creatures, but is part of a universal energy. Is this in any way 'scientific'? Of course not.

Kirlian photograph *Some people believe that Kirlian photography is evidence of the human 'aura'.*

In the light of what we now know about the slow emergence of stars and solar systems since the Big Bang and the eons-long unfolding of evolution, the fact that the universe has a curious capacity to create complex wholes seems undeniable. As scientists strive to understand this complexity, the possibility that life holds together because intelligence is built into our universe does not seem too far-fetched. In a post-modern world, perhaps we have to reinvent the idea of 'living energy' as a metaphor for the vast ocean of information, whose flow through matter organizes life. Here we are referring to energy as an idea rather than a fact.

The whole person

Complementary medical disciplines describe how this life energy flows through our bodies, and that illness or 'dis-ease' can be caused by blockages and imbalances in this flow. When it works well we are resilient, and if we become ill we bounce back. But if too much adaptation to stress and strain overloads the life energy, if it is asked to do too much or if it is weakened (by environmental factors, poor diet, trauma, stress, pollution or lack of sleep, for example), then the whole person – mind, body and spirit – may lose its equilibrium. This implies that if we are sensitive to these shifts, we will sense disharmony and imbalance long before an actual disease sets in. Accordingly, mind, body and spirit are all integral to good health and wellbeing, and therefore holistic approaches to treatment aim to engage all three to support the healing process.

Energy as therapy

These approaches are based on the idea that since the material body 'is energy', it will respond to treatments that use 'energy' to encourage the flow of 'energy' within our bodies. Unscientifically, these disciplines claim to work on a vibrational basis: tuning frequencies of our mind and body with the help of crystals, water, homeopathic remedies made from natural substances, colour, sound and light. Other therapies claim to detect energy flow and correct imbalances. None of the therapies in this section are based on science, but rather on something that can be felt and manipulated, and used as a tool for encouraging our innate ability to self-heal.

AROMATHERAPY

If you are interested in **Aromatherapy**, you may also like to read about:
- **Herbalism**, pages 152–153
- **Flower Essences**, pages 158–159
- **Swedish Massage**, pages 120–121
- **Chakras and the Aura**, pages 172–173

The term aromatherapy literally means **'treatment using scents'** and was coined by French chemist René-Maurice Gattefossé in the 1920s. It uses essential oils derived from flowers, herbs, plants, trees and spices for therapeutic purposes. The therapy has evolved as a branch of herbal medicine, and aromatherapists believe it works **pharmacologically, physiologically and psychologically.** Each **essential oil** is said to have particular properties and characteristics considered helpful for particular ailments and emotional problems.

Treatment using scents

Aromatherapists claim that each living plant has a unique life force or energy of its own, and aromatherapy aims to harness this energy by extracting the plant's essential oils that give it its scent. Oils are distilled from the leaves, flowers, fruit, wood, bark and roots. They are natural chemical compounds, generally more complex than pharmaceutical drugs, but slower-acting and, therapists believe, more profoundly healing.

Dr Gattefossé (1881–1950) discovered quite by accident that pure lavender oil healed his badly burned hand quickly, with no blistering, infection or scarring. As a result, he was prompted to research the medicinal properties of essential oils of other plants.

Pharmacological, physical and psychological effects

Essential oils can work in the body in three ways: pharmacologically, physiologically and psychologically. As pharmacological agents, the chemical constituents of the oils may act rather like any medicinal compound. Oil molecules absorbed through the skin are transported in the bloodstream to all parts of the body.

When aromatherapists refer to the physiological effects of essential oils, they mean how they affect different body functions. For example, oils such as black pepper, juniper and rosemary are described as having a warming or rubefacient effect on muscles and joints, and may be helpful with pain associated with arthritis. Oils such as basil, chamomile, peppermint and cardamom are described as 'carminative', meaning that they are thought to help settle the digestive system. They are used in many preparations today.

Aromatherapists claim that the scent of essential oils can also have particular psychological effects. Our sense of smell depends partly on nerve receptors in the nose that convert the scent molecules into electrical impulses. The olfactory (smell) nerve transmits these impulses to the brain, especially to the limbic system – an area of the brain associated not only with olfactory processes but also with emotion and long-term memory. Our animal cousins still rely far more on smell than humans do, and this may be a clue as to why

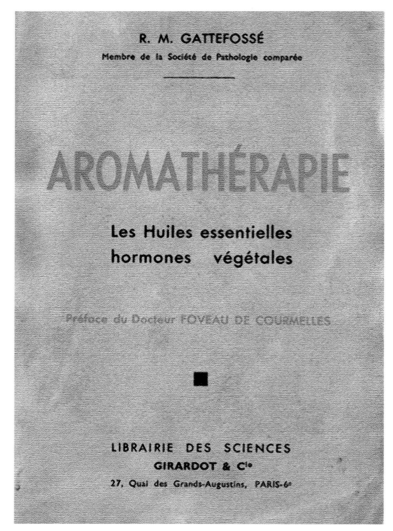

Aromathérapie *The word 'aromatherapy' was coined by René-Maurice Gattefossé in France, in 1928, to describe the science of using the oils of aromatic plants to heal the body and mind, and was the title of his seminal book on the subject.*

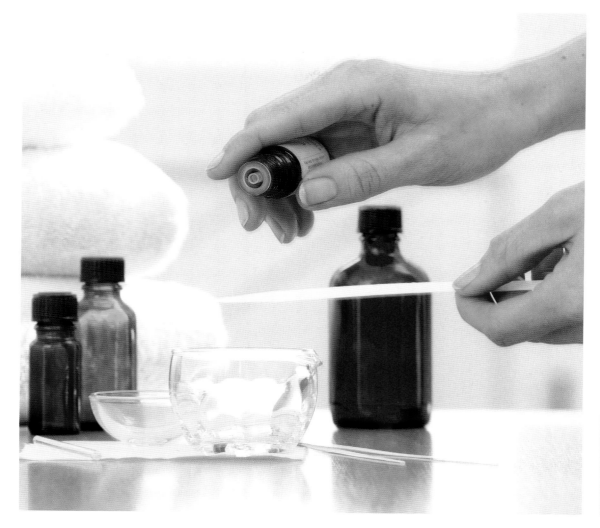

Essential oils *Many different parts of plants, including the seeds, petals, roots, bark, peel, berries and leaves, are used to produce individual oils, whose price will depend upon the cost of the raw ingredients and the amount required to produce the oil.*

smells can sometimes bypass the rational mind, strongly evoking memories and perhaps triggering particular emotions. Some smells seem more relaxing; others tend to make people feel more awake or mentally alert.

Essential oils

About 150 essential oils have been extracted for use in aromatherapy. Each has a unique fragrance and contains many different chemical components. All have antiseptic properties to some degree, and can have numerous other actions, including anti-inflammatory, pain-relieving, decongestant, antispasmodic, antibacterial or antidepressant. Each oil is said to have a dominant characteristic that classifies it as stimulating, relaxing or refreshing, for example.

It can take between 20 minutes and several hours for oils to be absorbed into the body. After some hours the oils leave the body; most are exhaled, while others are eliminated in urine, faeces and perspiration. Oils can be used in massage, baths, steam inhalations, creams, lotions and shampoos, gargles and mouthwashes and hot and cold compresses. They can also be put into candles or dispersed using sources of heat, such as a radiator or vaporizer, which encourages the volatile oils to be released into the atmosphere.

Diluting oils

Before being used for massage, essential oils are diluted with carrier oils, such as sweet almond, grape seed, olive or apricot kernel, or added to water or alcohol. For example, 10 drops of an essential oil may be added to 75 ml (2^1/$_2$ fl oz) of grape seed oil for massage, or 15 drops can be added to 400 ml (14 fl oz) of fresh water to use in the environment. One or 2 drops can be added to a bowl of hot or cold water to use as the basis for a compress; or 5–10 drops can be added to a full bath. Some oils, such as tea tree, lavender and sandalwood, are used neat on small areas of the skin for a local healing effect. Oils can also be blended to combine their therapeutic properties.

RESEARCH AND EVIDENCE

A systematic review of scientific evidence by the Natural Standard, an international research collaboration that produces scientifically based reviews of complementary and alternative medicine topics, concludes that aromatherapy may help reduce anxiety in the short term. Certain oils may help prevent bronchitis. Tea tree oil has been found to help relieve acne and there appears to be some strong evidence for the antibacterial and anti-inflammatory effects of tea tree and eucalyptus oils.

FLOWER ESSENCES

Flower essences provide the basis of a gentle healing therapy for the mind, body and spirit. These bottled essences are said to contain plant **vibrations** that can balance **negative emotions**, which are both the cause and product of ill health. **Bach Flower Remedies** and **Australian Bush Flower Essences** are the best-known flower essence therapies, but others from South Africa and the US are gaining in popularity.

If you are interested in **Flower Essences**, you may also like to read about:
- **Homeopathy**, pages 160–161
- **Crystal Healing**, pages 166–167

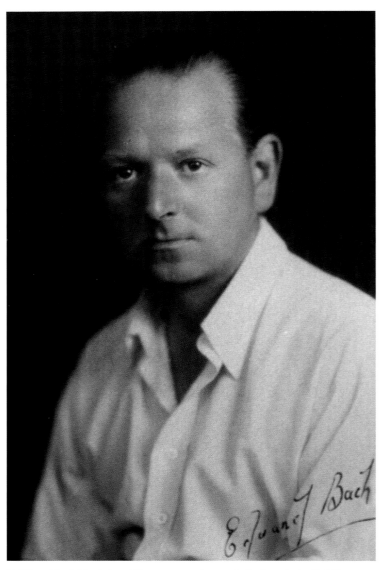

Dr Edward Bach *The father of flower essence therapy, Dr Bach sparked a discipline that is becoming increasingly popular around the world. Bach Flower Remedies use only British trees and flowers.*

Good vibrations

Flower essences are said to contain the vibration of the flower's energy, after the petals have been immersed in sun-warmed water. Essences do not work in a biochemical way, as herbs or essential oils do, because no physical extract of the plant remains in the essences. The theory is that the essences contain the vital energy of the plant, and that they work in a similar way to a homeopathic remedy by triggering the body's own healing processes.

Negative emotions

Dr Edward Bach (1886–1936) was a surgeon, pathologist and homeopathic physician. Having noticed that patients with the same illnesses often shared similar emotional states, he concluded that negative emotions and attitudes were a manifestation of deeper disharmony that predisposed people towards ill health. He subsequently identified seven basic negative states and created 12 healers from flowers or trees native to the UK.

Bach believed that when we harm others or act against our deepest nature we distort our most basic virtues. In this way, courage, love, mental equanimity, humility, strength and understanding can turn into negative qualities such as possessiveness, fear, indecision, depression, impatience, cruelty and hatred. These negative emotions, he maintained, contribute to ill health by depressing both the mind and the immune system. Dr Bach believed that his flower essences could go to the root of the illness, and improve emotional wellbeing, which in turn would restore physical health.

Flower essences are reputed to be effective ways of providing support in times of crisis. Practitioners claim that they can also help to change recurring behavioural patterns, and improve the negative emotional states that may be the precursors to ill health. They are safe for people and animals of all ages and states of health.

RESEARCH AND EVIDENCE

Although many individuals report the effectiveness of treatment with flower essences, to date there is a lack of detailed scientific research to support these claims.

BACH FLOWER REMEDIES

Dr Bach created 38 Flower Remedies in all, which reflected what he believed to be the 38 basic states of mind. They are sold as a liquid preserved in brandy. A few drops should be diluted in water and taken as four drops four times a day, or sipped at intervals throughout the day. The remedies may also be applied externally, to pulse points, a method often used for the treatment of babies, or in an emergency. A therapist may blend several remedies together to suit an individual, but people can also self-diagnose and treat themselves.

ESSENCE	USE	POSITIVE VIBRATION
Agrimony	For those who hide their feelings behind humour and put on a brave face	Joy
Beech	For a perfectionist who tends to be intolerant of other people's methods and experience	Tolerance
Clematis	For the absent-minded day dreamer who needs to stay awake and focus on the here and now	Creative idealism
Gorse	For those who suffer hopelessness and despair after a long struggle, and who are stuck in a negative pattern	Hope
Holly	For those who develop a victim mentality and suffer bouts of anger, jealousy and envy	Divine love
Impatiens	For impatience and irritability; for those who are always in a rush and are too busy to slow down	Patience
Mimulus	For fear of known things, such as fear of flying or public speaking	Unaffectedness
Wild Oat	For those who need help in deciding on the path and purpose in their lives	Purposefulness
Rescue Remedy	Comprised of Cherry Plum for desperation; Rock Rose for terror, fear or panic; Impatiens (see above); Clematis (see above); and Star of Bethlehem for shock and trauma	Calm, balance and relief of trauma or shock

Impatiens

AUSTRALIAN BUSH FLOWER ESSENCES

Australian naturopath Ian White created these essences using flowers indigenous to Australia. The essences are supposed to give clarity to people's lives, and also the strength, courage and commitment to follow and pursue their goals and dreams, developing a high level of intuition, self-esteem, spirituality, creativity and fun.

Combination essences are marketed to address specific health problems or periods of life, such as adolescence or childhood. Single essences can be blended for individual needs. Seven drops are normally taken directly from the bottle, morning and night, although they can be diluted in water and sipped throughout the day.

ESSENCE	NEGATIVE CONDITION	POSITIVE OUTCOME
Alpine Mint Bush	Mental and emotional exhaustion, lack of joy	Revitalization, joy, renewal
Black-eyed Susan	Impatience, being 'on the go', overcommitted	Stillness, slowing down, inner peace
Bush Gardenia	Stale relationships, self-interest, unawareness	Passion, renewed interest in partner, improved communication
Dog Rose	Fearfulness, shyness, insecurity, apprehension	Confidence, self-belief, courage, ability to embrace life
Kangaroo Paw	Gaucheness, unawareness, insensitivity	Kindness, sensitivity, enjoyment of people, relaxation
Mountain Devil	Hatred, anger, holding of grudges, suspicion	Unconditional love, happiness, healthy boundaries, forgiveness
Red Lily	Vagueness, disconnectedness, lack of focus	Groundedness, focus, living in the present, connection with life and God

Black-eyed Susan

HOMEOPATHY

If you are interested in **Homeopathy**, you may also like to read about:
- **Healing Water**, pages 164–165
- **Flower Essences**, pages 158–159

The term homeopathy comes from the Greek meaning 'similar suffering', in the sense that **'like cures like'**. Homeopaths believe that an extremely diluted form of a substance can cure the same **symptoms** in an ill person that it is capable of causing in a healthy person. Homeopathy is a form of **energy medicine** that claims to work with the body's vital force to encourage **emotional and physical healing**.

Like cures like

Hippocrates (c. 460–377 BCE), the 'father of medicine', referred to the fact that 'disease is produced and through the application of the like, it is cured'. Similarly, based on the idea that 'like cures like', in the late 18th century the German physician Dr Samuel Hahnemann (1755–1843) began developing a new system of medicine, which became known as homeopathy.

In his time many treatments involved purging and bleeding people. Consequently, the cures were very often more harmful than the diseases. Hahnemann, while investigating the medicinal effects of cinchona bark (quinine) on malaria, found that taking it caused him to experience thirst, throbbing in the head and fever – in fact the symptoms of malaria. He deduced that the drug's power to cure the disease arose from its ability to produce symptoms similar to the disease itself. He and his early followers administered herbs, minerals and other substances to healthy people, including themselves, and kept detailed records of what they observed. Hahnemann was careful to test these substances in a very dilute form. Paradoxically, he found that the effectiveness of the remedy increased as it became more dilute.

Energy medicine

Homeopathy uses substances that have been diluted so much that, in the commonly used 30c strength, no actual molecules of the original substance remain. It has been suggested, therefore, that homeopathic medicines rely on some kind of energetic effect.

At each dilution stage the liquid is vigorously shaken ('succussed'). Some homeopaths have suggested that in the process the water absorbs information from the medicinal substance present. Practitioners believe that these remedies rebalance the body's subtle energy system. If this is so, then homeopathic remedies would have to be more like radio signals than drugs. Homeopathy can be characterized as a form of 'vibrational medicine'.

Emotional and physical healing

Often confused with herbalism, homeopathic remedies use minerals and even some animal products as a base, as well as plants. Dilutions of drugs or

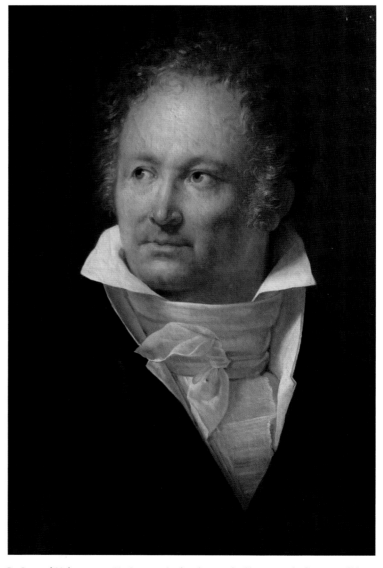

Dr Samuel Hahnemann *Having practised and researched homeopathy for most of his working life, Dr Hahnemann created the first materia medica for homeopathic remedies, which is still used today.*

products of illness are sometimes used too. Remedies are prepared using a process known as 'potentization' (serial dilution, with shaking at each stage), which homeopaths believe brings out a substance's subtle healing properties.

The kinds of health problems that homeopaths are commonly consulted for include eczema, asthma, psoriasis, migraine, irritable bowel syndrome, menstrual and menopausal difficulties, allergies, infertility, phobias, grief and depression. Perhaps its greatest strength is in treating conditions where conventional medicine has little to offer. Nonetheless many homeopaths believe there is no ailment that will not respond to homeopathy. They would, however, observe that treatment of deep-seated problems takes a long time, because according to homeopathic theory new symptoms are likely to appear as current ones are addressed. The reason for this is that long-term health conditions may have a multitude of different causative factors: genetics, trauma and injury, previous illnesses and emotional conflicts are all considered potential causes. Homeopaths claim that, in some cases, 'old' symptoms associated with past illnesses may manifest themselves as the remedy gets to work.

The importance of symptoms

The remedies have what is called a 'drug picture'. This comprises all the symptoms recorded during 'provings' (testing of the remedy on healthy volunteers) plus the symptoms noted over the last two centuries as having been cured by the remedy. These symptoms could be physical, mental, emotional or more 'general'. Therefore, when homeopaths ask about a patient's symptoms, they want to know not only about the chief complaint, but also about behavioural tendencies and personality traits, and every other symptom or experience, such as thirst, bowel movements, the times at which the condition appears improved, the precise nature of any pain, as well as anything else that the patient has noticed about his or her health while experiencing the problem. This total 'symptom picture' of a person's overall health and wellbeing forms the basis on which the homeopath selects the remedy whose 'drug picture' best coincides with the 'symptom picture'.

Homeopathy is only believed to be as successful as the skill of the homeopath; in other words, the wrong remedy will do no harm, but only the correct remedy will facilitate healing.

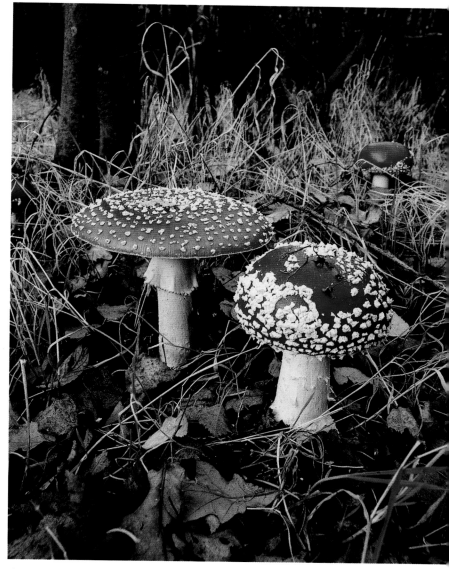

Fly agaric *This poisonous fungus is used in dilution to relieve chilblains, as well as twitching and jerking movements, neuralgia, headaches and sciatica.*

PRECAUTIONS

✖ Although homeopathy has been used for a very wide range of conditions, it should not be used to treat life-threatening conditions, nor should it be allowed to delay the use of established therapies for severe illness. Anyone with unusual or persistent unexplained symptoms should seek appropriate medical advice.

✖ Allergic reactions to low-potency essences are theoretically possible, but are extremely rare.

✖ Some homeopathic practitioners have recommended against immunization of children. There is no evidence to support homeopathy as a viable substitute. Patients or parents should discuss vaccination with a healthcare professional. There is no evidence to suggest that homeopathic remedies can prevent malaria.

RESEARCH AND EVIDENCE

In 1991, three professors of medicine from the Netherlands, none of them homeopaths, performed an analysis of 25 years of clinical studies using homeopathic medicines and published their results in the *British Medical Journal*. This analysis covered 107 controlled trials, of which 81 showed that homeopathic medicines were effective, 24 showed they were ineffective and two were inconclusive.

Homeopathy has been the subject of many research studies for the treatment of illnesses, including migraine, vertigo, upper respiratory tract infections, eczema, hay fever and asthma. According to a review of scientific studies of homeopathy by the Natural Standard (see page 157), early results for the treatment of some of these conditions have been considered promising. However, many studies have been criticized for their design and reporting, and further high-quality scientific research is needed before claims can be confirmed or refuted.

COLOUR THERAPY

Colour therapy focuses on **the impact of colour** and works on the premise that colour is a form of energy, that each colour vibrates at its own frequency and that a colour vibrating at the appropriate frequency can initiate **healing**. Research has shown that colour affects us mentally and emotionally.

If you are interested in **Colour Therapy**, you may also like to read about:
● **Chakras and the Aura**, pages 172–173
● **Crystal Healing**, pages 166–167
● **Acupuncture**, page 126
● **Healing Water**, pages 164–165

The impact of colour

Some colour therapists believe that the impact of colour is due to the effects of its vibrations on our energy fields, while others say that colour directly affects our cells or that it changes the way energy moves through the body. Some consider its primary impact to be on the mind and emotions.

Healing with colour and light

Colour therapists choose the colour they believe will balance weaknesses in a person's energy field. They may also focus coloured light on certain parts of the body, such as the chakras (energy centres). Some therapists use crystals, coloured water and oils or colour visualization to encourage harmony and healing. Others suggest wearing particular colours or eating foods of those colours. Colour therapists believe that colours can have both positive and negative effects, as shown in the chart below.

While sunlight and colour have a long history of use in healing, only recently have the therapeutic applications of light become the focus of medical research. Soft laser light has been found to help certain kinds of chronic pain; full-spectrum light can relieve depression.

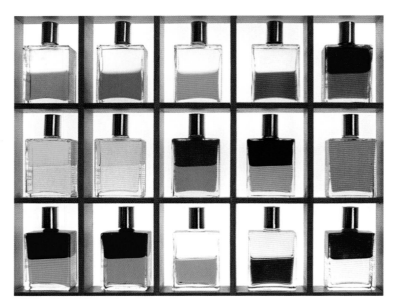

Coloured oils *Some colour therapists apply coloured oils to help alter the frequency of the light on the body. These may be produced from crystals or plants.*

COLOUR	POSITIVE EFFECT	NEGATIVE EFFECT
Red	Uplifting, increasing vitality, sexuality and ambition; good for blood and circulatory disorders	Agitation, anger, aggression
Orange	Energizing; good for gallstones, digestive ailments, chest and kidney disorders, depression	Agitation, restlessness
Yellow	Cheering, stimulating; good for digestion and skin problems	Exhaustion, depression
Green	Balancing, serene, hopeful, harmonious; good for heart conditions, healing broken bones, regenerating tissue	Lethargy, overcomplacency
Blue	Truthful, noble, serene, cool, soothing, calming; good for nightmares, fever, bleeding, burns, sore throats, shock, nervous conditions	Overly sedative; feeling cold, passive, sad and depressed
Indigo	Stimulates the intellect, courage, authority, inner calmness; good for purifying blood, ear, eyes, nose and throat, nervous system and skin disorders; relates to self-responsibility	Headaches and sleepiness
Violet	Creative, meditative; good for addictions and compulsions, agitation	Overstimulation of creative energy; contraindicated for depression

PRECAUTIONS
✖ Eyesight may be damaged by exposure to bright light, while strobe lights may cause seizures in susceptible individuals.

RESEARCH AND EVIDENCE

Scientific evidence on colour therapy has been studied by the Natural Standard (see page 157) for a number of conditions including high blood pressure and musculoskeletal pain, but the results have not been considered conclusive.

SOUND THERAPY

If you are interested in **Sound Therapy**, you may also like to read about:
- **Flower Essences**, pages 158–159
- **Chakras and the Aura**, pages 172–173
- **Colour Therapy**, page 162
- **Acupuncture**, page 126

Using sounds for healing has a long tradition. Sound therapy works on the premise that since all objects – including the human body, its organs and cells – have their own unique **resonant frequency**, it is possible to use sound to **'harmonize'** the mind and body and restore wellbeing.

Using sounds

Sounds, especially musical sounds and drumming, play a part in many healing traditions around the world, such as Buddhist chanting, choral singing, shamanic drumming and the sounding of Tibetan bowls. In a totally different way, sound waves are used in modern medicine for the disruption of kidney stones and gallstones, or in ultrasound therapy and imaging.

Resonant frequency

According to sound therapists, every cell in the body resonates at its own sound frequency, and in good health, this frequency is constant and even. But when there is illness, the affected area acquires a different resonance. In sound therapy, a practitioner claims to generate a sound that is identical to that of a healthy cell in the affected part of the body. The aim is to 'harmonize' the flow of regulatory information in the mind and body, and so restore good health. Interestingly, the sound required may not even be heard by the human ear. The field of cymatics was pioneered by Swiss scientist Dr Hans Jenny in the 1950s, and many practitioners use his techniques today.

Harmony

The concept of harmony occurs throughout vibrational medicine. This is no coincidence, since the body is in some ways like an orchestra. Music provides some useful metaphors for the beautifully organized coordination of body systems, mind and environment on which health depends, so when the body-mind lacks harmony and rhythm, we get ill.

In sound therapies this 'harmony' is imagined as a composite frequency set up by the vibrations of all the cells in the body. Vibrational therapists maintain that when an area of the body is 'out of tune', it affects the whole.

Sound healers use voice, musical instruments and modern technology to effect changes in wellbeing. The practice of cymatics involves using special equipment to generate frequencies and harmonics aimed at stimulating affected systems in the body. Some therapists use a modification of acupuncture, in which calibrated tuning forks are sounded at specific acupuncture points. Traditionally, each chakra (energy centre of the body) has its special sound and affinity with particular processes in the body, and some sound therapists try to make use of such properties.

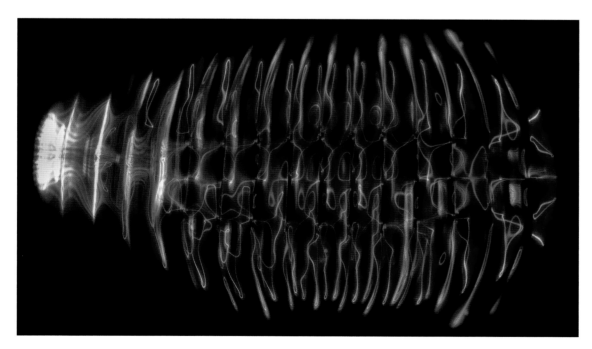

Cymatic imaging *Cymatics is a technique that uses fine particles such as those in smoke to make sound patterns visible. As the image shows, voice and music patterns can be very beautiful.*

RESEARCH AND EVIDENCE

Practitioners claim that sound therapy has been successfully used for the treatment of pain, inflammation, arthritis, rheumatism, back pain, post-operative healing, fractures and muscular injuries. It is also used for a wide range of physical and emotional conditions. However, to date there are insufficient clinical trials to support these claims.

HEALING WATER

Water has long been used both externally and internally to promote wellbeing and health. **Hydrotherapy**, **thalassotherapy** and **flotation therapy** are just some of the tools that modern therapists use to harness the healing power of water. In general these therapies use the physical force of water rather than its 'vibrational' possibilities.

If you are interested in **Healing Water**, you may also like to read about:
- Flower Essences, pages 158–159
- Crystal Healing, pages 166–167
- Chakras and the Aura, pages 172–173
- Sound Therapy, page 163

Hydrotherapy

This is literally treatment with water in each of its three forms: solid (ice), liquid and vapour (steam). Water can act as a natural stimulus, increasing energy and boosting resistance to disease, and improving body awareness. As warm-blooded beings we react sensitively to changes in temperature, and these reactions have been found to activate vital body systems. The nerves carry impulses felt at the skin deeper into the body, where they are said to stimulate the immune system, influence the production of stress hormones, invigorate the circulation and digestion, encouraging blood flow and lessen pain sensitivity.

Modern-day hydrotherapy can involve whirlpools, jacuzzis, hot tubs, saunas, steam rooms, pools, baths, showers (which also employ water massage techniques), compresses and internal hydrotherapy (such as colonic irrigation and douching) as well as sitz, spinal, head and foot baths.

Thalassotherapy

Based on the Greek word *thalassa*, meaning 'sea', thalassotherapy is a hydrotherapy treatment that utilizes sea water and other sea 'products', such as seaweed, sea salts, algae, mud and sand. Bathing in sea water is a purification ritual that is still undertaken in many countries around the world. Therapists believe that sea water is charged with negative ions and elements that help calm the mind and body.

According to thalassotherapists, contact with sea water opens up the skin's pores, allowing precious trace elements to be absorbed into the bloodstream. Various types of seaweed are reputed to have antibiotic, antiviral, anti-inflammatory, nourishing and other therapeutic qualities, and here once again we can recognize the language of vibrational medicine, because these substances are also said to convey the energy of the sea itself, and the healing power of water to restore and rejuvenate.

Flotation therapy

Originally undertaken as an experiment to gauge the effects of sensory deprivation, flotation tanks are now widely used for flotation therapy, which claims a host of therapeutic benefits. Dissolving large amounts of Epsom salts (magnesium sulphate) in water produces a solution so dense that the body floats on its surface. Once released from the pressures of gravity in a darkened flotation tank, muscles can achieve deep relaxation. People who find flotation helpful generally say that the benefits of this relaxation (though scientifically unproven) include feelings of rejuvenation, clarity of thought and enhanced physical and mental resilience.

Water and water memory

High-ranking immunologist Dr Jacques Benveniste (1935–2004) put forward the concept of 'water memory' after apparently demonstrating that water retains the 'memory' of molecules even at extremely weak dilutions, and suggested that this might explain the therapeutic properties of homeopathic medicines. Exciting though these ideas seem, researchers who tried to reproduce his results largely failed.

The ideas of Dr Masaru Emoto are even more revolutionary than Benveniste's. He claims to show that the molecular structure of water can be changed by thoughts, words, ideas and music. Emoto believes that his research shows that water has the ability to absorb, hold and even retransmit human feelings and emotions. Although he has promoted his work as demonstrating the interconnectedness of mind and matter, far more rigorous research will be needed before Dr Emoto's remarkable claims can be verified.

PRECAUTIONS

✻ Recipients should avoid sudden or prolonged exposure to extreme temperatures in baths, wraps, saunas or other types of hydrotherapy. This applies particularly to pregnant women and those with heart or lung disease.

✻ Heat can cause dehydration or low blood sodium levels. People with circulatory disorders such as chilblains or Raynaud's disease may find that their symptoms worsen in cold temperatures.

✻ High water temperatures should be avoided by those with temperature-sensitivity disorders, such as neuropathy, and by people fitted with pacemakers, defibrillators or liver infusion pumps.

✻ Some contaminants or additives in water (such as essential oils and chlorine) can irritate the skin. People suffering from dermatitis, eczema or open wounds may risk skin infections, or a worsening of their symptoms.

✻ Therapy with water jets is not recommended for those suffering from fractures, blood clots, bleeding disorders, severe osteoporosis or open wounds. Pregnant women should avoid water-jet therapy and therapies that use very hot water.

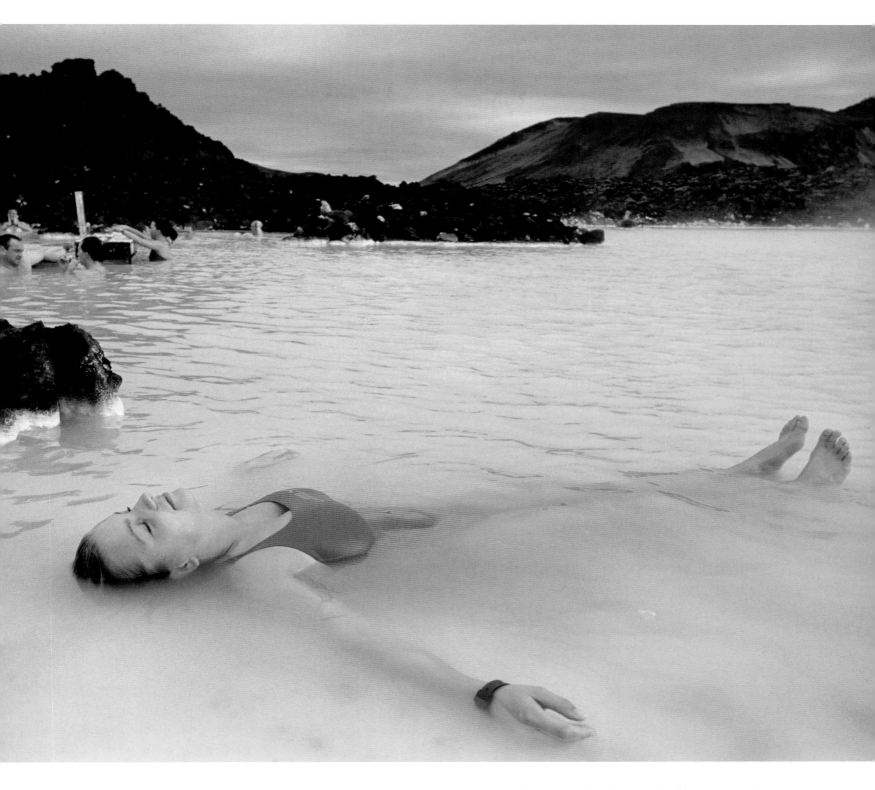

The Blue Lagoon, Iceland *The geothermal sea water found here is unique and contains minerals, silica and algae, which all exert positive influences on the skin.*

RESEARCH AND EVIDENCE

According to a review of scientific studies by the Natural Standard (see page 157), some studies indicate that mild back pain can be reduced by regular use of hot whirlpool baths with massaging jets. However, additional research is necessary.

CRYSTAL HEALING

If you are interested in **Crystal Healing**, you may like to read about:

- Flower Essences, pages 158–159
- Healing Water, pages 164–165
- Chakras and the Aura, pages 172–173
- Reiki, pages 174–175
- Spiritual Healing and Therapeutic Touch, pages 176–177
- Colour Therapy, page 162

The use of crystals in all their **forms** is a type of healing ritual that can be traced back to ancient times. Crystal therapists construe ill health (physical or emotional) as being due to disordered vibrations in the body and believe that specific crystals can encourage healing by correcting those vibrations. Healers also work with crystals on the body's energy centres (**chakras**) in various ways to nourish and balance them or to unblock the flow of energy. Crystals are also used for **meditation** and in **gem essences**, and certain **colours** of stones can be chosen and **worn** for psychological and/or physical benefit.

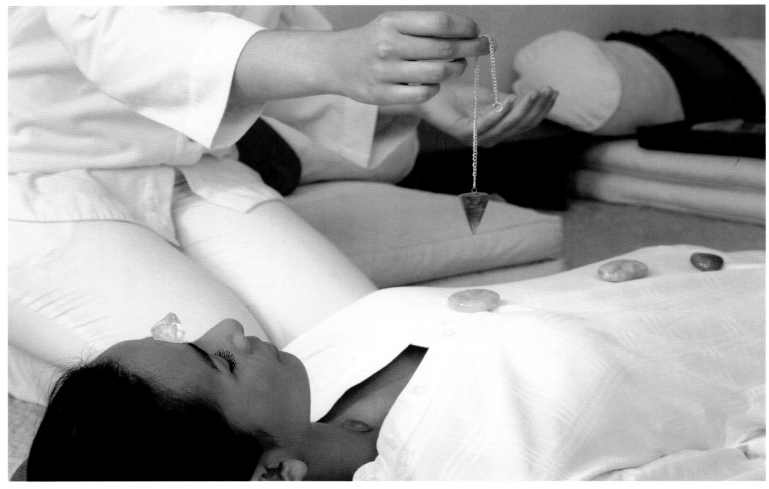

Crystal therapy *Crystals set in an energy field will collect and focus that energy, which is why they are so effective in balancing the energy of the various chakras.*

WEARING CRYSTALS

Many people are deeply attracted to wearing gems and crystals. If one believes in the healing power of a jewel or crystal, then wearing it with this intention may improve the wearer's sense of wellbeing. Crystal healers recommend a pendant that hangs down towards the heart as the most effective type of jewellery for healing purposes, because the heart is believed to be the 'bridging chakra' between spirit and matter. Crystals can be worn over the thymus (midway between the heart and throat chakra) as practitioner's claim that this can stimulate the immune system. Some crystals can be cleansed by holding them under running water and then placing them in the sun to 're-energize'.

Stone	Moonstone	Clear quartz	Amethyst	Rose quartz	Citrine	Iolite
Effect	Balances hormones	Keeps clear focus	Relaxes the mind	Enhances unconditional love	Energizes the mind	Inspires creativity

Crystal forms

Crystals were formed from the gases and minerals in the Earth's molten core rising to the Earth's mantle to cool and solidify. They are characterized by their geometric structure, conforming to one of seven basic shapes – hexagonal, cubic, triagonal, tetragonal, orthorhombic, triclinic and monoclinic. Crystals may be amorphic – lacking an inner structure.

Crystals and chakras

The chakras are conceived of as a kind of backbone of the 'energy body', and the vibrational frequencies of crystals are said to correspond to the different chakras. Crystal healers believe that crystals can unblock or transform the disordered flow of energy that they consider to be the cause of ill health.

Crystals may be selected according to the traditional colour of the chakra that is to be worked on. A practitioner might place them on the body over the chakra (solar plexus, heart, throat or forehead, for instance) while the client is encouraged to visualize their own energy flow in alignment with that of the crystal. Alternatively, they might be placed around the body, laid out in specific arrangements on the body or simply held in the hands. Although they are normally placed on chakras or organs that need specific healing, practitioners say they can also be used to expand spiritual awareness. For example, quartz is one of the most frequently used stones to heal and balance the seventh (crown) chakra, which is believed to bring the recipient closer to the divine. Pure white light passes easily through clear quartz, leaving all the colours of the spectrum unaltered.

Gem essences

These are said to capture the properties of crystals by immersing a cleansed stone in spring water and allowing sunlight to transfer the energy signature or 'vibration' of the stone, along with its healing properties, to the water. Some crystals are toxic and cannot be placed directly into the water. Essences can be used sublingually (beneath the tongue), rubbed on the skin, sprayed around a room or dropped into a bath.

Crystal meditation

Crystals are meditated with by holding the crystal, allowing the eyes to go slightly out of focus and gazing into the crystal while breathing gently with the out-breath slightly longer than the in. The eyes then explore the crystal until they are ready to close. This is supposed to bring an alignment between the meditator's mind and the vibrations of the crystal, inducing relaxation. Adherents of crystal meditation claim that it plays a dual role in opening the mind and encouraging the flow of energy. Healers recommend specific crystals to realign the energy imbalance that lies behind a specific ailment.

Crystal colours

There are obvious overlaps between colour therapy and crystal therapy. In both therapies colours are viewed as vibrations that affect various areas of the body and have different kinds of psychological impact. Both colour and crystal therapists believe that people feel an affinity with a certain colour or type of crystal because they need its vibration, and certain colours of gemstones (as in colour therapy) are said to have various qualities, as follows:

- Red crystals stimulate and strengthen
- Blue crystals ground and project energy
- Green crystals balance and provide healing
- White or clear crystals purify
- Orange crystals activate or construct
- Yellow crystals awaken and energize
- Pink crystals nurture and comfort.

PRECAUTIONS

✖ Crystal therapy should not be relied upon as the sole treatment for potentially dangerous conditions.

RESEARCH AND EVIDENCE

Although very popular, crystal therapy is based on non-scientific concepts and has not been studied scientifically. Its effectiveness is unknown.

APPLIED KINESIOLOGY

If you are interested in **Applied Kinesiology,** you may also like to read about:
- **Reiki**, pages 174–175
- **Crystal Healing**, pages 166–167
- **Polarity Therapy**, page 169

This therapy is based on a combination of Western science and Eastern principles of **energy flow.** Applied kinesiologists test **muscle strength** to identify imbalances in the body's structural, chemical and emotional energy. Some practitioners who use applied kinesiology for diagnosis also claim it can restore health.

Energy flow

US chiropractor George J. Goodheart (1918–2008) developed applied kinesiology (AK) in 1964. It is based on the idea that the body has a system of channels or meridians through which information in the form of energy flows. According to this theory we are healthy when energy flows freely, ensuring that every organ, cell and muscle along its pathways functions well. Conversely, when any of these organs is not functioning well, everything along the pathway is affected. Since this will include muscles associated with particular channels, it is supposedly possible to ascertain the health of organs by testing the strength of the related muscles. So, for example, according to AK theory, the muscles on the front of the thighs are linked energetically to the small intestine. Therefore, if someone has been eating a food to which they are intolerant, an AK practitioner would predict a problem with the energy in the entire small-intestine channel, including the front of the thighs. The AK method is said to be capable of diagnosing physical, mental and emotional problems.

Muscle strength

AK practitioners diagnose such problems by testing muscles on various meridians to establish the health of every organ and system along that meridian (see page 101). In most cases, they will touch a part of the body that links to a particular muscle, while quickly and gently pressing down on the limb itself. The practitioner will ask the patient to resist this pressure, and if they are unable to, this is said to be a sign that there is an energy imbalance in a related body part. If the patient can resist the pressure, the energy will be flowing normally. A kinesiologist may test the strength of the relevant muscles, and work backwards to find the cause of the problem.

Practitioners generally use the AK technique to identify the treatment required in order to correct the imbalance found. For example, the client

might be asked to hold samples of various homeopathic remedies, nutritional supplements or vials containing materials to which they might be allergic. Improvement in muscle strength is said to indicate a substance that would help restore health. Some practitioners of other therapies, such as osteopathy, chiropractic, nutritional therapy and acupuncture, claim that they find AK an effective tool and use it in combination with their main treatment modality.

Kinesiology treatment *When there is blocked, stagnant or excessive energy, the electrical signals of the muscles involved go weak and do not respond to pressure.*

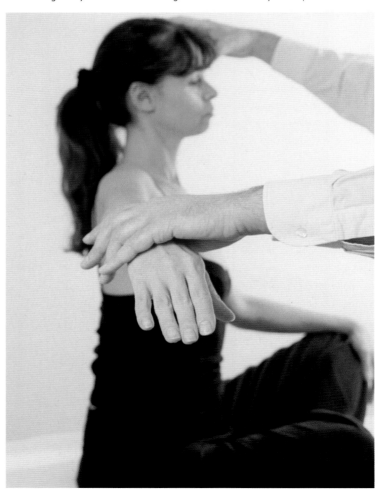

RESEARCH AND EVIDENCE
The conventional research and medical communities see AK as pseudoscience. Although AK's adherents and convinced users claim that the methods are effective, the available scientific research suggests otherwise.

POLARITY THERAPY

If you are interested in **Polarity Therapy**, you may also like to read about:

- Traditional Chinese Medicine, pages 98–101
- Chakras and the Aura, pages 172–173
- Yoga, pages 106–109
- Ayurveda, pages 94–97

Polarity therapy is based on the premise that the **flow and balance of energy** is the foundation of good health, and that this is governed by five energy centres, known as chakras. Therapists use **four healing techniques** to resolve energy blockages and restore good health.

Energy flow and balance

Polarity therapy was invented by naturopath and chiropractor Dr Randolph Stone (1890–1981), who believed that the human energy field is affected by a multitude of factors, including diet, touch, movement, sound, attitudes, relationships, trauma and the environment. He coined the term 'polarity therapy', which borrowed the notion of opposing forces (yin and yang) from Chinese philosophy. The theory is that 'energy' flows from the universe into the body through the chakras (see page 172), which distribute energy throughout the body. The name 'polarity' was given to convey the image of electro-magnetic energy flowing between the body's positive and negative poles.

Polarity therapists believe that energy flows in three currents to and from an energy source in the brain: negative, positive and neutral. These currents, known as *gunas*, run vertically from 'north to south', transversely from 'east to west' and outwards in spirals that start at the navel. Where the positive and negative *gunas* cross, they create a vortex of energy known as a chakra. Neutral *gunas* flow up and down the spine, linking and earthing the chakras. Each chakra is linked to particular body parts and certain emotional patterns. All body parts and chakras are said to be associated predominantly with one of the five elements: air, fire, water, earth and ether – ideas borrowed from Ayurvedic medicine.

Four healing techniques

Polarity therapists see their work as balancing opposing energies in the body, and they employ four main techniques: touch, awareness skills, diet and yoga postures. Three kinds of touch can be used – neutral (light), negative (deep) or positive (stimulating) – to remove blockages and balance the energy flow. Awareness skills are taught to encourage resolution of emotional issues that are said to cause energy flow to stagnate. Diets are prescribed to address specific energy problems. Finally, yoga postures are prescribed to stimulate particular chakras or release energy blockages.

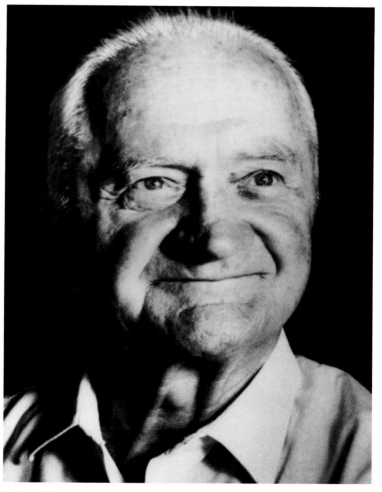

Dr Randolph Stone *Naturopath and chiropractor Dr Randolph Stone believed that a blockage of physical energy results in illness and unhappiness, and that this energy can be harnessed for spiritual development.*

PRECAUTIONS

✖ Polarity therapy should not be solely relied upon for the treatment of a potentially severe medical condition.

RESEARCH AND EVIDENCE

According to the review of scientific studies by the Natural Standard (see page 157) there is no evidence for the effectiveness of this therapy, nor scientific grounds for its theories.

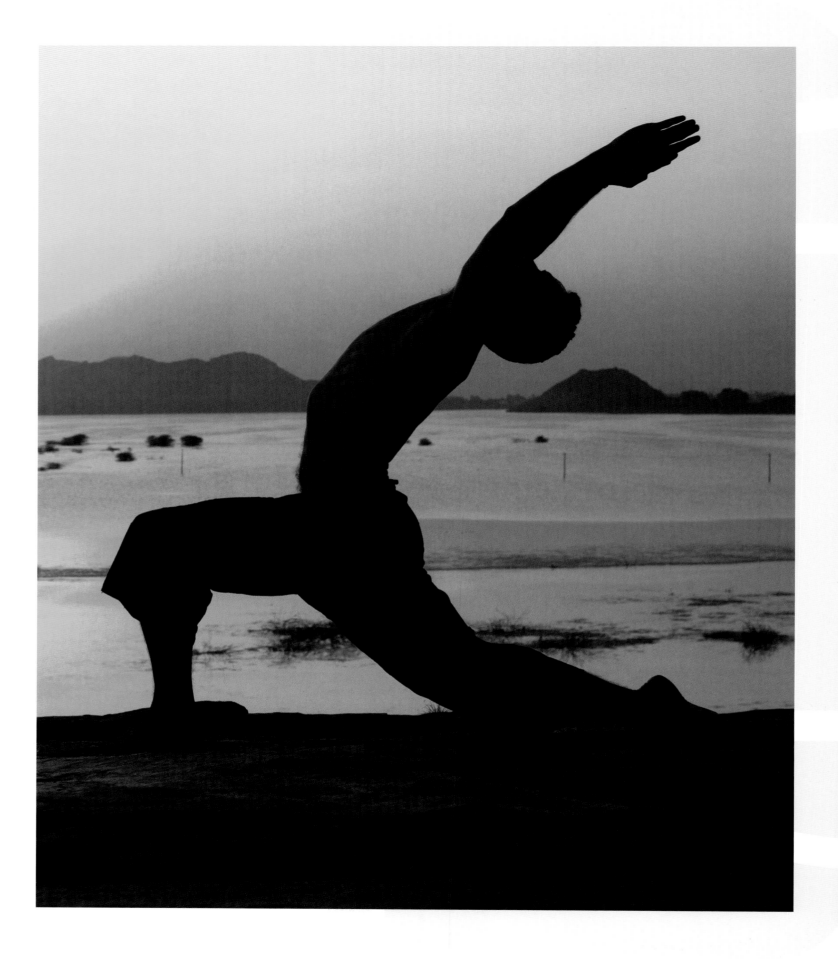

BODY AND SPIRIT

Eastern systems of healing, such as ayurveda, have long recognized the concept of 'spirit' as a fundamental building block of health. In Eastern philosophy we are viewed first and foremost as a spirit experiencing existence, and there is a belief in a universal order – a cosmic consciousness – that pervades all life. We can access this cosmic consciousness through our inner wisdom, and it is the aspect of our individuality that cannot be swayed by the demands of daily life or our ego. This cosmic consciousness is manifested in the physical world, in the five elements – wood, fire, earth, metal and water – of which the material world consists, as well as in our physical bodies. Ultimately, therefore, our health and wellbeing are part of, and interconnected with, the physical manifestation of cosmic consciousness.

Western separation of spirit from body

In Western religious traditions, by contrast, spirit and flesh have been separated, and the spirit is considered to be definitively non-material. St Paul was one of the key theologians to define this dichotomy. In the Epistle to the Romans 8:13 he wrote: 'For if you live according to the flesh you will die, but if by the Spirit you put to death the deeds of the body you will live.' And in Galatians 5:24 he continued in the same vein: 'Those who belong to Christ Jesus have crucified the flesh with its passions and desires.' This separation has influenced Western culture ever since, including the approach to health. With the demise of the concept of the four humours – that is, the relative proportions of blood, phlegm, yellow bile and black bile as the determinant of a person's physical and mental qualities (see also pages 15 and 75) – and its impact on healing from the Renaissance onwards, Western medical science has gradually come to reject any notion of subtle energy or the concept of spirit playing a role in health, and has instead relied on the development of the understanding of the physical body alone to determine a system of healthcare and wellbeing.

Yoga *Originally an Eastern tradition, yoga is now widely practised in the West as a method of synchronizing body and spirit. It instils practitioners with a feeling of peace and wellbeing.*

Yet in recent years this separation of spirit from body has come to be questioned. In part due to an increased recognition of the role that the mind plays in influencing health via the science of psychoneuroimmunology (see pages 76–77), health practitioners have become more accepting of the importance of spirituality in achieving good health and wellbeing. American doctor and author Larry Dossey is one of the chief advocates of spirituality-based medicine. In his bestselling book *Reinventing Medicine* (1999), he writes: 'I used to believe that we must choose between science and reason on one hand, and spirituality on the other, in how we lead our lives. Now I consider this a false choice. We can recover the sense of sacredness, not just in science, but in perhaps every area of life.'

The healing power of spirit and spirituality

Although it has proved difficult to conduct rigorous scientific studies on the effects of spirituality and prayer on health, some studies do show benefits to patients. According to the US-based CentraState Medical Centre, 'the psychological benefits of prayer may help reduce stress and anxiety, promote a more positive outlook and strengthen the will to live'.

Increasingly, individuals have turned to healing approaches such as reiki and spiritual healing based on the concept of accessing healing energies. Others have focused on healing via the chakras (energy centres of the body identified in ancient Indian texts) and the aura (the body's energy field) as a visual manifestation of our 'animating energy'. Although such concepts may lack scientific evidence to support them, many people consider the balancing of these subtle energies to be an integral part of their approach to health. There is a range of therapies claiming to work directly on the energy field.

All cultures have traditionally understood that we possess a spirit, animating energy or vital force that links to a universal energy or spirit that governs all life. According to Larry Dossey, we may be about to enter a third era of medicine that recognizes spirit as a powerful healing tool. He describes the first era of medicine as 'physical medicine', based on treating the body primarily with drugs, the second era as 'mind–body', dealing with psychological impacts on health, and the third era as 'eternity medicine', where patients are affected by intercessory prayer.

CHAKRAS AND THE AURA

Traditional healing systems tell us that our mind lives not just in the brain, but in the body too, and in the biosphere. Increasingly, neuroscientists and 'deep ecologists' would agree. Spiritual traditions also remind us that we are part of an intelligent, evolving universe. **Chakras** and the associated idea of an **aura** round the body may help us imagine, or even embody these important 21st-century ideas.

If you are interested in **Chakras and the Aura**, you may also like to read about:
- **Traditional Chinese Medicine**, pages 98–101
- **Yoga**, pages 106–109
- **Theosophy**, pages 270–271
- **Polarity Therapy**, page 169
- **Crystal Healing**, pages 166–167
- **Ayurveda**, pages 94–97
- **Reiki**, pages 174–175

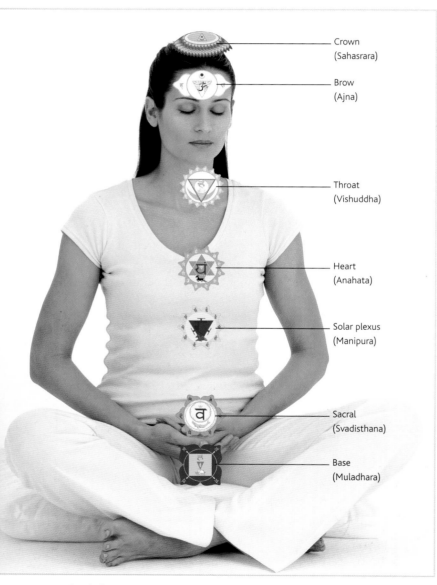

Crown
(Sahasrara)

Brow
(Ajna)

Throat
(Vishuddha)

Heart
(Anahata)

Solar plexus
(Manipura)

Sacral
(Svadisthana)

Base
(Muladhara)

The chakras *According to sacred texts, the chakras form a profound formula for wholeness and a template for transformation on all levels.*

The development of chakra theory

In the oldest-recorded descriptions of the chakras found in the Hindu sacred texts, the *Upanishads*, dating back at the earliest to c. 600 BCE, they are considered to be places occupied by the soul and characterized by a particular state of consciousness. During the 19th and 20th centuries Western contact with Indian culture led to a melding of spiritual traditions with Western insights into endocrine physiology, resulting in the quasi-scientific notions of chakras that we have today.

From the original discussion of the chakras in the *Upanishads*, chakra theory was extensively developed by Shaktism, a religious sect that arose in India in the 5th century BCE, which described the seven major chakras that are recognized today, aligned from the base of the spine to the top of the head. According to the Shakta tradition, the chakras are centres of pure consciousness and focal points for meditation. Shaktism also identified associations for each chakra: its element, visual symbol, mantric sound, deity and colour.

In Shakta theory the seven chakras are strung along the primary *nadi*, or channel of energy, in the body – the *sushumna nadi*. In addition there are two secondary *nadis* on either side of the *sushumna*: the *ida* on the left (containing descending life force) and the *pingala* on the right (containing ascending life force). The aim of Shakti practice was to awaken powerful kundalini energy, a vital life force unleashed during the creation of the world. Kundalini was considered to lie dormant at the base of the spine. By directing the energy of the secondary *nadi* into the central *nadi*, kundalini could be raised through each chakra in turn until it reached the highest crown chakra, at which point a state of enlightenment could be reached. Kundalini energy remains an important focus for many people today in the practice of meditation and yoga.

The West was first introduced to the concept of chakras and kundalini through the publication of *The Serpent Power* (1919) by Arthur Avalon, a pseudonym of Sir John Woodroffe (1865–1936), translator of nearly 20 ancient Sanskrit texts. Our understanding also owes much to the Theosophist Charles W. Leadbeater (1854–1934), whose book *The Chakras* was published in 1927. Leadbeater developed the concept that the chakras could be seen

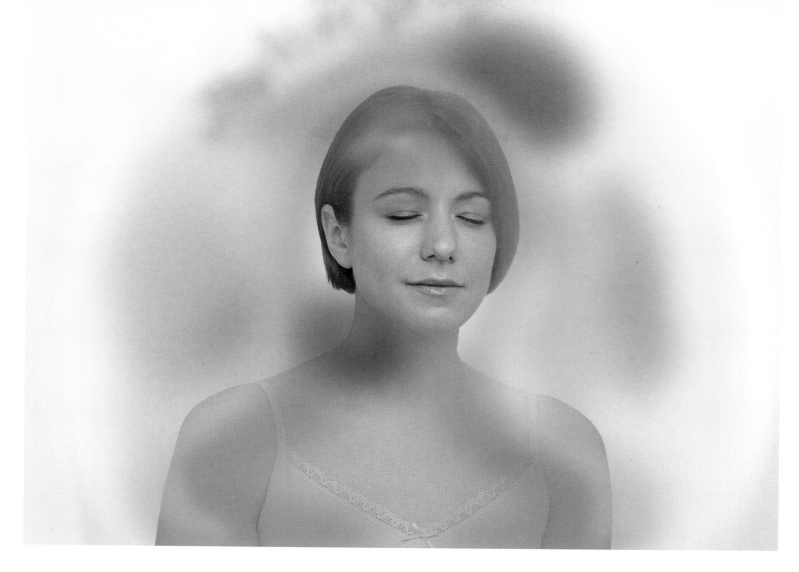

psychically as rotating discs or wheels and that subtle energies are centred in and moved by the chakras. He was the first person to suggest a link between the chakras and the various subtle layers of the aura. His notion of the chakras as being crucial in helping to maintain healthy energy flow is now a central aspect of the contemporary understanding of the chakras.

Alice Bailey (1880–1949), another member of the Theosophical Society, together with Leadbeater associated the chakras with particular endocrine glands and the sympathetic nervous system. Many people have observed that the traditional position of the chakras corresponds to the positions and functions of the glands of the endocrine system and the positions of the nerve ganglia along the spinal column. Whether Indian mystics intuited this link is unknown, but this correspondence forms the basis of the contemporary view that the chakras profoundly influence health and govern the effective functioning of particular systems of the body.

The aura

Related to the chakra system is the concept of the aura: a form of energy field that is the external manifestation of our physical and psychological energy. People who claim a paranormal ability to see auras report that they constantly shift in size, shape and colouring in response to thoughts and

The aura *Auras look something like this according to clairvoyants. The aura is said to reflect the emotional and energetic field of people and objects. It is claimed that the colour spectrum varies with our physical, emotional, mental and spiritual states.*

emotions, and believe that the qualities of a person's aura can provide information about their spiritual health and wellbeing. They also alter in response to external stimuli, such as sound, colour and light, as well as environmental electromagnetic energy. However, when aura-reading psychics have been tested in experiments, for instance in darkened rooms or with subjects behind screens, evidence of their ability has not been forthcoming.

Scientific interest in the aura was given a boost in the 1970s by Kirlian Photography (KP). Developed by Russian scientist Semyon Kirlian (1898–1978) in 1939, KP involves placing objects on a highly charged photographic plate. Kirlian discovered that beautiful patterns of light appear around the objects when photographed — especially living creatures. But the case for KP as evidence for auras has been overstated: they are products of the electric field's interaction with living tissue rather than emanations from the body itself. Sceptics, who point out that even coins or paper clips generate a Kirlian 'aura', assert that there is no scientific evidence that KP patterns have diagnostic or psychic significance.

REIKI

If you are interested in **Reiki**, you may also like to read about:

- **Traditional Chinese Medicine**, pages 98–101
- **Polarity Therapy**, page 169
- **Chakras and the Aura**, pages 172–173
- **Spiritual Healing and Therapeutic Touch**, pages 176–177

The word 'reiki' is compounded from two Japanese words: *rei*, meaning 'universal higher power', and *ki*, which translates as 'energy' or 'life force'. From its **origins** as a Japanese meditational practice in the 1920s, reiki has since become a prominent form of complementary therapy based on the idea that **energy for healing** is **channelled** through a **reiki practitioner's** hands. The theory is that illness occurs when 'vital energy', or *ki*, is low or 'out of balance' and that reiki **treatment** works to restore *ki*.

The origins of reiki

Reiki is said to have been revealed to Japanese scholar Dr Mikao Usai (1865–1926) after 21 days of fasting and meditation on a holy mountain in Japan. According to legend he stood under a sacred waterfall, undertaking a meditation to open and purify the topmost chakra. Upon his return, Usai claimed he could heal 'without energy depletion', a method he developed into the system now known as reiki. Only in the last 15 years has this therapy been widely practised in the West.

Channelling energy for healing

Reiki practitioners channel 'healing energy' in particular patterns, with the aim of encouraging a deep sense of relaxation, unblocking the flow of *ki* and 'detoxifying' the body, thus providing a new vitality. Most reiki treatments do not involve actual touch; the reiki master holds his or her hands several centimetres away from the recipient's body and controls the energy field from there. The energy is said to flow from a universal source through the practitioner, who transfers it to the recipient. It is believed that the reiki energy enters the body of the practitioner at the throat chakra and is released through the hands. According to reiki practitioners, recipients take an active and responsible part in the healing process, instinctively drawing in the energy and directing it to where it is needed through the chakras (energy centres), meridians (energy channels) and the nervous system.

Reiki practitioners

Reiki energy is transferred to students, who require no special abilities or training, by reiki masters through a series of 'attunements'. During the process of attunement a series of symbols is 'sealed into the student's energy field' in order to open the student permanently to reiki energy, which they can then use to treat themselves or others.

Reiki has much in common with other forms of spiritual or energy healing. It has been observed that energy healers may inadvertently be drained of their own life energy or unknowingly take on the pain and dysfunction of

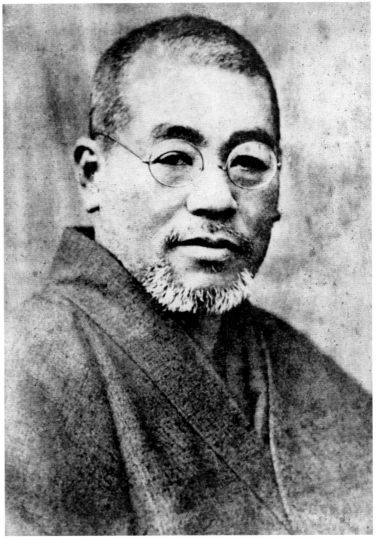

Dr Mikao Usai *During his mystical experience on Mount Kurama, Dr Mikao Usai received the ability to perform reiki and subsequently developed a system of healing.*

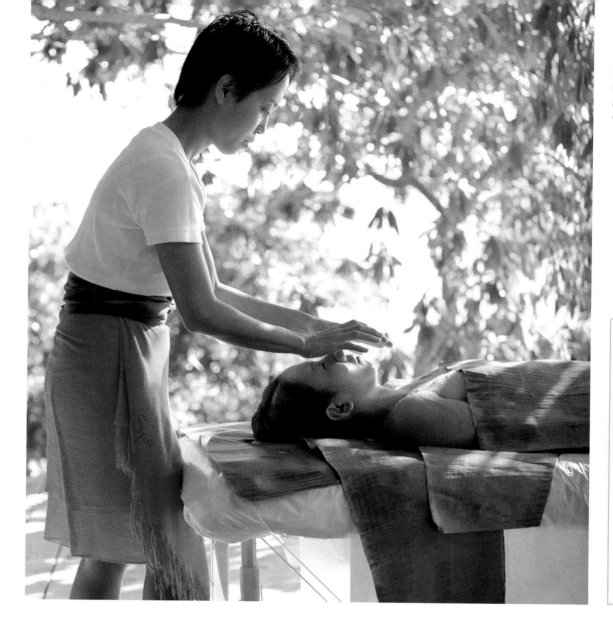

Reiki treatment *A reiki practitioner is a channel for directing energy to wherever healing is needed, but it is the recipient who is the actual healer.*

others while dispensing treatment. However, reiki practitioners, it is claimed, are not only protected from these hazards, but actually replenish their life energy by practising reiki.

There are three degrees of training, and in the second one practitioners are equipped to perform reiki from a distance. This method involves using symbols to form a connection between practitioner and recipient, regardless of location, to facilitate the transmission of energy. In the third degree of training practitioners become reiki masters, capable of attuning other people to reiki and teaching the three degrees. It normally takes at least six months of training and supervised experience before an individual can set up as a professional reiki practitioner.

Treatment

Recipients normally lie down for treatment, which can take between 45 and 90 minutes, although some practitioners target and channel universal energy to particular areas of the body, which takes less time. The recipient may experience feelings of warmth or tingling, and a state of deep relaxation and general wellbeing. It is not uncommon for there to be a reported release of emotions, which is believed to reflect the unblocking and balancing of energy within the body.

Reiki aims to stimulate healing processes rather than effect a cure. Several sessions are normally required, and there are said to be no side effects from the treatment. Reiki is becoming increasingly popular in the West for pain management, stress-related health conditions, insomnia and skin disorders. Reiki practitioners believe that it encourages optimum emotional and mental health, improves creativity, encourages focus and inspires self-confidence.

RESEARCH AND EVIDENCE

According to the Natural Standard, an international research collaboration that produces scientifically based reviews of complementary and alternative medicine topics, reiki has been studied for its effects on the nervous system, including heart rate and blood pressure, pain management, depression and memory. However, the results are not conclusive. As with all 'energy therapies', science rejects the theory on which reiki is based.

SPIRITUAL HEALING AND THERAPEUTIC TOUCH

If you are interested in **Spiritual Healing and Therapeutic Touch**, you may also like to read about:
- Traditional Chinese Medicine, pages 98–101
- Chakras and the Aura, pages 172–173
- Reiki, pages 174–175

Spiritual healing involves channelling a 'divine' or universal **healing energy** from its **spiritual source** to a recipient via a 'healer'. According to adherents, spiritual **healing treatment** has the power to balance the mind, body and spirit, thus achieving **benefits** to the recipient's wellbeing. Less overtly spiritual in approach, **therapeutic touch** involves the use of the 'energy field' to heal and restore balance.

Healing energy

Spiritual healing is based on the premise that our bodies are designed to heal themselves when there is a natural flow of healing energy through the body. However, if poor diet, negative emotions, trauma, injury, stress and other adverse factors block this healing process or impede the flow of energy around the body, it leads to illness and imbalance. Spiritual healing is said to provide the energy required to restore balance so that the body, mind and spirit can create and maintain positive health and wellbeing.

Spiritual healing may be the oldest form of medical treatment, since this type of approach to healing has been practised in virtually every culture the world over throughout recorded history. In traditional cultures, where it is administered by shamans and medicine men, it is very much a part of the fabric of society. In the Western world, where body, mind and spirit have long been considered as separate, conventional medicine, which focuses on material intervention, has viewed spiritual healing with great scepticism.

Spiritual source

Although the energy channelled by spiritual healers is believed to come from God or a higher being, it does not necessarily involve religion or religious ritual. Many spiritual healers view spirituality as distinct from religion, and believe that 'spirit' is the common experience behind organized religion's different dogmas and belief systems; an experience involving awareness of and a relationship with an 'entity' that transcends the personal self. Some healers refer to this 'entity' as God; others regard it as a universal energy.

In theory at least, all of us have the power to heal should we choose to develop it. However, some spiritual healers appear to have the ability to receive this healing 'energy' or 'spirit' and successfully guide it to recipients. An element of belief would seem to be required – an indication of the strong link between mind and body – since spiritual healing fails to work for some people, perhaps because they consciously or unconsciously block the experience. Some spiritual healers appear to absorb 'negative energy' and illness from their client, which then needs to be cleared through meditation or prayer.

Treatment and benefits

Treatment normally begins with a healer 'attuning' to the healing energy. Healers will scan the body with their hands, sensing energy levels and locating areas of low or blocked energy. Some therapists work on the chakras (energy centres). Spiritual energy is then said to be transferred to the requisite areas of the body. It is common for recipients to experience feelings of heat or tingling at the site.

Spiritual healing has been used to help a variety of mental, physical and emotional problems, and has been integrated into conventional medical settings in some hospitals and general practices. It has been found to encourage relaxation, acceptance and calm, and reduce pain, alleviate physical symptoms and lift mood. There is evidence suggesting that whether or not spiritual healing proves effective at a physical level, patients' ability to cope with their health problems may improve. The reason for this is unclear, though it may be that the relaxation response and positive expectancy encourage the body to heal itself. Some research studies have found that prayer can have a positive impact on the health of ill people.

Therapeutic touch

This system of using the hands to alleviate pain and promote healing was developed in the 1960s by Dolores Krieger, Professor of Nursing at New York University, USA, and Dora Kunz, who was believed to have a natural ability to perceive unseen human energy fields. Based on the ancient ritual of the laying-on of hands, but without the specifically spiritual aspect, Krieger and Kunz believed that anyone could be taught the principles. They began running classes at Pumpkin Hollow Farm in the Berkshires, in New York State, where patients were referred by their physicians. Therapeutic touch has since spread throughout the world and is increasingly used by the nursing profession.

During the healing session the practitioner adopts a relaxed and meditative approach, using his or her hands to sense areas on the body that the patient feels are imbalanced. Most patients report a deep sensation of relaxation after the treatment.

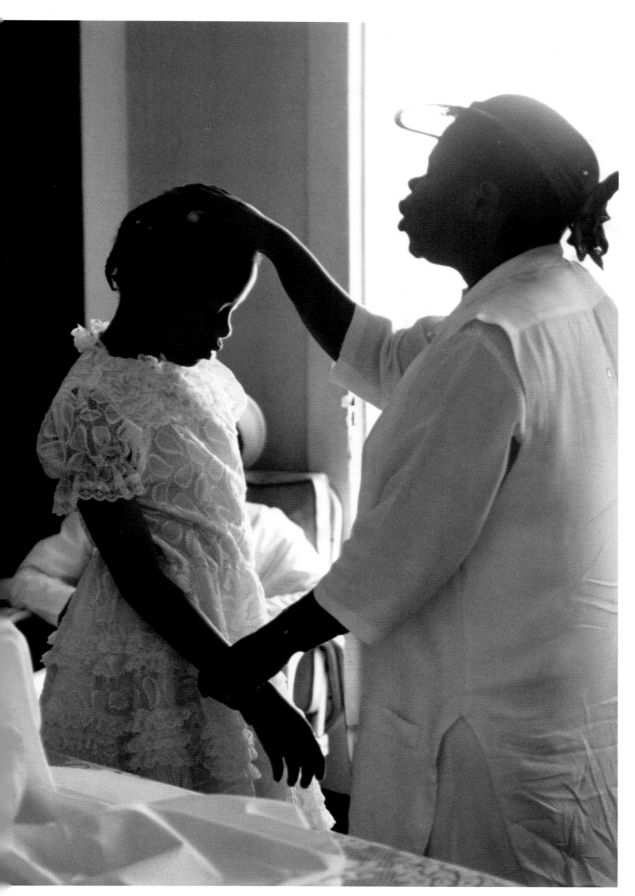

Laying-on of hands *In Kingston, Jamaica, at the Prayer Tower, the Minister asks God to heal a sick child.*

PRECAUTIONS

✖ Spiritual healing may not be appropriate for those with psychiatric conditions such as schizophrenia, or for people who may self-blame or feel ashamed if the results are not as they had hoped.

RESEARCH AND EVIDENCE

According to the Natural Standard's (see page 175) review of research, spiritual healing has been investigated for many conditions, including chronic pain, high blood pressure, rheumatoid arthritis, eczema and psychiatric disorders. Despite many positive results, the overall benefits remain scientifically unclear. However, there are many examples of qualitative research and case studies that suggest that spiritual healing can be a useful adjunct to conventional treatment.

PART THREE
SPIRIT

WESTERN FAITHS 182

EASTERN FAITHS 202

TRIBAL, SHAMANIC AND ANIMIST TRADITIONS 224

EARTH MYSTERIES 244

SPIRITUAL, SECRET AND OCCULT SOCIETIES 262

ANCIENT MYSTERIES 274

PATHS TO OTHER REALMS 288

PART THREE
SPIRIT

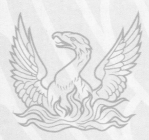

When I was 23 years old I lived in central London, in an old house divided into apartments. Some new tenants moved into the flat directly above me and then once a week had an evening of drumming and chanting. At first the noise annoyed me, but after a few weeks I began to enjoy it and started to hum along. What had started as a disturbance became a pleasure.

One day I spoke to my neighbour and asked what was going on at the weekly gathering. I also told her that I enjoyed the sound. She replied that it was a weekly meeting of a Sufi group. Sufis, she explained, were Muslims who particularly enjoyed using music to connect directly with God and love.

She then invited me to join them for a session, and I accepted. They were a very relaxed and friendly group. Their drumming and chanting touched me. I liked the ambience. It helped me to connect with the good and beautiful things in life. It also reminded me of the magical atmosphere that can often happen with Christian Holy Communion, when the wine and bread are blessed and then shared.

After the session they asked me what I thought of the evening, and I expressed my appreciation. I then took a risk and shared with them that it reminded me of the Christian sacraments. I was concerned that this might offend them. Instead they smiled. One of them told me there was a legend that the founder of their particular Sufi group was a reincarnation of Jesus.

What a surprising idea. Whether it was actually true or not did not matter. I liked it. In one stroke it melted all kinds of religious division. Islam and Christianity were entwined. Eastern ideas about reincarnation were integrated into Western faiths. In a world where religious belief is so often the cause of conflict, these Sufis presented an approach that was relaxed, loving and inclusive.

As I continued exploring the many different spiritual traditions, I increasingly met people and groups who celebrated diversity and spoke a language of oneness and interconnection. They told of a benevolent ocean of energy or consciousness in which we all live, whatever our culture and beliefs.

I stopped seeing the different faiths and traditions as being in competition with each other. We have the only path to God! Believe or go to hell! I began to see this sparkling tapestry of spiritual jewels, each offering its own valuable perspective.

Nowadays when people who are beginning their spiritual exploration come to me and ask what they should do, I always advise them to spend a couple of years tasting around. Our spiritual development is best served, I believe, if we do not restrict ourselves to the beliefs of a single faith but take time to explore the different pathways. In the contemporary world, in our global village, this kind of general enquiry is an adult and intelligent strategy. Having surveyed and understood the different approaches, we can then make decisions about what will best serve our growth and development. This, for me, is one of the great values of an encyclopedia like this one. It provides an overview and guidance for all our journeys.

May all our journeys be blessed, safe and inspiring.

William Bloom

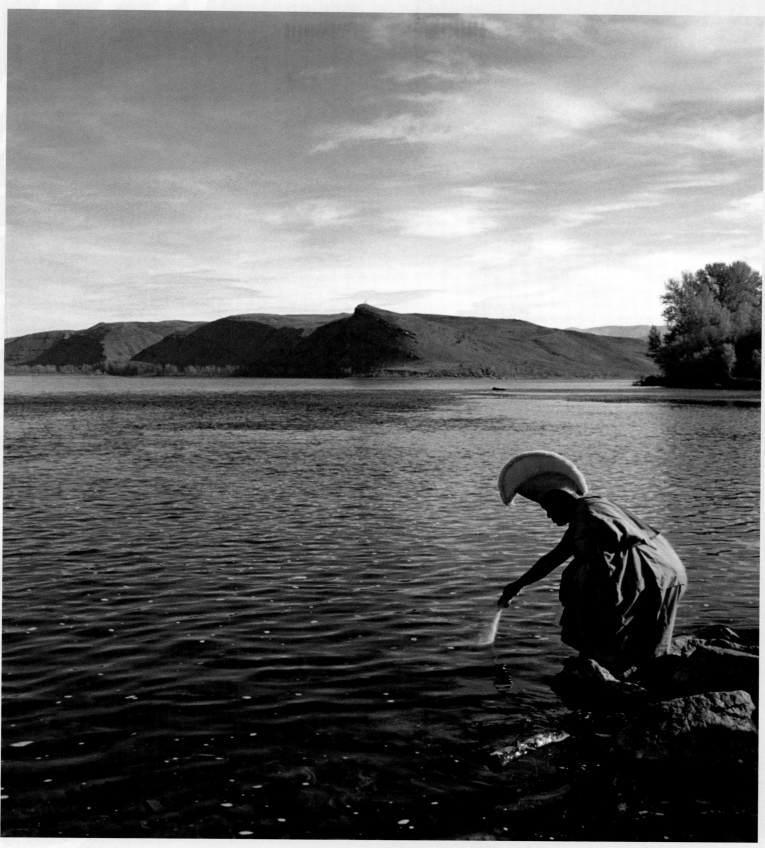

Buddhism *A Buddhist monk pours sand from a destroyed Mandala into the Ulug-Hem River in Russia.*

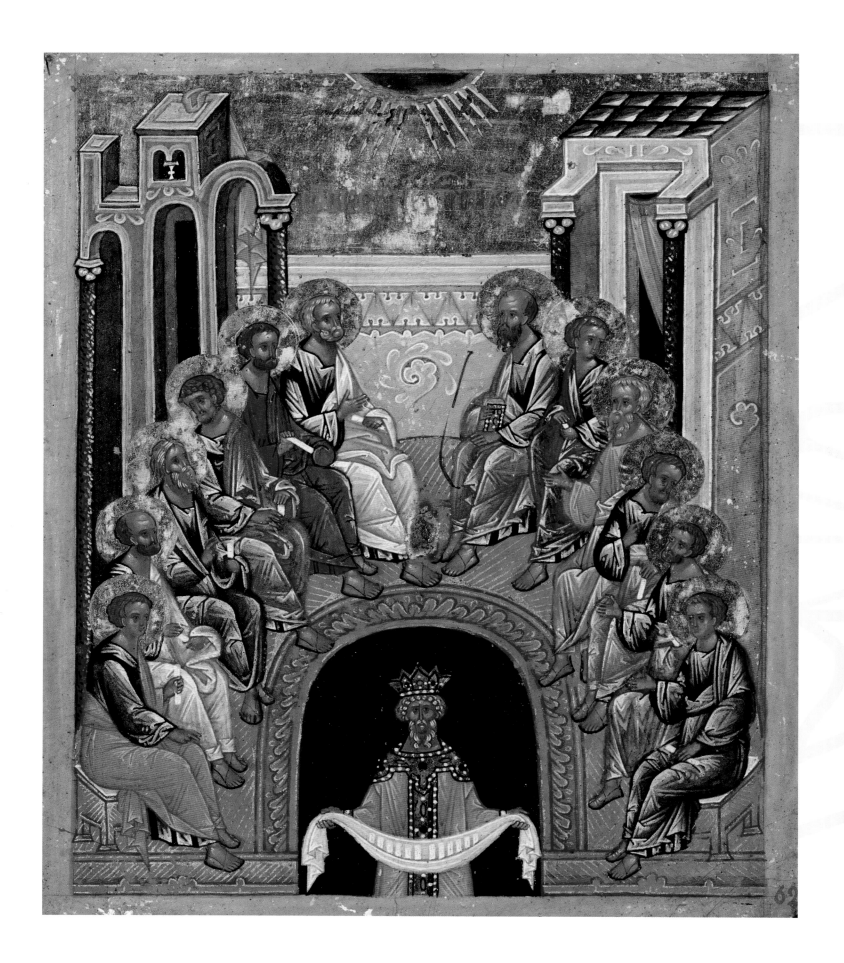

WESTERN FAITHS

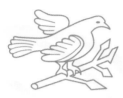 Western spirituality has been greatly influenced by the three main faiths of Judaism, Christianity and Islam. Over time, each of these faiths has grown into a major world religion, sustained by a thriving community and an accepted canon of holy scripture. Significantly, each faith also has its own inner or mystical tradition, which points to a radically different understanding of spirituality and also offers an alternative approach to reading sacred texts.

A common heritage

Judaism, Christianity and Islam developed in historical sequence, each new faith evolving from its predecessor, while also adding to the body of holy scripture. All three faiths are considered to be monotheistic, in that they all subscribe to a belief in one God, who is all-powerful and all-knowing, and who created the world and everything in it. They are also described as Abrahamic, since they each believe that Abraham gave rise to the faith when he entered into a covenant with God. This common heritage has been a source of both unity and conflict.

The significance of the sacred texts

According to Judaism, God revealed to Moses the written and spoken Torah, which includes God's laws and commandments. The Torah is thus the most sacred scripture in Judaism. According to Christianity, God sent his only son, Jesus Christ, to earth to atone for the sins of mankind. Jesus's life and teachings are described in the New Testament, which was subsequently combined with the Torah and other Jewish texts to create the Christian Bible. According to Islam, Jesus Christ was not the Son of God, but a prophet of great standing, like Moses. Islam contends that the last prophet was Muhammad, and that the Koran – the revelations given to Muhammad – is the final word of God, thus making the Koran the most important sacred text, superseding all others.

The Holy Spirit *The descent of the Holy Spirit is depicted in this 15th-century Russian icon from the Cathedral of St Sophia in Novgorod.*

Holy scripture plays a pivotal role in each of the main faiths. At one extreme it is viewed as the actual word of God to be read literally without exception; at another it is the word of God in the mouths of humans, and thus needs careful interpretation before it can be applied, leaving the door open to wide disagreement. What all three faiths do agree on, however, is that God must be worshipped and His laws obeyed if we are to gain His favour and thus be rewarded with eternal life in the heavenly hereafter. For Judaism, Christianity and Islam, spiritual practice as described in holy scripture is essential if we are to make that journey.

Spiritual traditions in contrast

The inner traditions of the three faiths – Kabbalah, Gnosticism and Sufism – see things quite differently. Much more closely associated with the Western Mystery Schools, these spiritual traditions do not see God as an abstract being to be worshipped from afar, but believe that God is in everything. Kabbalists, Gnostics and Sufis do not think that heaven is a place we go to when we die, but an ecstatic experience of the divine in the here and now. Sacred scripture is not the word of God, but a guidebook to mystical experience. They were written not to tell us God's laws, but to help us to develop the god within.

In the main faiths, God is seen as masculine, not because He is viewed as a male Being, but because God is understood to be the primal mystery that initiates everything we experience. The female principle or Goddess, by contrast, refers to what we actually experience, meaning that the universe and everything in it is female. From this mystical perspective, God is viewed as the great Mystery or Spirit; and the Goddess is viewed as the great Manifest or Matter. For followers of the inner traditions, the goal of the spiritual journey is not to reject the female world of experience, but to conjoin the male and female principles, so that Matter becomes infused with Spirit. When this is achieved, everything that we experience is imbued with mystery, or a profound sense of wonder, which is the simple recognition that God is everything and everyone. This is why so many followers of the inner traditions have proclaimed their own divinity, often causing outrage to adherents of the main faiths, who see God as a separate being.

WESTERN MYSTERY TRADITIONS

If you are interested in **Western Mystery Traditions**, you may also like to read about:

- **Numerology**, pages 66–67
- **Western Astrology**, pages 56–57
- **The Gnostic Gospels**, pages 192–193

In recent years, there has been a resurgence of interest in the Western mystery traditions of the ancient world. In particular, **Pythagoreanism** (the belief that there is an underlying order to the cosmos, which we can study to acquire profound spiritual insights) and **Gnosticism** (the view that the goal of spiritual activity is to attain experiential knowledge of our sacred self) together with **Hermeticism** (characterized by the conviction that 'All is One and All is God') have attracted special attention. What unites these traditions is a celebration of the primal mystery at the heart of life.

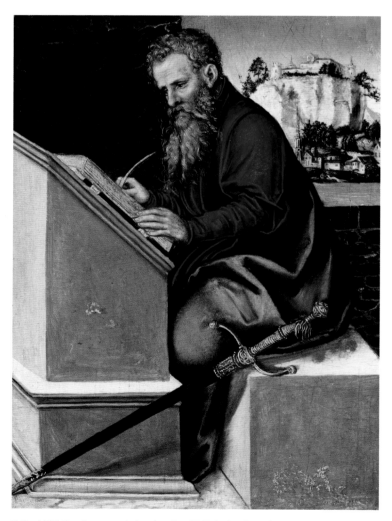

St Paul *This Renaissance painting dated to 1547 depicts St Paul, writing with a sword by his side. He was venerated by both Gnostic and orthodox Christians.*

Pythagoreanism

Pythagoras was a pagan philosopher born on the Greek island of Samos in the 6th century BCE. Although he is remembered today as one of the world's foremost mathematicians, he was renowned in his own time as a great sage with godlike powers. He was described as being dressed in flowing white robes and wore a golden coronet, travelling from place to place, healing the sick and raising the dead.

In 530 BCE Pythagoras moved to southern Italy, where he founded one of the most influential mystery schools of the Western world. There he swore his students to secrecy, before initiating them into the sacred study of mathematics and science, the occult arts of numerology and astrology, and the theory of the transmigration of souls (reincarnation). Pythagoras died around 500 BCE, but his school lived on, and a sect known as the Pythagoreans rapidly spread and flourished around Asia Minor, over time incorporating the ideas of philosophers such as Socrates (c. 469–399 BCE). As well as contributing greatly to the foundations of modern science and mathematics, the Pythagoreans laid a foundation for much contemporary spiritual practice. In particular, they recognized the need for an ethical approach to life, they believed in spiritual community, they performed purification rituals to enhance their spiritual sensitivity and they were committed vegans, considering all living creatures to have immortal souls.

Gnosticism

This term refers to the beliefs and practices of a diverse group of spiritual seekers from the Mediterranean and Middle East, who practised *gnosis*, which is Greek for 'knowledge' in the sense of enlightenment. Although Gnosticism pre-dates Christianity, many Gnostic scriptures are overtly Christian, making direct reference to a mythical Christ. This has led some modern-day scholars to argue that there never was a historical Jesus Christ, and that the stories of Jesus's life were actually composed by Jewish Gnostics as a way of conveying the secret teachings of gnosis, a belief that was given increased credibility following the discovery of the Gnostic Gospels at Nag Hammadi in Egypt in 1945.

The early Gnostics formed mystery schools where followers were initiated via sacred ceremonies and secret rites. Instead of pursuing intellectual knowledge, these dedicated men and women were seeking transcendence of the individual self in order to experience their essential oneness with the Great Mystery, or God. As the influential Roman Gnostic, Valentinus (c. 100–160 CE), wrote:

> 'Through Gnosis we are purified of diversity and experience the vision of unity. Those who have realized Gnosis know the source and the destination. They have set themselves free by waking up from the stupor in which they lived, and become themselves again.'

The Gnostics did not see heaven as a place that you go to when you die, but rather as an experience of life when you transcend your personal self. Similarly, the Christian Gnostics did not see themselves as followers of Christ; instead, they aimed to transcend the personal self so that they could become a living Christ. In this, the Gnostics revered Paul as their great apostle – it was Paul who said: 'The secret is this: Christ in you!'

Hermeticism

This term denotes a mystery tradition based on the teachings of Hermes Trismegistus, reputedly a wise sage and Egyptian priest who was generally regarded as an incarnation of the Egyptian god Thoth. The most important Hermetic texts are known as the Corpus Hermeticum, and they are believed to have been written in the 2nd century CE, although the philosophies and practices they describe go back to pharaohic Egypt. There is much in Hermeticism that is similar to Gnosticism; however, there is no reference to Judaism or Christianity in the Hermetica.

The most common literary device is for Hermes Trismestigus to enter into a dialogue with a perplexed pupil, and thereby reveal to him the secret wisdom. One of the central themes is the unity of God with all things, as in the following passage:

> 'He is hidden yet obvious everywhere.
> He is bodiless yet embodied in everything.
> There is nothing which He is not.
> He has no name because all names are his name.
> He is the unity of all things,
> So we must know him by all names
> And call everything "God".'

As in other Western mystery traditions, God was viewed as a direct experience of the primal mystery rather than an abstract being to be worshipped from afar:

> 'God is the root and source of all.
> Everything has a source,
> Except this source itself,
> Which springs from nothing.'

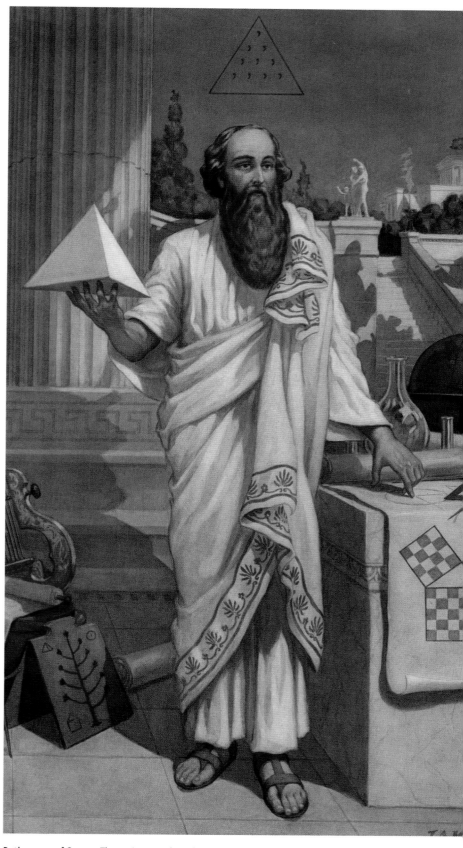

Pythagoras of Samos *The ancient Greek mathematician Pythagoras is shown working on triangle formulas in this 1928 drawing by J. Augustus Knapp.*

JUDAISM

If you are interested in **Judaism**, you may also like to read about:
● **The Kabbalah**, pages 188–189

Judaism is currently practised by approximately 13 million Jewish people worldwide, with more than 40 per cent living in Israel. Modern-day Judaism centres around a belief in **holy scripture**, acceptance of **principles of faith**, the practice of religious **observances** and the celebration of Jewish **festivals**. There is no historical evidence for the precise emergence of Judaism, but the language of ancient Jewish scriptures suggests that they were composed between the 10th and 2nd centuries BCE. The long history of the Jewish people has been marked by exile and persecution, culminating in the **Holocaust**.

Holy scripture

According to Jewish theology, Judaism began around 2000 BCE, when Yahweh or Jehovah (the Jewish God) made a covenant with Abraham and his descendants, the Jews. Yahweh subsequently revealed His laws to Moses on Mount Sinai, in the form of both a written and spoken Torah. The written version of the Torah became the first section of the Tanakh, the Jewish Bible, and it contains the Five Books of Moses: Genesis, Exodus, Leviticus, Numbers and Deuteronomy. The Torah is regarded as the most holy and important of all Jewish scriptures, and according to Jewish scholars it contains 613 commandments. Their interpretation is the subject of the Talmud, generally thought to be the second most important scripture in Judaism.

Principles of faith

The Jews have no central governing body that prescribes the exact nature of Judaism. For this reason, many influential Jewish scholars have attempted to articulate a set of principles that encapsulates the essence of Judaism. Arguably the most important figure is Maimonides (1135–1204), whose 13 principles of faith are largely accepted by Jews as the foundation of their religion. Below are five of his key principles:

1. I believe with perfect faith that the Creator, Blessed be His Name, is the Creator and Guide of everything that has been created; He alone has made, does make and will make all things.
5. I believe with perfect faith that to the Creator, and to Him alone, it is right to pray, and that it is not right to pray to any being besides Him.
6. I believe with perfect faith that all the words of the prophets are true.
11. I believe with perfect faith that the Creator, Blessed be His Name, rewards those who keep His commandments and punishes those that transgress them.
12. I believe with perfect faith in the coming of the Messiah; and even though he may tarry, nonetheless, I wait every day for his coming.

Observances and festivals

In the Book of Genesis it is written that Yahweh completed the whole of Creation in six days, and on the seventh day He rested. In commemoration, Jews keep the Sabbath (from *Shabbat*, meaning 'cease') as a day of rest. The Sabbath observance begins at sundown every Friday and is judged to have ended on Saturday night, when three stars appear in the sky.

Jews observe a number of High Holy Days, such as the festivals of Rosh Hashana(h), the Jewish New Year, which involves blowing the *shofar*, a trumpet fashioned from a ram's horn, and also Yom Kippur, arguably the most important Jewish festival, a solemn day of fasting and prayer.

In addition, Jewish people celebrate three foot festivals: Passover, Sukkot(h) and Shavuot(h). Passover is a week-long festival to commemorate the Exodus from Egypt; Sukkot(h) (or Tabernacles) is a week-long festival to commemorate the 40 years that the Israelites spent wandering in the desert; and Shavuot(h) is a joyous festival to celebrate Moses receiving the Torah on Mount Sinai.

Probably the most well-known Jewish festival to non-Jews is Hanukkah, sometimes referred to as the Festival of Lights. The observance of Hanukkah involves lighting the menorah – a specially crafted nine-branched candle-holder – for eight consecutive nights on particular days, which vary from year to year. An extra candle, known as a *shamash*, is also lit, to ensure that no one accidentally uses the light of the menorah for any purpose other than celebrating Hanukkah.

Practising Jews also observe a number of religious practices, for example 'keeping kosher', which requires that all foods forbidden by, or not prepared in accordance with, Jewish law must never be consumed. As a consequence, Jews do not eat birds or animals that prey on other animals, and they observe a strict prohibition against eating shellfish and pork. In addition, there is a prohibition against consuming blood, which had led to the observance of *melihah* for the preparation of meat.

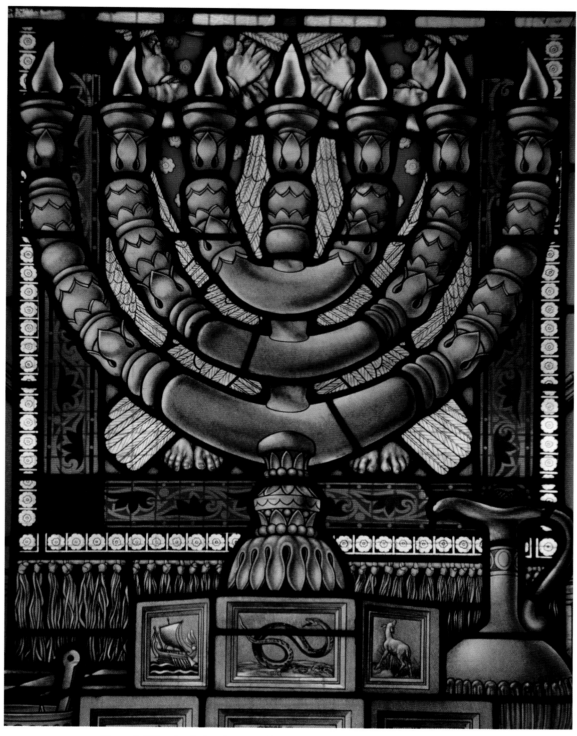

Menorah *This stained-glass depiction of a menorah, a symbol of the Jewish faith, can be found at the Rabbinate Synagogue, Jerusalem, Israel.*

The Holocaust

Throughout history Jewish people have suffered extreme persecution. Indiscriminate and brutal attacks on Jews have been widely documented in Europe since medieval times. This widespread persecution culminated in the Second World War, when the ruling Nazi Party of Germany, led by Adolph Hitler, began a systematic attempt to exterminate all Jews living in Europe. This resulted in the Holocaust, the wholescale murder of six million Jews. The colossal genocide only ended in 1945, when Germany was defeated. As a direct consequence, the State of Israel was founded in 1948 on contested lands referred to in Jewish scripture.

THE KABBALAH

The **Kabbalah** – also written Kaballah, Quaballa and Caballa – is the mystical tradition of Judaism. Its foremost sacred writings are the **Zohar**. For believers, these holy books reveal the hidden meaning of the Torah, and the true significance of the Jewish observances. The insights of Kabbalah are expressed through the **Tree of Life**.

If you are interested in **The Kabbalah**, you may also like to read about:
● **Western Mystery Traditions**, pages 184–184
● **Judaism**, pages 186–187

Kabbalah

Little can be said about the precise origins of Kabbalah – literally meaning 'receiving' – although we do know that the practice enjoyed a flowering in France, Germany and Spain in the 12th and 13th centuries. Isaac the Blind (c. 1160–1235) is reputed to have written the Bahir, a seminal work, and at the end of the 13th century Moses de Leon is believed to have composed the Zohar, a detailed explication of the purported ancient oral tradition.

In keeping with other Western mystical traditions, the primary focus of Kabbalah is to discover the divine self within, as opposed to worshipping an all-powerful Supreme Creator without. Traditional Kabbalists achieve this by cultivating a mystical union of Spirit and Matter in consciousness. When this goal is reached, Kabbalists become like living gods, an idea that has much in common with gnosis and other mystical traditions.

The Zohar

The Zohar is generally regarded as the primary sacred text of Kabbalah. Many Kabbalists believe that the Zohar was first written in the 1st century CE, while others hold it to be a medieval work. Many Jews consider the Zohar to be heretical; others consider it to be a cornerstone of their religion.

The primary aim of the Zohar is to reveal the hidden, or occult, meaning of the Torah, the first section of the Jewish Bible. Those who read the Torah and see only the literal meaning of the stories and the commandments are thus cautioned:

> 'The narratives of the Torah are its garments. He who thinks that these garments are the Torah itself deserves to perish and have no share in the world to come. Woe unto the fools who look no further when they see an elegant robe! More valuable than the garment is the body which carries it, and more valuable even than that is the soul which animates the body. Fools see only the garment of the Torah, the more intelligent see the body, the wise see the soul, its proper being; and in the Messianic time the "upper soul" of the Torah will stand revealed.' Translation from On Jewish Law and Lore (1955) by Louis Ginzberg (1873–1953).

Kabbalah teaches that holy scripture is meant to be studied not to better understand the Creator's laws and His Commandments, but rather because sacred texts map out a spiritual pathway towards the experience of divinity within. In practice, the Kabbalist must go on a spiritual journey of awakening, and the scripture will help guide him or her on their way; for example, the seven heavens referred to in the Torah are seven distinct ecstatic states of consciousness to be attained through contemplation and prayer, rather than seven different places that we may ascend to in the afterlife. Each of these experiences is a necessary stage along the way to the ultimate realization of the divine self.

The Tree of Life

In Kabbalah, there is a pictorial representation of the different stages of the spiritual journey and it is referred to as the Tree of Life. The tree is composed of ten 'sephiroth' (emanations), represented by ten spheres, and each sphere refers to a different aspect of divine emanation. Above the tree (but never pictured) is Aur Ain Soph, meaning 'Light Without End', and from this limitless light each of the ten divine emanations flows:

1. Keter – Crown
2. Chokmah – Wisdom
3. Binah – Understanding
4. Chesed – Kindness
5. Gevurah – Strength
6. Tipheret – Adornment
7. Netzach – Resilience
8. Hod – Splendour
9. Yesod – Foundation
10. Malkuth – Kingdom

In many traditions, there is a mysterious 11th sephiroth, referred to as Daath, meaning 'Knowledge' in the sense of transcendent enlightenment, the ultimate goal of Kabbalah.

Different Kabbalists approach the teaching of the Tree of Life in different ways, giving each sephiroth a slightly different interpretation, but it is customary to approach the journey along the Tree of Life from the bottom up – that is, from Malkuth to Keter. Traditionally, Malkuth (Kingdom) refers to worldly or material consciousness, and Keter (Crown) to that which is above the head, meaning beyond all human comprehension; in other words, to the ultimate experience of the divine. By making this journey, we can transform our ordinary, earthly consciousness into a truly liberating experience of our own divinity in the here and now.

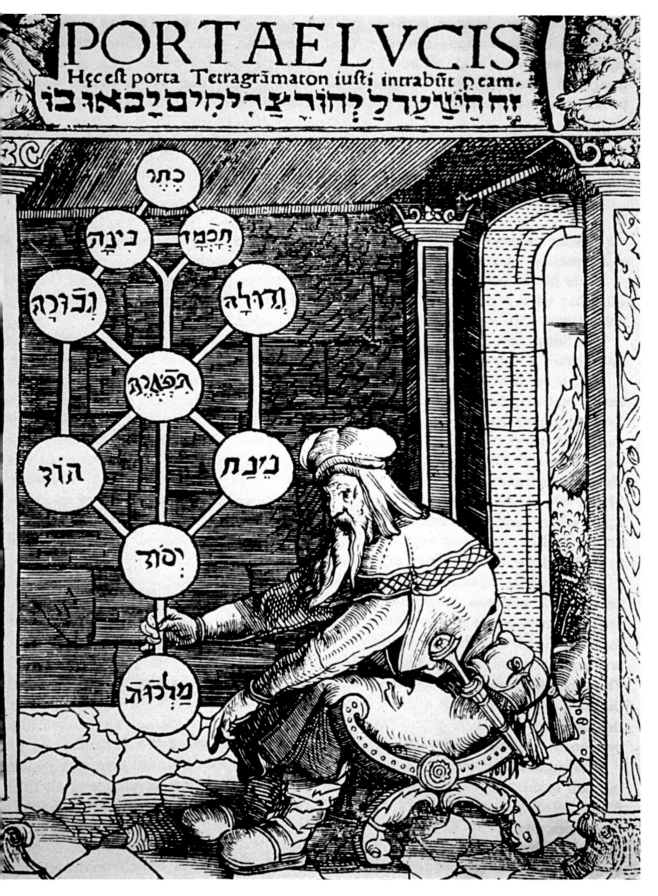

The Tree of Life *Paul Ricci's 1516 artwork entitled the* Sephirotic Tree of Life *pictorially represents the ten divine emanations with ten spheres or sephiroth.*

CHRISTIANITY

If you are interested in **Christianity**, you may also like to read about:
● **The Gnostic Gospels**, pages 192–193

Christianity is the world's largest religion, practised by billions of believers around the globe. Its most holy scripture is the **New Testament**, which early Christians combined with the Jewish Tanakh to create the Christian Bible. The principles and practices of Christianity are inspired by the gospel story of **Jesus**, whom most Christians regard not as a prophet, but as the Son of God made flesh. Contemporary Christianity encompasses a vast variety of traditions, including **Catholicism**, **Protestantism** and the **Eastern Orthodox Church**.

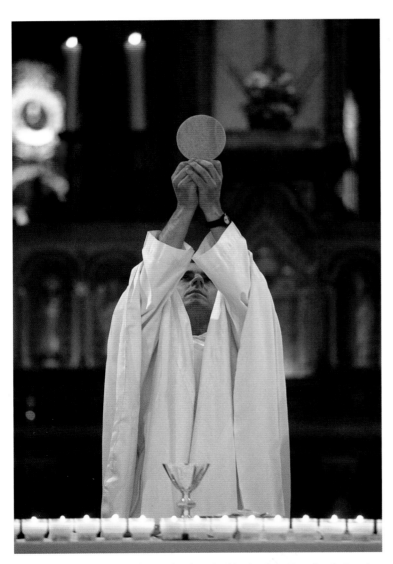

Holding the host *In Saint Ambroise Church, Paris, this priest is consecrating the bread, or host, for communion, which becomes, for believers, the actual body of Christ.*

The New Testament

This consists of four gospels – Matthew, Mark, Luke and John – which collectively describe Christ's life and teachings; an additional 'gospel' – Acts – which recounts the ministries of Christ's apostles; 21 early letters, commonly called Epistles; and an apocalyptic prophecy, known as the Book of Revelation, which foretells the second coming of Christ. Collectively, these sacred texts are some of the most influential writings in the Western world. They have helped to shape Western culture, and they continue to provide moral guidance and spiritual insight for Christians worldwide.

In the four gospels, we learn that Jesus is the long-promised Messiah of the Jewish Bible. We are told that Jesus was born to a virgin, Mary, and that he spent his life performing miracles and teaching a new spirituality. Jesus's radical new message brought him many enemies, and he was put to death by crucifixion, but after three days he was resurrected, at which point he returned to his disciples as promised, before ascending to be with his heavenly Father. The crucifixion and subsequent resurrection of Jesus are the most important events in the story of Jesus, since Christians believe that Christ died on the cross to atone for the sins of mankind, so that we could all enjoy eternal life in the hereafter.

Contemporary Christianity is divided on the subject of the historical truth of the New Testament. Some believe it is the word of God and thus cannot be questioned, while others believe it is an all-too-human attempt at recording an oral tradition, complete with mistakes and embellishments. Modern scholars continue to search for evidence of the events described. Archeology and linguistic analysis of the gospels are among the many tools being used.

The teachings of Jesus

At the heart of the Christian message is the experience and practice of love: love of God and love of others. In Matthew, when Jesus was asked by a Pharisee to state God's greatest commandment, he gave him the following reply:

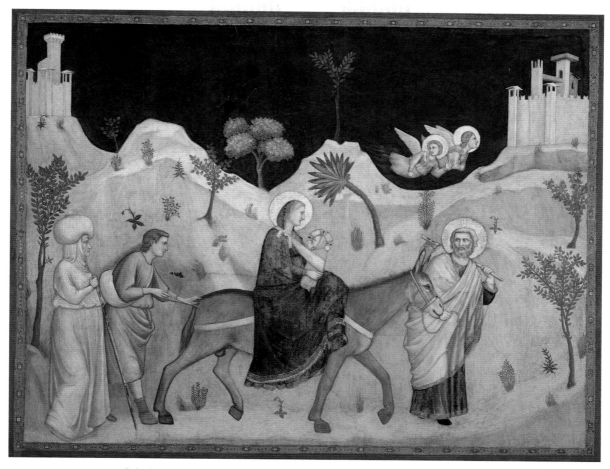

Flight into Egypt *This 14th-century painting by Giotto di Bondone portrays the flight into Egypt that Joseph and Mary made with the infant Jesus.*

'"You shall love the Lord your God with all your heart, and with all your soul, and with all your mind." This is the greatest and foremost commandment. And a second is like it, "You shall love your neighbour as yourself." On these two commandments depend the whole Law and the Prophets.'

In John, Jesus tells his disciples that love is the new spirituality he has come to teach, and that to be a follower of Christ is to practise love:

'I give you a new commandment to love each other, as I have loved you. By this commandment everyone will know that you are my disciples, if you love each other.'

The new teaching of love put Jesus at odds with much traditional lore. In the Old Testament it is written 'an eye for an eye', but in Matthew Jesus explicitly rejects this retributive doctrine, instead counselling his followers to forgive: 'If you forgive others for their wrongs, then your heavenly Father will forgive you.'

Catholicism and Protestantism

The early Christians suffered extreme persecution until Christianity became the official religion of Rome in the 4th century CE, with the formation of the Roman Catholic Church. Catholicism is now the largest denomination.

One of the most important sacraments in Catholicism is the Eucharist. It involves the celebration of Mass and the ingesting of consecrated bread and wine, which – for believers – become the actual body and blood of Christ.

In the 16th century, a major doctrinal split emerged within Christianity with the advent of Protestantism. These early reformers sought to bypass the papal hierarchy of the Catholic Church, claiming that the Bible was the word of God and needed no theological interpretation, and that faith in Christ was sufficient for eternal salvation, meaning one no longer needed the blessing of a Catholic priest.

Eastern Orthodox Church

The Eastern Orthodox Church emerged during the period of the Holy Roman Empire from the 3rd century CE when the empire had two emperors and two administrative centres, one in Rome, the other in Istanbul, then Constantinople. When the Western Roman Empire fell, the split between East and West grew and in the 11th century CE the 'Great Schism' occurred when the two churches fully separated. Despite attempts to reconcile the two communions they remain separate today. Specifically Western concerns with original sin, predestination and purgatory are of less importance in the Orthodox Church. Today there are an estimated 225 million Orthodox Christians worldwide.

THE GNOSTIC GOSPELS

If you are interested in **The Gnostic Gospels**, you may also like to read about:
- **Western Mystery Traditions**, pages 184–185
- **Christianity**, pages 190–191

The extraordinary find of a vast amount of early Gnostic writings in 1945 at Nag Hammadi in Egypt has led modern scholars to completely rethink the origins and meaning of Christianity. Instead of just four gospels – Matthew, Mark, Luke and John – we now know that there were many other gospels, for example the Gospel of Mary, **Thomas**, **Philip**, Judas and **Truth**, which were suppressed by the early Roman Catholic Church.

The Gospel of Thomas

In 1898 a partial version of the Gospel of Thomas was found in Oxyrhynchus in Egypt, and then a second more complete version was found at Nag Hammadi. This gospel is unlike the four canonical gospels, which give an account of the life of Jesus; instead, Thomas relates the teachings of Jesus as words he spoke to his followers in 114 separate sayings. These profound sayings are strikingly similar to what is found in the New Testament. However, a major difference is that in Thomas we find a rejection of the idea of bodily resurrection and an emphasis on spiritual resurrection.

In keeping with the basic tenets of Gnosticism, the Gospel of Thomas claims that our salvation will come not from blind faith but by direct experience of the Christ within. The sayings of Jesus that Thomas shares with us point to this mystical experience, and if the reader 'has ears to hear' – that is, if he or she can correctly interpret the teachings – then the secret of eternal life will be revealed:

> 'These are the hidden words that the living Jesus spoke. And Didymos Judas Thomas wrote them down.
> And he said: "Whoever finds the meaning of these words will not taste death."'

The promise of eternal life in the here and now is the central theme of the Gospel of Thomas. Not surprisingly, the disciples plead with Jesus to describe the promised kingdom. Jesus responds with a timeless saying that speaks directly to the mystical experience at the heart of all Gnostic teaching:

> 'The kingdom is like a person who has a hidden treasure in his field, of which he knows nothing.'

According to Gnosticism, the way to God is to 'know' who we truly are.

The Gospel of Truth

This was another of the gospels found at Nag Hammadi. Scholars had long suspected its existence because it was referred to by Iranaeus (c. 130–203 CE), a highly influential Christian theologian and historian, who emphatically rejected it as part of the orthodox Christian canon, claiming it was written by followers of the Gnostic philosopher Valentinus. Iranaeus damned it as heresy, complaining: 'It agrees in nothing with the Gospels of the apostles.'

Unlike the Gospel of Thomas, the Gospel of Truth does not list any of Jesus's sayings; instead, it reads more like a philosophical treatise, with emphasis on clarifying the nature of the Father, and the relationship of the Father to the Son, so that the reader can 'know' the truth that leads to salvation. In keeping with many other spiritual traditions, those who seek the truth are compared to the blind who cannot see, or to dreamers who need to awaken. They are cut off from their Father, so that life on earth has become a living hell:

> 'This ignorance of the Father brought about terror and fear. And terror became dense like a fog, so that no one was able to see.'

The solution the gospel offers is gnosis, or knowledge of our sacred self, which is eternally one with God the Father:

> 'They consider knowledge of the Father to be the dawn. It is thus that each one has behaved, as if he were asleep, during the time when he was ignorant and thus he comes to understand, as if he were awakening. And happy is the man who comes to himself and awakens. Indeed, blessed is he who has opened the eyes of the blind.'

The Gospel of Philip

Another extremely important gospel recovered at Nag Hammadi, the Gospel of Philip, is particularly concerned with marriage; that is, the mystical union of male and female rather than the physical marriage of husband and wife, which is variously expressed as the relationship of Father and Mother, Christ and Mary, and Adam and Eve.

In Gnostic philosophy, the Father always represents the primal mystery and the Mother the material world. According to Philip, because we have lost sight of the mystery, we have been cut off from the experience of heaven on Earth, which only gnosis can restore:

> 'If the woman had not separated from the man, she should not die with the man. His separation became the beginning of death. Because of this, Christ came to repair the separation… and again unite the two, and to give life to those who died as a result of the separation, and unite them.'

Attaining the mystical union of male and female, mystery and manifest, heaven and earth, is the goal of Gnostic practice.

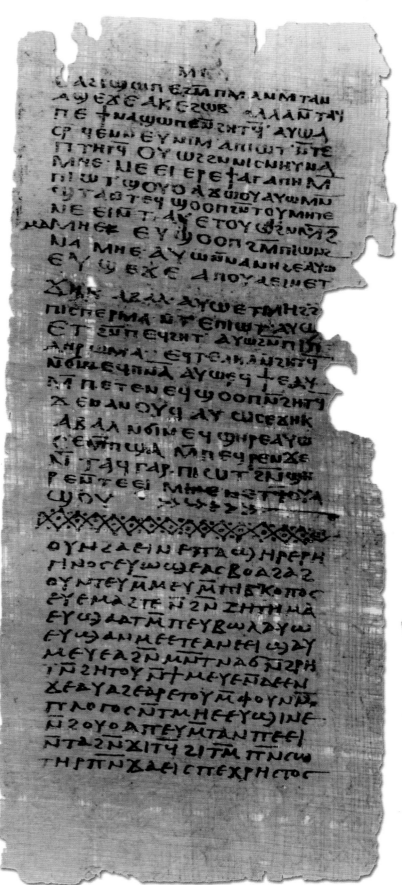

Gnostic gospels *These fragments of manuscripts were discovered in Nag Hammadi in Egypt in 1945. They are gospels about the secret teachings of gnosis, and are viewed by orthodox Christians as heresy.*

If you are interested in **Spiritualism**, you may also like to read about:
● Channelling, pages 42–43

SPIRITUALISM

Followers of Spiritualism tend to believe in Jesus Christ, but they differ from the main Christian churches in that they believe that the spirits of the dead can be contacted by sensitive individuals, known as **mediums**. There are today many active Spiritual traditions inspired by Spiritualism, including **Spiritualist churches**, **White Eagle**, **Alice Bailey** and *A Course in Miracles*. Spiritualism today is most widely practised in Britain and the USA.

Mediums

In the claim that they are in direct contact with people who have died, mediums are rare. They may be born with this ability – or 'gift', as it is known – or it may arise suddenly for no apparent reason. Alternatively, it may be

Spiritual healing *Prayer plays an important part in faith healing. Here, two healers are seen praying for a patient at a demonstration of spiritual healing held by the UK's National Federation of Spiritual Healers.*

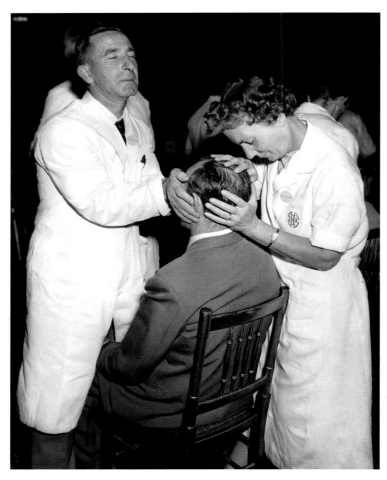

developed and refined over the course of many years. In some circles it is believed that all small children have this ability to communicate with spirits, but that most grow out of it or are actively taught to suppress it by adults who are scared by the phenomenon.

Spiritualist mediums typically seek to help people by receiving and passing on messages from loved ones who have died. Some mediums hear voices, others have visions, while yet others may experience certain feelings, which they translate into messages for the bereaved. This practice gives emotional support to a great many people. Spiritualists recognize that there have, unfortunately, always been a number of fake mediums, who pretend to communicate with the dead as a way of extracting money from vulnerable people. In Britain and America in the mid to late 1800s this complaint became so widespread that Spiritualists were forced to organize in churches in order to keep out the charlatan element.

The Spiritualist churches

The first Spiritualist church in Britain was founded in 1855. By the late 1800s, many thousands of Spiritualist churches and groups had formed throughout Britain and the USA. Today there are Spiritualist churches practically everywhere in the English-speaking world.

Just like orthodox Christian churches, Spiritualist churches are places of worship; however, in a Spiritualist church the service is conducted by a medium rather than an ordained minister. As well as the usual hymns and prayers, time is also set aside for communicating with the spirit world. In the UK it is customary for the medium to acquire some sort of evidence from the dead person that they are who they say they are, before relaying messages to members of the congregation. This information might consist of the first letter of the deceased's name, the place where they lived or worked, a favourite hobby or even the illness from which they died. Once contact has been verified, the medium will begin to pass on messages that are often helpful to the bereaved.

Many Spiritualist churches also offer spiritual healing. Typically, this involves the minister, or medium, placing his or her hands on a member of the congregation who is ill, then directing healing energy to them.

Some mediums are in regular contact with what they call 'spirit guides', who assume the role of helping the medium to develop their gift. On occasion, spirit guides will use the medium to communicate spiritual teachings to the wider world. This process is known as channelling and has led to the development of a number of significant and popular movements in Britain and the USA today.

White Eagle

In 1936 the British medium Grace Cooke founded the White Eagle Lodge after making contact with her spirit guide, White Eagle. Cooke subsequently published a great deal of spiritual guidance channelled through her. Much of White Eagle's teaching consists of advice for the spiritual traveller, for example:

> *'There is no restriction on a person's soul other than that which it places upon itself... Therefore think of having a pair of wings on your shoulders, of a winged disc, the latter being the symbol of the sun; and the sun, of course, being the Christ Spirit; the wings, indicating the power of the soul to fly – to rise above your limitations.'*

Alice Bailey

Alice Ann Bailey (1880–1949) was a highly regarded and influential writer on occult, Theosophical and other spiritual matters. She claimed that the majority of her written work had been channelled from a 'Master of the Wisdom', whom she initially referred to as 'The Tibetan', and later as 'Djwhal Khul'. Her work is still attracting attention today.

A Course in Miracles

In 1976 Dr Helen Schucman (1909–1981) and Dr William Thetford (1923–1988) published what went on to become an extremely popular book, *A Course in Miracles*, claiming that it was a transcription of an inner voice that Dr Schucman had heard, whom she referred to as Jesus Christ. Many readers regard it as scripture, claiming that it is more coherent than the Bible because it comes from a single source. The book itself urges the reader to cultivate awareness of love of self and others as a foundation for spiritual practice.

Spiritual materialization *This painting commemorates the materialization of Annie Morgan, said to have been dead for 200 years, as she revealed herself to mediums in 1870.*

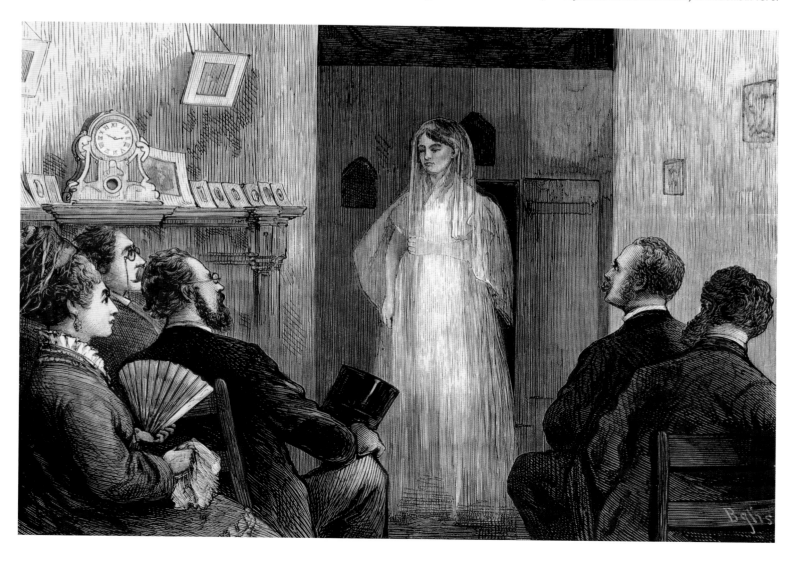

ISLAM

The religion of Islam was born of the mystical revelations given to the Prophet **Muhammad**. Islam literally means 'submission', and its adherents are called Muslims, meaning 'those who submit to God'. The holy scripture of Islam is the **Koran** (or Qur'an) and it forms the basis of all Islamic spiritual practice. There are more than a billion Muslims in the world today, comprising both **Sunni** and **Shia** traditions. Most Muslims believe that there are five fundamental duties – or **pillars** – to Islam. The day-to-day life of Muslims is governed by **Sharia** law.

If you are interested in **Islam**, you may also like to read about:
- Judaism, pages 186–187
- Christianity, pages 190–191
- Sufism, pages 198–199
- Pilgrimage and Retreats, pages 298–299

Muhammad

The Prophet Muhammad is thought to have been born in Mecca in Arabia in 570 CE. At the age of 40, disillusioned with life, he retreated to a cave, where he received the first of many divine revelations from the angel Gabriel. Muhammad returned to Mecca to share the word of God, but he was persecuted, so he moved to Medina, where he attracted many thousands of followers. After much fighting with warring tribes, Muhammad succeeded in conquering Medina. He continued to receive revelations from Gabriel, and each of these revelations subsequently became a verse in the Koran. Muhammad died in 632 CE, having successfully converted most of the Arabian peninsula to Islam.

Importantly, Muslims do not view Muhammad as the founder of a new religion, but rather as the last in a long line of prophets in the Jewish–Christian tradition of Adam, Abraham, Moses and Jesus. According to Islam, Muhammad was God's last prophet, and his task was to clarify mistakes and misunderstandings from earlier teachings. For that reason, the Koran is seen as the ultimate and most authoritative word on the true religion of God.

The Koran

This holy scripture is said to have been written down during Muhammad's own lifetime by his followers, and Muslims believe that it is the direct word of God.

The Koran consists of 114 chapters, or *suras*, and each *sura* is composed of separate verses, or *ayats*. The first *ayat*, Al-Fatiha, is translated:

'In the name of Allah, the Most Gracious, the Most Merciful:
All Praise is due to Allah, Lord of the Universe,
The Most Gracious, the Most Merciful,
Sovereign of the Day of Recompense.
You alone we worship, and You alone we ask for help.
Guide us to the straight path;

The way of those on whom You have bestowed your grace,
not the way of those who have earned Your anger,
nor of those who went astray.'

Sunni and Shia

There are two main denominations within Islam, Sunni and Shia, with Sunni being the larger of the two. The split can be traced back to the death of Muhammad, when most Muslims agreed that Islam should be led by elected men who had been followers of the Prophet, while another group, the Shia, wanted the leader of Islam to come from Muhammad's family. Shia Muslims claim to take their lead from a long line of imams descended from Muhammad's cousin and son-in-law, Ali. In practice, the difference today is largely political, as each group acknowledges a different religious authority.

The five pillars

Sunni Muslims believe that there are five pillars – or spiritual duties – to Islam, while Shia Muslims hold the view that there are eight. In practice, the duties of Sunni and Shia largely overlap.

The first pillar is Shahadah, meaning 'statement of faith', which Muslims are required to repeat in prayer: 'I testify that there is none worthy of worship except God and I testify that Muhammad is the Messenger of God.'

The second pillar is Salah, meaning 'ritual prayer', which must be performed five times a day. In many Muslim countries, a call to prayer is sung or broadcast from mosques inviting Muslims to worship. Salah is always performed facing towards Mecca and involves reciting verses from the Koran.

The third pillar is Zakat, the practice of giving alms. Muslims consider it a spiritual duty to give to the poor, and to help to pay for the spread of Islam.

The fourth pillar is Sawm, which involves fasting during daylight hours for the duration of Ramadan, a holy month in the Islamic calendar. Fasting is believed to help focus the mind on God and to atone for past sins.

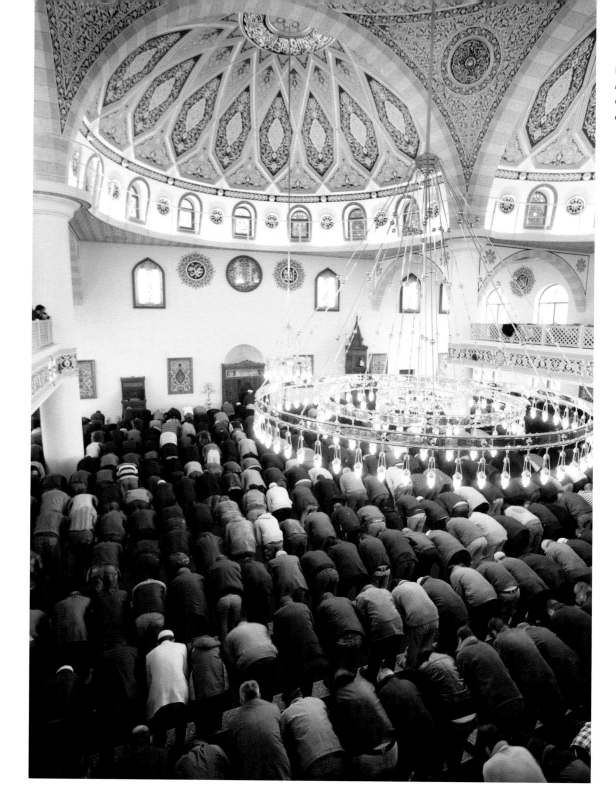

Mosque *The Merkez Mosque in Duisburg-Marxloh is the biggest mosque in Germany. This picture shows the mosque during Friday prayer.*

The fifth pillar is Hajj, or holy pilgrimage. Every Muslim who can reasonably make the trip is expected to travel at least once in their lifetime to the holy city of Mecca in Saudi Arabia. At the great mosque – al-Haram – the pilgrim performs many rituals, including walking seven times around the Kaaba and touching the Black Stone. Every year several million Muslims converge on Mecca for these sacred rites, making it the largest pilgrimage in the world.

Sharia law

An extensive legal and moral framework derived from the Koran, Sharia governs all aspects of life, including family, business, money, dress, sex, hygiene and food. In relation to the last, for example, vegetables and seafood are *halal*, meaning allowed, whereas meat is only *halal* if the animal has been killed 'kindly'. By following Sharia law, Muslims maintain spiritual purity and ensure that they act in accordance with God's will.

SUFISM

Sufism is the mystical tradition of Islam, and its adherents are known as **Sufis**, or dervishes. Sufism embodies a profound **philosophy** and diverse spiritual **practices**, designed to awaken the adherent to an ecstatic experience of God. Sufism has been popularized in the West by modern-day teachers such as G. I. Gurdjieff (c. 1866–1949) and Idries Shah (1924–1996).

If you are interested in **Sufism**, you may also like to read about:

- **Islam**, pages 196–197
- **Western Mystery Traditions**, pages 184–185
- **Hinduism**, pages 204–205
- **Tantra**, pages 214–215

Sufis

Almost all Sufis trace their roots within Islam to Muhammad via his cousin and son-in-law, Ali. However, it was not until 1000 CE that the first major texts on Sufism were composed, with a number of different Sufi orders emerging in the early Middle Ages. From the 13th to the 16th centuries, Sufism helped spread Islam into Africa, south Asia and Turkey, and contributed to a golden age of Islamic culture.

Sufis have often been regarded as dangerous heretics by fundamentalist Muslims. While the goal of Islam is to attain such spiritual purity that we are fit to meet God in the afterlife, Sufis believe that it is possible to become one with the divine in this life. As a consequence, Sufi masters will sometimes proclaim their own divinity, provoking outrage in the hearts and minds of more orthodox believers. Many Sufis, such as the celebrated 9th-century Sufi master Al Hallaj, were put to death for proclaiming this spiritual conviction. Some Sufis refer to themselves as 'lovers of God'.

Unlike other Muslims, Sufis do not think of the Koran as a text to be studied in order to find spiritual and moral guidance and follow God's law; instead, they see the Koran as a sacred text, which, if correctly read, offers a pathway to God in the here and now. For many Sufis, jihad is not a call to war but an internal battle with the personal self, which we can transcend to attain intimate and direct experience of God.

Sufis believe that it is important to gain spiritual insight and experience for oneself, and not to rely too heavily on a spiritual teacher. According to Idries Shah, a highly successful writer and modern-day proponent of Sufism in the West: 'As soon as possible the teacher should dismiss the pupil, who becomes his own man of wisdom, and then continues his self-work.'

Sufi philosophy

This is primarily concerned with understanding the unity of self with God. Some of the best tools for understanding the mystical philosophy of Sufism are the teaching stories and poems of the Sufi masters, such as the celebrated Persian poet Rumi (1207–1273):

> *'Your task is not to seek for love, but merely to seek and find all the barriers within yourself that you have built against it.'*

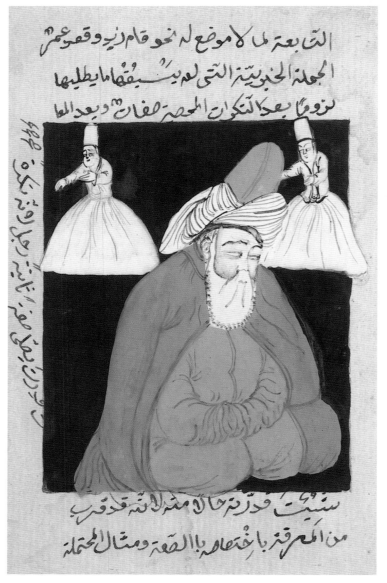

Rumi *This drawing of the famous Persian poet and Sufi master Mevlana Celaleddin i Rumi, features whirling dervishes in the background.*

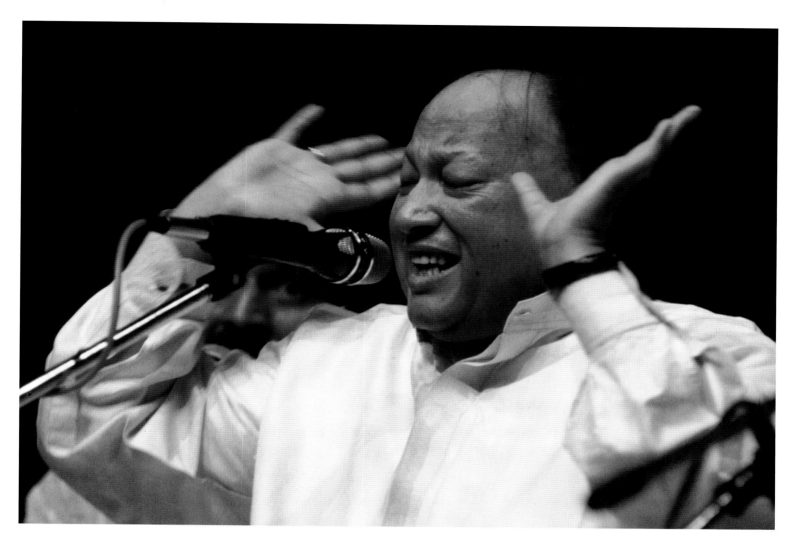

Sufi masters often celebrate the experience of the mystical union of self and God by writing sacred poetry. Sometimes this poetry is so sublime that in reading it many people claim to be transported far beyond the narrow confines of the rational mind into an immediate and ecstatic experience of the unity of all with God. To quote again from Rumi:

'I drank You down in one,
Collapsing intoxicated by purity.
Ever since, I can't tell if I exist or not.'

Sufi practices

An important spiritual practice in Sufism is the silent *dhikr*, which is the unspoken repetition of Allah, the name of God. When Sufis practise the *dhikr*, they are not just repeating a word; they are seeking to invoke an experience of God with each and every breath.

According to the mystic Kabir (1398–1448), 'The breath that does not repeat the name of God is a wasted breath.'

Sufis have developed a number of celebratory and often ecstatic practices for cultivating a direct experience of the divine. In Pakistan, there is a tradition of devotional Sufi music known as Qawali. During a performance,

Qawali singing *Nusrat Fateh Ali Khan, The King of Qawali, singing on stage. Qawali, a form of ecstatic and often improvised singing, is seen as a way to get closer to the divine.*

the musicians typically play the harmonium and drum, and chant for long periods, taking themselves and their audience into a deeper and deeper trance. They wait for the devotional singer to be consumed by the experience of God, at which point he will burst forth into improvised ecstatic song, taking everyone a step closer to the divine. One of the greatest exponents of Qawali singing was Nusrat Fateh Ali Khan, who died in 1997 after achieving fame in the West.

There is an old Sufi saying: 'There are two ways a person can be blessed by Allah. The first is to be able to sing Qawali. The second is to be able to appreciate someone singing Qawali.'

In Turkey, followers of the celebrated 13th-century poet Rumi founded the Mevlevi Order of Sufism. These Sufis, known as dervishes, practise a form of dancing called whirling, which enables the dancers to attain a state of profound spiritual intoxication in which they are able to become one with God. Whirling dervishes take both themselves and their audiences closer to an ecstatic experience of God.

BAHAI

The Bahai faith is a modern spiritual tradition founded by Persian nobleman **Baha'u'llah** in the 19th century. Today Bahai is practised by approximately six million people in more than 200 countries around the world. The **spiritual beliefs** of the Bahai faith are based on the idea of the fundamental unity of all things.

If you are interested in **Bahai**, you may also like to read about:
- **Hinduism**, pages 204–205
- **Buddhism**, pages 208–209
- **The Gnostic Gospels**, pages 192–193
- **Western Mystery Traditions**, pages 184–185

Baha'u'llah

Born in Tehran (the capital of modern-day Iran) in 1817, Baha'u'llah was offered a government position soon after his father's death. He declined and instead became a follower of a young man known as the Bab (1819–1850), who claimed to be the promised Mahdi, or Messiah, of Islam. The Bab further proclaimed that the great Promised One was about to come and establish the kingdom of God on Earth. These heretical claims brought the Bab and his

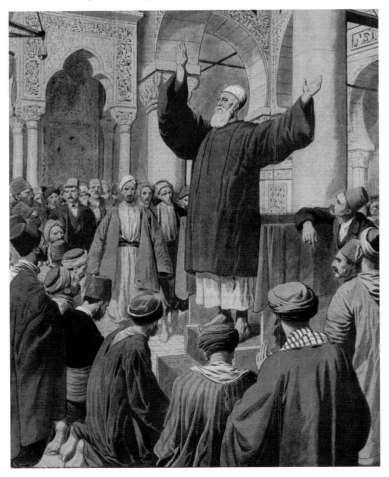

Abdul Baha *This illustration from* Le Petit Journal *shows Abdul Baha (1844–1921), the son and successor of Baha'u'llah, preaching the Bahai faith.*

followers into direct conflict with the Islamic authorities, which led to Baha'u'llah being briefly imprisoned and tortured by having the soles of his feet beaten with sticks.

In 1850 the Bab was arrested and executed by firing squad, which resulted in a small group of his followers plotting to assassinate the Shah, a course of action opposed by Baha'u'llah. The plot failed and the plotters were duly rounded up and executed. In the chaos that followed, all other Babists in the region were hunted down. Most were killed, but Baha'u'llah was sent instead to Siyah Chal, which literally means 'black pit', a hellish underground dungeon in Tehran.

It was while he was incarcerated in Siyah Chal that Baha'u'llah later claimed he was visited by God's maiden, who told him that he was the last in the long line of divine messengers, including Krishna, Moses, Buddha, Christ and Muhammad, and that he was the Promised One of whom the Bab had foretold. It was also revealed to Baha'u'llah that each of the world's religions was representative of a stage in the development of God's overall plan and purpose for humanity, and that we had finally entered the age when the peoples of the world were ready to come together as one.

After four months Baha'u'llah was released, but he was then forced into exile. He arrived in Baghdad with his wife and family in 1853, and although he continued to practise and teach the Babist faith, he kept his mystical revelations secret. In 1854 he left his family to live in the mountains of Kurdistan, where he disguised himself as a dervish and lived as a hermit. During this time he wrote many books, including *The Four Valleys*, an important text for Bahais.

Two years later the Babist community in Baghdad was in disarray, and so Baha'u'llah's family tracked him down and pleaded with him to return to lead the Babist movement. Baha'u'llah spent the next seven years teaching and writing in Baghdad, before he and a group of his followers visited the Garden of Ridvan on the River Tigris just outside the city. They stayed there for 12 days, during which time Baha'u'llah finally revealed his divine status and spiritual mission. This event in 1863 is recognized by Bahais as the birth of the Bahai faith, and is celebrated by the Festival of Rivdan.

Soon after, the Ottoman authorities ordered Baha'u'llah to move to Istanbul, and from there he was exiled to Edirne (Adrianopolis) in northern Turkey. While in Edirne, Baha'u'llah wrote letters to world leaders, inviting

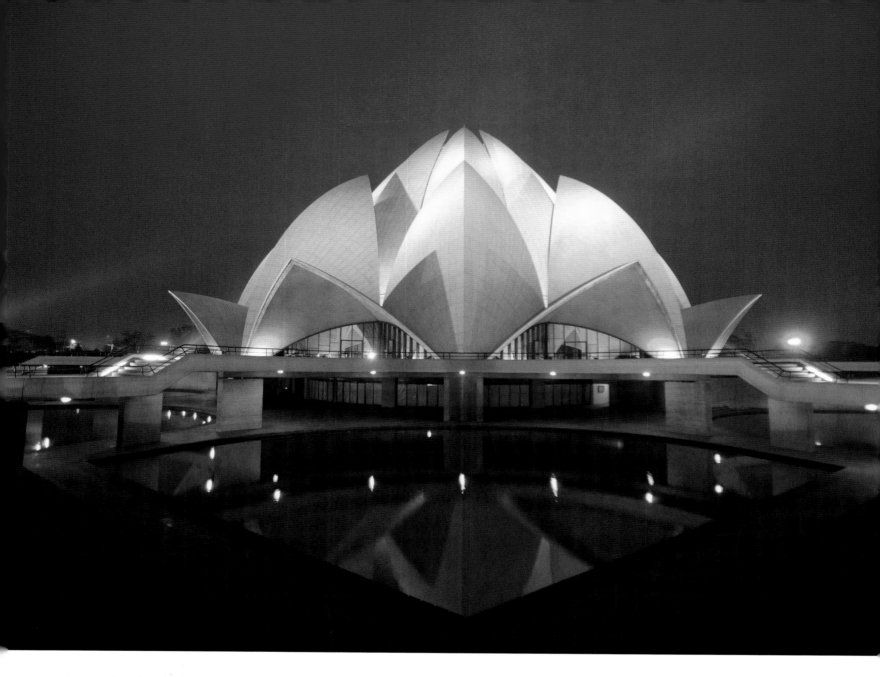

them to adopt the Bahai faith, to give up their material possessions and to work together for the betterment of humanity.

After a further four and half years of writing books and teaching, Baha'u'llah was exiled to the penal colony of Akka (Acre) in Palestine, where he remained for the next 24 years, writing prolifically and preaching the new religion of unity. Initially, he was incarcerated and poorly treated, but over time the authorities and local people came to respect him, and in 1879 he was rehoused in the Mansion of Bahji, where he wrote *The Book of Laws* and other important works. Baha'u'llah continued to write and teach until his death in 1892, naming his son Abdul Baha as his successor in his will.

Spiritual beliefs

Bahais believe that the goal of spiritual practice is to attain the realization of the unity of all things, including all religions and our oneness with each other.

The Lotus Temple *Also known as the Bahai House of Worship, the Lotus Temple in Delhi was designed by architect Farborz Sahba and completed in 1986. It is made of 27 free-standing 'petals' and surrounded by nine ponds.*

Following Baha'u'llah, the view of the Bahais is that the collective realization of unity will result in the experience of heaven on Earth, but to achieve that requires overcoming all forms of prejudice, the elimination of extreme poverty and wealth, the attainment of balance between nature and technology, worldwide education for all, and for the peoples of the world to recognize that they all belong to the same human family.

Bahais seek personal and community transformation. In practice, this is achieved by a combination of daily prayer – which is viewed as an intimate communion with God – and assisting with small-scale, social and economic development projects around the world.

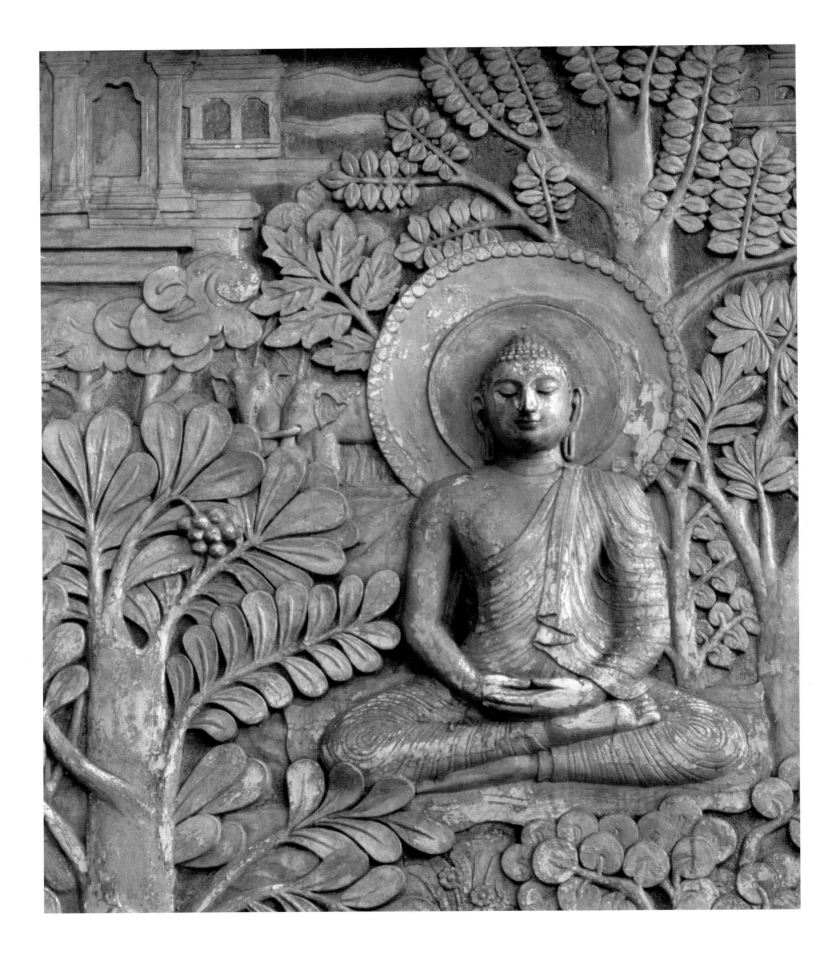

EASTERN FAITHS

The main Eastern traditions of Hinduism, Buddhism and Taoism have a common approach to spirituality that is different from the Western traditions. While the Western Abrahamic faiths, Judaism, Christianity and Islam, have developed to serve and worship God, Eastern traditions have held the purpose of spirituality to be enlightenment in the sense of transcendent knowledge of our true nature.

Shared spiritual aspirations

The spiritual aim of Hinduism, Buddhism and Jainism is to attain *moksha* or *nirvana*, Sanskrit terms that are generally understood to mean liberation from the personal self in order to achieve an ecstatic union with God, or final freedom from the karmic cycle of death and rebirth. To that end, most forms of Eastern spirituality are concerned with making an individual spiritual journey, often described as an 'awakening'. Hindus seek to see through the personal self to their true nature, which is one with Brahman or God; Buddhists seek to awaken from the illusory world of the senses to experience their true Buddha nature; Sikhs aim to 'grow towards and into God'; and Taoists seek to reunite with the Great Mystery, known as Tao. In each tradition the most revered sacred texts emphasize that our everyday experience of life hides a deeper reality, and that it is possible to awaken to an experience of the divine – often characterized as blissful liberation from the ordinary self – by adopting spiritual practices. The Taoist Master Chuang Tzu (4th century BCE) claimed: 'Only after we are awake do we know that we have dreamed. But there comes a great awakening, and then we know that life is a great dream.'

Origins and evolution

Eastern traditions have extremely ancient origins. Elements of Hinduism can be traced back to between c. 2500 and 1500 BCE, while the Vedas, the great body of Hindu sacred literature, is dated to between c. 1500 and 500 BCE,

Buddha *This relief carving depicts a scene from the life of the Buddha and is found at the Buddhist Gangarama Temple in Sri Lanka.*

and the earliest of these texts are probably based on oral traditions pre-dating them by some thousands of years. Following the birth of the Buddha in India c. 560 BCE, Buddhism arose as a tradition distinct from Hinduism, even though it shared many of Hinduism's central ideas. Although Buddhism subsequently declined in India, Buddhist missionaries successfully instituted Buddhism as a religion in what is now Sri Lanka during the 2nd century BCE, in South East Asia and China c. 500 CE and in Tibet c. 600 CE. Taoism is believed to have begun in China around the same time that Buddhism arose in India. Although Taoism shares many of Buddhism's principles, it too has its own unique expression of spiritual insight.

East meets West

The encounter of the cultures of the West and East during the period of Western colonial expansion beginning in the 18th century led to a further transmission of and interest in Eastern traditions. During the 19th and early 20th centuries many key Sanskrit texts were translated into European languages for the first time, and several prominent spiritual seekers, such as Madame Blavatsky (1831–1891), the founder of Theosophy, one of her successors, Charles W. Leadbeater (1854–1934), and the eminent Swiss psychologist, Carl Jung (1875–1961), among others, brought Eastern spiritual principles to the awareness of the West. In more recent years psychologists have become interested in the application of Eastern principles of meditation and detachment to the treatment of anxiety and depression, while the development of quantum physics has led many people to an appreciation of the points of connection between Eastern philosophies and modern physics. In his bestselling book *The Tao of Physics* (1975), Fritjof Capra explored these links in such concepts as the unity of all things, the relativity of space and time, and a sense of physical things and phenomena as transient manifestations of underlying energy.

Despite these unique aspects of Eastern traditions there are also many spiritual points of connection with Western faiths in terms of compassionate behaviour and the principle of developing what Buddhists term *metta-bhavana* or loving kindness. According to the Dalai Lama of Tibet, 'Every religion has more or less the same viewpoint and the same goal.'

HINDUISM

If you are interested in **Hinduism**, you may also like to read about:
- **Hindu Sacred Texts**, pages 206–207
- **Yoga**, pages 106–109
- **Meditation**, pages 78–79
- **Past Lives and Past-Life Therapies**, pages 50–51

Hinduism is one of the world's oldest religions. There are roughly one billion practising Hindus in the world today, the overwhelming majority living in India. Hinduism is a truly **eclectic religion**, embracing many pathways to **enlightenment**. Each separate pathway is known as a **yoga**, and they are customarily taught or revealed to the devotee by a **guru**. Hinduism acknowledges One Supreme God, but also has many other gods, or **Devas**.

Eclectic religion

Hinduism has gradually emerged and evolved over many thousands of years, first arising in the Indus Valley in modern Pakistan between c. 2500 BCE and 1500 BCE. It is hard to define for the simple reason that it is eclectic, celebrating many divergent spiritual philosophies and practices. Some important concepts within Hinduism include dharma, karma and

Hindu pilgrimage *Thousands of pilgrims flock to the ghats (slopes or steps into sacred water) during the annual Hindu pilgrimage to the holy Pushkar lake in Rajasthan, India.*

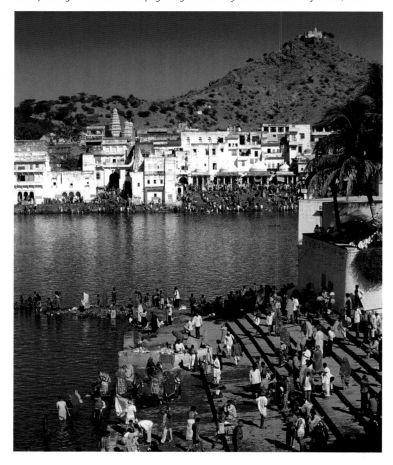

reincarnation, ritual, devotion and the idea of one and many gods. The Vedas (meaning 'knowledge') is the great body of sacred Hindu literature, which is revered as revelation and which includes such important texts as the Upanishads and the Yoga Sutras. The Vedas provides guidance on a key Hindu concept, dharma, a term that comprises a range of meanings including religion, truth, duty, ethics and law. Adherents of Dharmic Hinduism focus particularly on karma, the idea that every action has an effect that must be accounted for in this and future lifetimes. Karma is closely linked with the concept of reincarnation (*samsara*), the cycle of death and rebirth. Liberation from *samsara* is achieved by becoming free of karma that we have built up over many lifetimes. Another important approach to Hinduism is *bhakti* (meaning 'devotion'), which focuses on ritual and the honouring of deities via icons and holy people. *Bhakti* is widely known as the path of love.

What binds the many different strands of Hinduism together is their common quest for ultimate or transcendent truth. This is why Hindus call their religion Santana Dharma, a Sanskrit term which means 'eternal doctrine'. According to the Hindu sage Sri Aurobindo (1872–1950): 'That which we call the Hindu religion is really the eternal religion because it embraces all others.'

Enlightenment

Almost all Hindu traditions incorporate the idea of *atman*, meaning 'true self', together with the idea of Brahman, meaning 'supreme spirit'. For most Hindus, the goal of spiritual practice is to unite the *atman* with Brahman so that the devotee can experience their fundamental oneness with deity. In the Upanishads, sacred scriptures composed between c. 600 and 300 BCE and forming part of the Vedas, we are told that whoever becomes fully aware of their true self will realize their identity with Brahman and experience *moksha*. This is an ecstatic experience of the divine, characterized by freedom from *jiva*, or personal self.

The yogas

In the West yoga typically refers to what Hindus know as hatha yoga, a purification of the body brought about by the practice of *asanas*, or postures.

In India the term yoga – literally translated as 'union' – has a much wider application, referring to spiritual practice in general. Jnana yoga, for example, differs greatly from hatha yoga in that it emphasizes meditation and the study of sacred scripture in order to attain profound spiritual insights into the true nature of God. Bhakti yoga, by contrast, is a path of the heart, with a focus on devotion and unconditional surrender. Bhaktas practise ritualized worship to lose all sense of their personal self in order to experience an ecstatic union with God.

Ashtanga yoga is another form of yoga, focusing largely on spiritual purity and the practice of meditation as a pathway to enlightenment. Ashtanga literally means 'eight-limbed', and the eight limbs are:

1. Yama – abstaining from violence, lying, covetousness, sensuality and possessiveness
2. Niyama – cultivating purity, contentment, austerity, study and surrender
3. Asana – practising meditation in the seated posture
4. Pranayama – developing breath control
5. Pratyahara – withdrawing attention from the sensory world
6. Dharana – focusing awareness on a single object
7. Dhyana – focusing awareness on a single object and on awareness itself
8. Samadhi – a heightened consciousness that recognizes the oneness of all.

The role of the guru

A guru is a spiritual teacher or guide, recognized as possessing special insight or wisdom. For many Hindu devotees, finding a true guru is an essential step on their individual path to enlightenment. Some particularly well-known gurus who have influenced the West include Maharishi Mahesh Yogi (1917–2008), who was guru to the Beatles in the late 1960s and popularized Transcendental Meditation, and Mata Amritanandamayi Devi, known as Amma, who teaches love and service, and blesses all with holy hugs.

The Devas

As well as acknowledging One Supreme God, Hinduism recognizes a pantheon of lesser gods who each embody different aspects of the divine. The three most important are: Brahma – the Creator; Vishnu – the maintainer; and Shiva – the Transformer or Destroyer.

One of Hinduism's most popular deities is Ganesha, the elephant-headed god. Hindus refer to him as the 'the overcomer of obstacles'. He is frequently invoked at the start of projects in order to bring good luck.

Maharishi Mahesh Yogi *This picture shows the renowned guru with British music group The Beatles in the 1960s.*

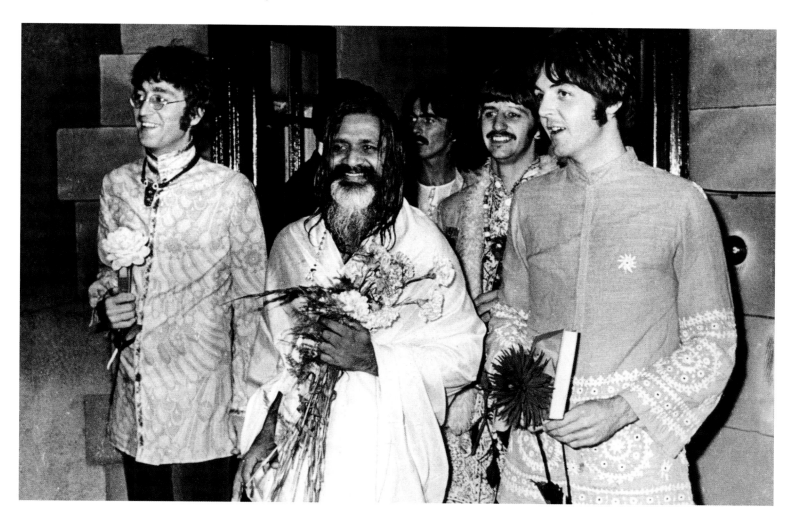

HINDU SACRED TEXTS

If you are interested in **Hindu Sacred Texts**, you may also like to read about:
● Hinduism, pages 204–205

Hinduism encompasses a vast wealth of sacred scripture, beginning with the ancient **Vedas** (c. 1500–500 BCE). Each Veda has its own commentaries, known as the **Brahmanas** (c. 900–600 BCE), describing how Vedic rituals should be performed. **The Upanishads** (c. 600 BCE–300 CE) convey the mystical heart of Hinduism. The **Ramayana** (c. 400–200 CE) tells the story of Lord Rama, while the **Mahabharata** (c. 700 BCE–300 CE) recounts the epic tale of the Bharata dynasty. The **Bhagavad Gita** (c. 400–100 BCE) is a poetic account of Hindu philosophy, especially revered by the followers of Krishna.

The Vedas

These are a collection of mantras, recited or chanted by 'priests' at Hindu rituals. There are four primary Vedas (*samhitas*), comprising some 20,000 verses. According to orthodox Hinduism, the Vedas were not created by humans, but were 'revealed' and subsequently written down. The Vedas are the fertile soil from which the great works of Hindu scripture have grown.

The Brahmanas

Each Brahmana comments on one of the Vedas, containing both guidance on the performance of holy rites and an accompanying explanation. These texts are extremely important for many practising Hindus, for whom proper observance of ritual is necessary in order to attain spiritual purity, essential for fostering union with God.

The Upanishads

These texts convey the essential teachings of Vedanta, of which there are three major schools. The first is Advaita (meaning 'not two'), and it holds that Brahman is indivisible unity, having no qualities that can be defined. In Advaita, the *atman* – the essential self – and Brahman – the supreme spirit – are experienced and celebrated as one. The Isha Upanishad states:

'What ignorance or sorrow is there for one who sees unity?
It has filled all. It is radiant, beyond any thing, and completely safe…
Wise, intelligent, encompassing, self-existent,
It organizes everything for all eternity.'

The second school of Vedanta is Dvaita (meaning 'dualism'), and it holds that the *jiva* – the personal self – and Brahman – the supreme spirit – are separate beings. In Dvaita, Brahman is represented in the form of Krishna (an avatar of Vishnu) as a personal God. The Dvaitic school is expounded more fully in the Brahma Sutras and the Bhagavad Gita.

The third major school of Vedanta is Vishishtadvaita (meaning 'not two, but with qualifications'), and it seeks to reconcile the seeming contradictions between Advaita and Dvaita. Vishishtadvaita holds that Brahman is the indivisible unity but that Brahman can be experienced in a multiplicity of forms. According to the Katha Upanishad:

'Beyond the senses are the objects; beyond the objects is the mind; beyond the mind, the intellect; beyond the intellect, the Great Atman; beyond the Great Atman, the Unmanifest; beyond the Unmanifest, the self of the Universe. Beyond the self of the Universe there is nothing: this is the end, the Supreme Goal.'

The Ramayana

This is an ancient Sanskrit poem consisting of some 24,000 verses in seven separate books. It tells the epic story of Lord Rama, whose wife, Sita, is abducted by the demon Ravana, the King of Lanka. At the end of the story Lord Rama is helped by his great devotee, the monkey god Hanuman, to vanquish and kill Ravana.

The narrative of the Ramayana repeatedly explores the nature of dharma (see page 204), and reveals the wisdom of the Hindu sages.

The Mahabharata

This is another great epic of Hindu literature, which recounts the long history of the Bharata dynasty, and it has played a major role in shaping Indian culture. The Mahabharata is formed of 18 books describing an 18-day war between 18 armies. The Mahabharata is eight times as long as 8th-century BCE Greek poet Homer's famous epics *The Iliad* and *The Odyssey* combined, making it one of the longest poems ever to have been written. It develops many important Hindu concepts, such as dharma and karma (see page 204), and introduces important Hindu figures like Arjuna and Krishna. Krishna dies at the very end of the story, thus marking the beginning of the age of Kali, the fourth and final period in the history of mankind. During the story, the author Vyasa promises the reader: 'If you listen carefully, at the end you'll be someone else'.

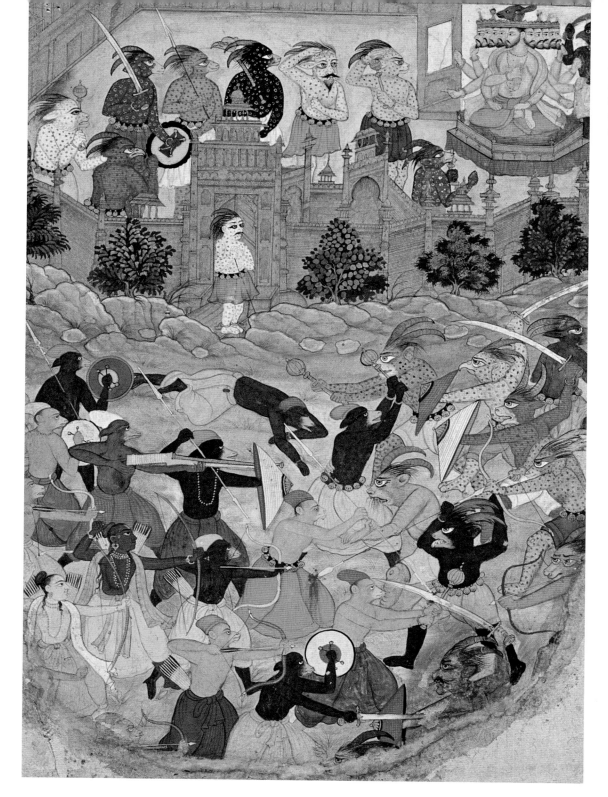

The Bhagavad Gita

Meaning 'Song of God', the Bhagavad Gita is taken from the Bhishma Parva, a single chapter of the Mahabharata. The Gita, as it is known, comprises a conversation between the prince Arjuna and Krishna, his charioteer, on the eve of battle at the outset of the Kurukshetra civil war. Arjuna laments: 'How can any good come from killing one's own relatives? What value is victory if all our friends and loved ones are killed?'

During the ensuing dialogue, Krishna explains to Arjuna the true meaning of dharma, pointing out that one person's duty may be another person's sin. Krishna goes on to reveal his true identity as an incarnation of Vishnu, the Supreme Being, telling Arjuna he has nothing to fear. Krishna states:

> *'I am the goal, the sustainer, the master, the witness, the abode, the refuge and the most dear friend. I am the creation and the annihilation, the basis of everything, the resting place and the eternal seed.'*

BUDDHISM

If you are interested in **Buddhism**, you may also like to read about:
- **Tibetan Buddhism**, page 212
- **Zen Buddhism**, page 213
- **Buddhist Sacred Texts**, pages 210–211

There are approximately 400 million adherents to Buddhism throughout South East Asia and the Far East, in countries as diverse as Sri Lanka, Thailand, Tibet, China and Japan. Unlike followers of most other religions, many Buddhists do not believe either in a personal God or in many gods. Instead, what unites Buddhists is that they 'take refuge' in the three 'jewels' of Buddhism: the **Buddha**, the **Dharma** – including the **Noble Eightfold Path** – and the **Sangha**. Buddhism has divided into two main **traditions**: Theravada and Mahayana, with sub-divisions such as Tibetan and Zen Buddhism.

The Buddha

This is the name given to the great sage Siddhartha Gautama, the founder of Buddhism. It is believed that he was born a prince around 560 BCE in what is now Nepal. Siddhartha grew up enjoying great wealth and privilege, shielded from suffering by his protective father. At the age of 29, he is said to have grown tired of his lavish life, and he left his royal palace to see the world. Despite his father's best efforts to keep all evidence of human suffering hidden from him, he met an old man and learned that old age was the fate awaiting everyone. He was deeply shaken, and resolved to learn more about life. On subsequent trips he saw a sick man, a decaying corpse and an ascetic. Deeply distressed, he abandoned his wife and son, determined to find a way to escape the horrors of existence. Buddhists refer to this event as the Great Departure.

Siddhartha searched far and wide, studying under many teachers and practising meditation and extreme fasting with other young seekers. After a long, exhaustive and frequently futile quest, Siddhartha sat down under a Bodhi tree and resolved never to get up until he had attained enlightenment. After 49 days of continuous meditation, Siddhartha achieved a complete awakening. He saw that the cause of human suffering was ignorance, and he recognized the necessary steps to eliminate it. From then on Siddhartha was known as the Buddha, or 'awakened one'. Buddhists refer to this event as the Great Awakening.

The Dharma

After his great awakening, the Buddha spent the rest of his life teaching the Dharma, which has come to mean the teachings of Buddha. The Dharma begins with the Four Noble Truths:

1. There is suffering.
2. There is a cause to suffering.
3. There is an end to suffering.
4. There is a path to the end of suffering.

Put simply, the Dharma teaches that we suffer because of our attachments to worldly pleasures, and that we can only be free of our suffering if we see through the illusion of the separate self to our true nature. This leads to an ecstatic state of enlightened liberation known as nirvana, and the way to attain enlightenment is to follow the Noble Eightfold Path.

The Noble Eightfold Path

This represents a founding stone of the Dharma. It consists of a profound philosophy of being, a compassionate moral code with accompanying precepts and a set of meditative practices to perfect and transform the mind. The eight paths are:

1. Right Seeing – recognizing how things truly are (that is, the Four Noble Truths)
2. Right Intention – aiming to overcome desire; to do good; to develop compassion
3. Right Speech – not lying; not slandering; not offending; not speaking idly or with good purpose
4. Right Action – not harming; not stealing/deceiving; avoiding sexual misconduct
5. Right Livelihood – not producing/trading in weapons, sentient beings or poisons
6. Right Effort – seeking to cultivate, maintain and perfect wholesome states of mind
7. Right Mindfulness – contemplation of body, feeling, mental states and phenomena
8. Right Concentration – meditating on wholesome thoughts and deeds.

In conjunction with the Noble Eightfold Path, Buddhists also observe the Middle Way, a guiding principle of Theravada Buddhism developed by Siddhartha during his long search for enlightenment. In practice, this means avoiding the extremes of self-indulgence and self-denial, adopting a middle path of moderation instead.

The Sangha

Soon after his awakening, the Buddha travelled to North India where he encountered five men who had been his companions during the ascetic phase of his long quest for enlightenment. The Buddha taught them the Dharma – an event referred to by Buddhists as 'the Turning' or 'the First Turning of the Wheel of Dharma' – and the five men immediately apprenticed themselves, becoming the first Buddhist monks. Together with the Buddha, they formed the first Buddhist community, or Sangha, which became the third jewel of Buddhism. In time, the Sangha would grow as the Buddha's teachings spread throughout India and beyond. Today all practising Buddhists belong to a community, pursuing the Noble Eightfold Path individually and as part of a group. According to Buddhist teacher Thich Nhat Hanh, 'The essence of a sangha is awareness, understanding, acceptance, harmony and love.'

Different traditions

Buddhism quickly spread in many directions. To the south it became Theravada Buddhism, a form of Buddhism associated solely with the Buddha's teachings and easily identified by monks who wear distinctive orange robes and who shave their heads. To the north and east it became Mahayana Buddhism, a more inclusive tradition that has embraced many outside influences. This subsequently led to Tibetan Buddhism, whose monks wear distinctive maroon robes, and Zen Buddhism, which focuses on the achievement of enlightenment through meditation or the work of a teacher. Zen Buddhist monks dress in black or grey.

Buddhist monks *Thai Buddhist monks pray in front of the giant Buddha statue at a royal temple in Wat Suthat. They are chanting for the Thai King Bhumibol Adulyadej.*

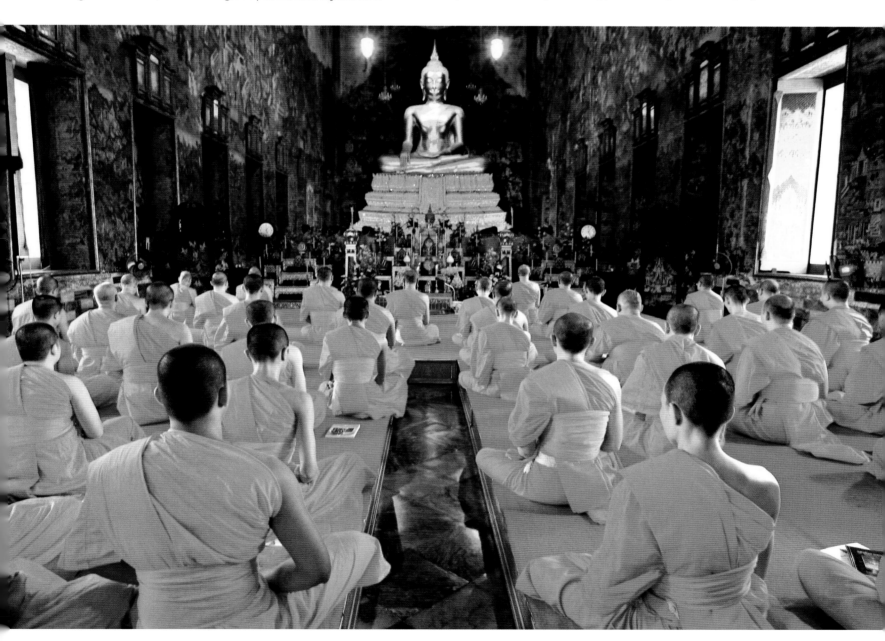

BUDDHIST SACRED TEXTS

If you are interested in **Buddhist Sacred Texts**, you may also like to read about:
- **Buddhism**, pages 208–209
- **Tibetan Buddhism**, page 212
- **Zen Buddhism**, page 213
- **Tantra**, pages 214–215

The first Buddhist scriptures, the Tripitaka, were composed in the 3rd century BCE. In the Theravada tradition, the most revered of these is the **Dhammapada**. During the following 400–500 years, the Mahayana tradition developed in Tibet and the east, and many **Sutras** were added, including the **Lotus**, the **Pure Land** and the **Heart** Sutras. In the 8th century CE, the **Tibetan Book of the Dead** became part of the Mahayana canon.

The Dhammapada

According to Buddhist tradition, the verses of the Dhammapada were spoken by the Buddha on a number of occasions and carefully memorized by his disciples. The text offers a complete explication of the Four Noble Truths and the Noble Eightfold Path. It consists of 423 verses divided into 26 chapters, with each chapter addressing a subject at the heart of Buddhism, for example: thought, pleasure, right living, the self, meditation and the Buddha. Typically, the verses contrast virtuous living with the path chosen by fools:

'All that we are is the result of what we have thought: it is founded on our thoughts, it is made up of our thoughts. If a man speaks or acts with an evil thought, pain follows him, as the wheel follows the foot of the ox that draws the carriage.

All that we are is the result of what we have thought: it is founded on our thoughts, it is made up of our thoughts. If a man speaks or acts with a pure thought, happiness follows him, like a shadow that never leaves.'

The Lotus Sutra

This was composed in Kashmir in the 1st century CE. It is believed to be one of the very last spoken discourses of the Buddha, which was written down and preserved for 500 years. It presents the idea that the Buddha is immortal, but that he willingly chose to enter the cycle of rebirth so that he could teach the Dharma to mankind over and over again. Such a person is called a Bodhisattva. Much of the Lotus Sutra text focuses on the 'skilful means' for attaining enlightenment.

The Lotus Sutra portrays Buddhahood as being much more than achieving the experience of emptiness; it is an ecstatic state of bliss characterized by a deep and abiding love for all, which leads to a longing to share enlightenment with others.

'One who upholds this Sutra should bring forth kindness and compassion for those at home, those who have left home and those who are not Bodhisattvas, thinking, "Those who do not hear or believe this Sutra suffer a great loss. When I have gained the Buddha Way I shall use whatever means I can to speak this Dharma so they may benefit from it."'

The Pure Land Sutra

In the Far East one of the most popular sacred texts of the Mahayana tradition is the Pure Land Sutra, known also as the Infinite Life Sutra. This Sutra begins as a conversation between the Buddha and his attendant, Ananda, and goes on to describe in poetic fashion the land of bliss inhabited by the Buddhas, and how sentient beings may enter there:

'…always in the realm of bliss, that pure Buddha land, there are wondrous winds blowing through the treasure trees and the treasure nettings, producing a fine and wondrous sound, like hundreds of thousands and thousands of heavenly musical instruments playing simultaneously…
In the myriad beings of that land, who have heard this sound, there arises the thought of the Buddha, Dharma and Sangha, with the intention of infinite goodness.'

The Heart Sutra

This is one of those rare scriptures in Buddhism not attributed to the Buddha himself. The Heart Sutra is believed to have been composed in the 1st century CE and it is one of the most loved of the Mahayana Sutras, as well as one of the shortest: it consists of just 14 verses in Sanskrit. It points to the blissful state of nirvana, in which our normal modes of experiencing are completely transcended:

'The Bodhisattva experiences no obstruction in his mind.
Because there is no obstruction, he has no fear.
And he passes far beyond confused imagination,
And reaches ultimate nirvana.'

The Tibetan Book of the Dead

Popularized by the celebrated Swiss psychologist Carl Jung (1875–1961), who attributed to it some of his most fundamental insights, the Tibetan Book of the Dead deals with death and rebirth, outlining what happens to us when we die. In many religions a person travels to a different realm when they die, but this book differs in that it describes how a new consciousness is born according to the karma we have built up during our last incarnation (see page 204), moving us ever closer to enlightenment, the goal of all sentient beings.

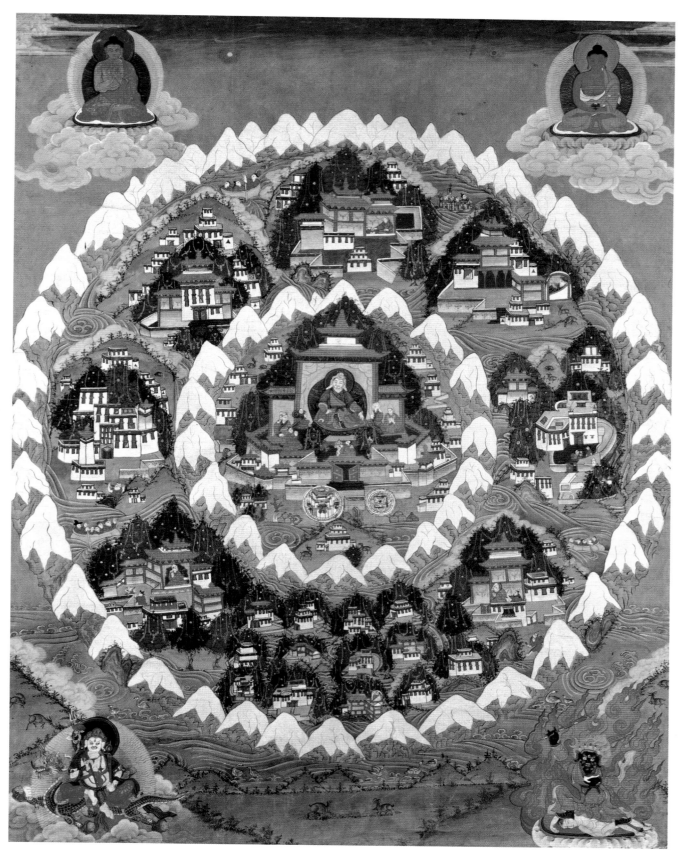

Shambhala *This Tibetan painted silk banner depicts Shambhala, the kingdom of Bliss described in the* Tibetan Book of the Dead.

TIBETAN BUDDHISM

If you are interested in **Tibetan Buddhism**, you may also like to read about:
- Buddhism, pages 208–209
- Zen Buddhism, page 213
- Buddhist Sacred Texts, pages 210–211
- Tantra, pages 214–215

Tibetan Buddhism is practised not only in Tibet, but also in Nepal, Bhutan, Mongolia and in parts of Russia and India, and in small pockets in the West. Tibetan Buddhism is in the Mahayana tradition, but also includes **Vajrayana**. The political leader of the Tibetans is the **Dalai Lama**, widely regarded as one of the world's foremost spiritual teachers. Tibetan Buddhists have developed their own **unique customs** and **sacred art**.

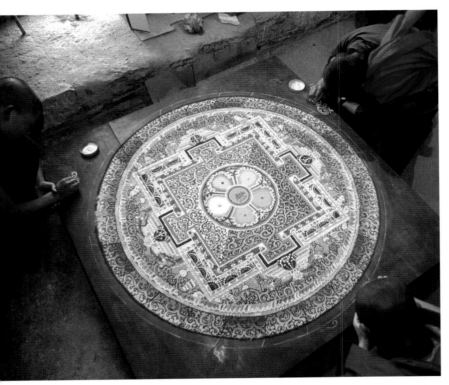

Sand paintings *These novice monks are creating a sand painting at the Semtoka Monastery in Bhutan.*

The Dalai Lama

Tibetan Buddhism has attracted particular interest in the West in recent years, especially since the invasion of Tibet by China in 1959 and the subsequent exile of His Holiness the Dalai Lama. The present Dalai Lama is the 14th Dalai Lama, and Tibetans believe him to be the most recent incarnation in a long line of Buddhist masters who have chosen to re-enter the cycle of death and rebirth in order to teach the Dharma (see page 208) to humanity.

When asked to explain his religion, the present Dalai Lama responded: 'My religion is simple. My religion is kindness.'

Vajrayana

While the Theravada tradition of Buddhism emphasizes the Dhammapada, and the Mahayana tradition the Perfection of Wisdom Sutras in addition, Tibetan Buddhism goes further by embracing a third *yana*, meaning 'vehicle', known as Vajrayana – the Diamond vehicle, or way.

The Vajrayana is a set of powerful tantric practices designed to elicit direct mystical experiences. The tantras themselves are transmitted via sacred lineages whose precise origin it is impossible to discern. They are 'taught' to advanced students by highly evolved Buddhist masters, because merely reading about a particular tantric practice (see page 214) is thought to be inadequate to ensure a proper awakening. Because of the esoteric nature of these sacred rites, the novice must find a teacher who is suitably qualified to transmit them. Tibetans advise scepticism in picking a teacher, but once chosen they expect the initiate to express complete reverence and devotion.

The tantras may involve deep meditation upon images and sounds, as well as creatively visualizing a personal connection to a particular deity. According to Tibetan Buddhist Lama Thubten Yeshe (1935–1984): 'Self-visualization empowers us to take control of our life and create for ourselves a pure environment in which our deepest nature can be expressed.'

Unique customs

Tibetan Buddhism is uniquely associated with the hanging of prayer flags, designed to bless people and nature. Another characteristic custom involves the creation of intricate coloured sand paintings that are then ritually destroyed, often as a gift to a river, to demonstrate the illusory nature of desire and life.

Sacred art

Tibetan Buddhists have developed their own unique religious iconography, which is given exquisite expression in traditional painting. Sacred art often depicts beautiful and blissful deities, but also angry and frightening ones as well. The role of the wrathful deities is to protect the true teaching of the Dharma from corruption.

ZEN BUDDHISM

If you are interested in **Zen Buddhism**, you may also like to read about:
● **Buddhism**, pages 208–209

Zen Buddhism was founded in the 6th century CE by **Bodhidharma**, a Buddhist of the Mahayana tradition. It is taught by **Zen masters** who employ unique spiritual techniques, such as **Zazen** and the contemplation of **Koans**, designed to create a direct and immediate experience of enlightenment. Zen Buddhism originated in China, and subsequently spread to Vietnam, Korea and Japan.

Bodhidharma

His name literally meaning 'Knower of the Way', Bodhidharma is said to have spent several decades staring at a cave wall in deep meditation before travelling from India to China to found a school of Buddhism known as Ch'an, which means 'meditation'. The familiar name Zen was acquired when the school arrived and settled in Japan.

Bodhidharma's teachings are said 'not to stand upon words', since they do not originate from or depend upon the study of sacred texts, as in orthodox Buddhism. Instead, Bodhidharma's calling was to teach a set of spiritual techniques that generate an experience of enlightenment in the here and now. As a consequence, rather than developing a body of sacred scripture, Zen has instead relied on the transmission of profound insight from one master to the next.

The Zen masters

With no holy scripture, a rich oral and written tradition in Zen has evolved, revolving mainly around stories of the great Zen masters, who are renowned for acting in unusual and unexpected ways in their attempts to enlighten their pupils, as in the following story:

> *'One day a young student visited the great Master Dokuon, hoping to show off his understanding of Zen. He spoke at length, before proudly proclaiming: "In reality, nothing exists." Master Dokuon sat silently smoking, before suddenly rising from his chair and whacking the student with his bamboo pipe. "If nothing exists," he said with a smile, "then where did this anger come from?"'*

Zazen

The practice of Zazen is central to Zen Buddhism. It is a form of meditation practised in the sitting position, the lotus position being popular. Its purpose is to bring a person so fully into the present moment that they transcend their usual sense of self. In this experience, the normal conception of self as a separate being in space and time dissolves and the student comes face to face with their own true nature, which is pure bliss. According to Zen Master Bassui (1327–1387): 'Seeing one's own nature is Buddhahood.'

Koans

These are anecdotes or questions posed by Zen masters designed to provoke a sudden transformation in consciousness that leads to enlightenment, for example: 'What is the sound of one hand clapping?'

Zen Buddhists *Monks of the Soto School, one of the three branches of Zen Buddhism, meditate at the Seiryu-ji Temple in Hikone City, Japan.*

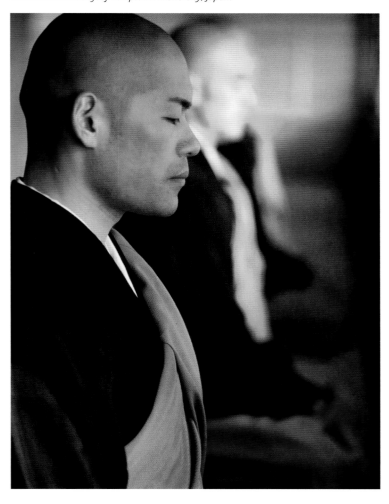

TANTRA

If you are interested in **Tantra**, you may also like to read about:
- **Hinduism**, pages 204–205
- **Tibetan Buddhism**, page 212
- **The Collective Unconscious**, pages 20–21
- **Chakras and the Aura**, pages 172–173

Tantra refers to a set of spiritual **beliefs** and **practices** originating in India and embraced by many Hindus, Buddhists and followers of the Bon and Jain faiths. Tantra has been practised in various forms in India, Pakistan, China, Tibet, Bhutan, Nepal, Sri Lanka, Korea, Burma, Cambodia, Indonesia and Japan. It has achieved a particular fame in the West because it encompasses **sexual rites**.

Tantric beliefs

Tantra is characterized by the belief that the universe we experience is a manifestation of divine energy (prana), and that we can channel this divine energy in order to attain spiritual goals. In the words of Lama Thubten Yeshe:

> 'Each one of us is a union of all universal energy. Everything that we need in order to be complete is within us right at this very moment. It is simply a matter of being able to recognize it. This is the tantric approach.'

Followers of Tantra often refer to the world we experience as *maya*, a dream-like illusion that we mistake for reality. Instead of rejecting *maya*, tantrists believe we must see through the illusion of *maya* to a deeper level of experience, where we recognize our own divine nature. For Tantrists, *maya*

is not an enemy to be fought and overcome; on the contrary, *maya* is the doorway to the divine. Swami Nikhilananda (1895–1973) stated: 'The very poison that kills becomes the elixir of life when used by the wise.'

To see through the illusion of *maya* is a profound mystical awakening, and the purpose of tantric practices is to take the initiate to this place.

Tantric practices

Highly specialized tantric techniques evolved in India, Tibet and beyond over many thousands of years. These practices include meditating upon mantras and yantras, practising special yogas such as kundalini and engaging in sacred sexual rites. In all cases, the role of the guru, or teacher, is central, since without proper guidance the effects of tantra will be negligible or, in a worst-case scenario, positively harmful.

Meditation upon mantras is one of the most widely used techniques employed by tantrists. A mantra is a sacred verbal utterance, imbued with the power to bring about change. However, it is important to recognize that mantras by themselves have no power to induce mystical experience, but when they are evoked with the correct mental and emotional attitude, which may require extensive preparation, they can act as a catalyst for profound spiritual transformation. As Lama Anagarike Govinda (1898–1985) explained:

> 'Mantras are not "spells", as even prominent Western scholars repeat again and again... Mantras do not act on account of their own "magic" nature, but only through the mind that experiences them.'

Yantras are sacred symbols that are used by tantrists to evoke visions of deities, such as Shiva in Hinduism or any number of Bhodisattvas in Tibetan Buddhism. Some of the most potent and inspiring yantras are mandalas, complex circular patterns (see left) whose intricate designs can evoke a profound spiritual awakening. Eminent psychologist Carl Jung believed that mandalas were representations of the unconscious self, and he advocated that we make our own mandalas in order to connect with our higher self. Yantra meditation facilitates direct personal contact with specific deities, which often provokes an ecstatic experience of blissful liberation from the personal self, the stated goal of most Eastern traditions. At such moments, the tantric yogi enjoys a direct and immediate experience of the divine.

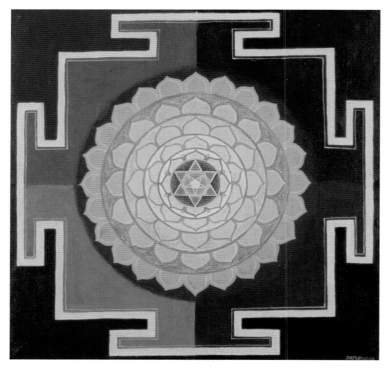

Yantra *This holy diagram, drawn up with pigment on board, is known as the Gayatri Yantra. The artist chants a mantra whilst painting in order to summon Gayatri Devi.*

Tantric Buddhism *The Lukhang Temple in Lhasa depicts the most sacred and esoteric practices of tantric Buddhism.*

Tantra includes a number of yogas, the most well-known being kundalini, meaning 'the unlimited energetic potential in every human being'. Kundalini is an extremely potent tantric practice designed to awaken the energy lying dormant in the spine. Tantric yogis advise Westerners to approach kundalini yoga with great care.

Sexual rites

There is a tradition in Hindu tantra that has sought to channel the powerful force of sexual energy in the service of spiritual goals. During tantric sex, men and women abstain from the pursuit of purely sexual ecstasy in order to achieve a spiritual awakening. In certain ceremonies the man represents Shiva – the god known as the Transformer or Destroyer – and the woman Shakti –

the goddess known as the Great Divine Mother – and when they come together in sexual union, each experiences a fusion of their own Shiva and Shakti energies, leading to a profound spiritual transformation.

By contrast, in Vajrayana Buddhism, novices are sometimes encouraged to have as much sex as possible, as a way of exhausting the desire for pleasure, so that they are better placed to attain spiritual enlightenment.

Many in the West mistakenly believe that the *Kama Sutra* is a tantric text, when in fact it is a 2nd-century CE Sanskrit work compiled by the scholar Vatsyayana, which dispenses a wealth of guidance on sex, from relationships to positions and techniques. By contrast, tantric sexual rites are not remotely concerned with pleasure but are instead exclusively focused on transcending the personal self in order to commune with the divine.

TAOISM

If you are interested in **Taoism**, you may also like to read about:
- **Taoist Sacred Texts**, pages 218–219
- **Traditional Chinese Medicine**, pages 98–101
- **T'ai Chi**, pages 112–113

Taoism is an ancient Chinese spiritual tradition that first emerged c. 500 BCE, although some Taoists believe that Taoism has much older roots. It is characterized by surrender, spontaneity and compassion. To be a Taoist means simply to follow the way of **Tao**. Taoist philosophy embraces the idea of polarity, which it expresses as **yin and yang**. Taoists cultivate a state of being known as *wu wei*.

Tao

The word Tao is Chinese for 'way', but in Taoism Tao has a much bigger meaning, in the sense of 'the way things are in themselves', 'the underlying reality' or 'the primal source'. According to the great Taoist master Lao Tzu (604–531 BCE):

'Tao is like an empty space,
That can never be filled up.
Yet it contains everything:
Blunt and sharp,
Resolved and confused,
Bright and dull,
The whole of Creation.
Hidden, but always present.
Who created it?
It existed before the Creator.'

Tao is sometimes described as 'the way of water' because Taoists seek to embody the yielding qualities of water. Like water, which flows round any obstacle it meets, Taoists look to accommodate problems rather than confront them head-on. Like water, which is soft and weak, yet has the power to wear away hard rocks, they trust in the strength of acceptance and perseverance as opposed to effort and brute force. Like a river flowing down to the ocean, Taoists seek to transform their lives into a fluid journey back to Tao, as in the words of the famed Chinese poet T'ao Ch'en (365–427 CE):

'Just surrender to the wave
of the great Change.
Neither happy nor afraid
And when it is time to go,
then simply go –
Without any unnecessary fuss.'

Yin and yang

One of the Taoist teachings best known in the West is that of yin and yang. This teaches that everything that exists contains polarities. In general, yin is associated with a way of being that is more passive, contracting and female.

Yang, on the other hand, tends to be associated with a more active, expanding and male quality. Both yin and yang are necessary for creation and life. This understanding of polarities can then be applied to other aspects of life, as Lao Tzu explained:

'Something can be beautiful if something else is ugly.
Someone can be good, if someone else is bad.
Presence and absence.
Long and short.
High and low.
Before and after.
Gibberish and meaning.
They can only exist together!'

Taoists call this ever-present polarity yin and yang, and they represent it with the famous yin/yang symbol, in which the dark yin segment is shown with a white spot of yang, and vice versa. In the words of Lao Tzu:

'Yin is form, the container,
Yang is essence, the contained.
Like the in-breath and the out-breath of Life
These two are one.'

Importantly, within everything yin there is some yang, and within everything yang there is some yin. Nothing in life is ever one thing only; it is always on a journey towards its opposite, a constant ever-changing flux, which we can either resist or accept.

Many people seeking spiritual growth find the Taoist teaching of yin and yang hard to employ, because their inclination is to try to exclude a given pole from their experience. They want success without failure, good without bad, insight without ignorance. But this is not in keeping with the Taoists' view, which is that everything contains its opposite; everything is inherently paradoxical. Living in harmony with Tao means accepting the paradoxes at the heart of life, for they are simply an expression of the mystery of the Tao.

Wu wei

At the heart of Taoist spiritual practice is the cultivation of the state of *wu wei*. This is usually translated as 'not-doing', which can create the misleading

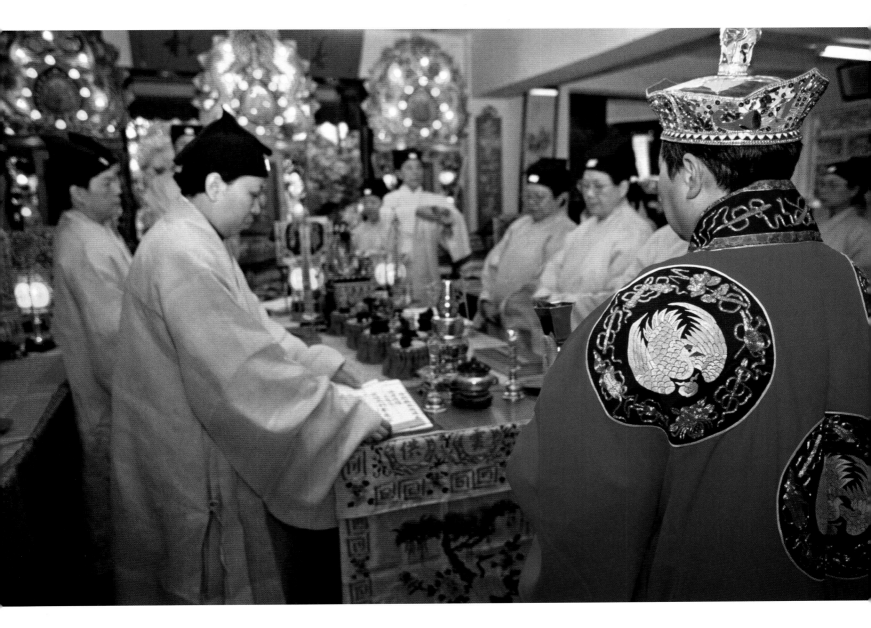

idea that being a Taoist involves doing nothing. A better translation would be 'doing by just being', since *wu wei* is about allowing actions to arise from a deep source inside rather than trying to control them with the rational mind. This can be achieved by seeing through the illusion of the separate, autonomous self, recognizing instead that all individual actions are simply an expression of Tao, arising in one particular body-mind.

Taoist practitioners who attain this deep level of insight are able to experience themselves as part of the natural unfolding of the universe, and so they give up trying to control what happens. This is the essence of *wu wei*. It leads to natural spontaneity, not to apathy. It means living in harmony with Tao. Lao Tzu counselled:

> '*The wise can act by just being,*
> *And teach without speaking.*
> *Things come to them, because they let them go.*
> *They create by not trying to possess.*

Taoist ritual *Whilst ancient Taoist texts, such as the* Tao Te Ching, *are very philosophical, in practice Taoism has become a religion that involves much ritual.*

> *They succeed by not seeking reward.*
> *What needs to be done is done — and then forgotten.*
> *They are always moving on.*'

When a person practises *wu wei* and surrenders his or her life to the Tao, they give up worrying about their own selfish concerns, and discover a deep longing to be of service to others. As in many other spiritual traditions, the guiding principle of life for the enlightened Taoist becomes compassionate love. According to Lao Tzu:

> '*If you have love,*
> *It is as if Heaven itself*
> *Were keeping you safe.*'

TAOIST SACRED TEXTS

The primary sacred text in Taoism is the **Tao Te Ching**, sometimes written as *Dao De Jing*, attributed to the legendary Taoist master Lao Tzu. Other important Taoist texts are the *Chuang Tzu* and the Leih Tzu, ancient collections of spiritual sayings and stories.

If you are interested in **Taoist Sacred Texts**, you may also like to read about:
- Taoism, pages 216–217
- Zen Buddhism, page 213

The *Tao Te Ching*

According to Taoist tradition, the *Tao Te Ching* was composed in the 6th century BCE by a cleric who worked in the Zhou Dynasty court in the state of Chou and went by the name of Li Erh Tan. The story goes that this incomparably wise man became so disillusioned with the lack of wisdom in the people around him that he gave up his job and travelled west on a water buffalo. After a very long journey he arrived at a mountain pass that marked the end of China, where he met a gatekeeper. The two men chatted and the gatekeeper was so impressed by the wisdom of the visitor that he begged him to write a single text that he could leave behind before travelling on. During the night Li Erh Tan set to work, and in the morning he handed the gatekeeper a copy of the *Tao Te Ching*. Then Li Erh Tan saddled up his water buffalo and was never seen again. In his absence he assumed the honorary title Lao Tzu, which means 'Old Master'.

Whatever its true origins, the *Tao Te Ching* is undoubtedly a timeless classic. In the space of 81 brief sections it distils the ancient wisdom of Taoism into a concise, poetic and directly accessible form, as relevant today as when it was first written.

The *Tao Te Ching* addresses many Taoist themes: emptiness, surrender, yin and yang, wisdom, compassion and natural goodness, with occasional comments on politics. It begins by introducing the ineffable idea of Tao:

> 'Tao is not a way that can be pointed out.
> Nor an idea that can be defined.
> Tao is indefinable original totality.
> Ideas create the appearance of separate things.
> Always hidden, it is the mysterious essence.
> Always manifest, it is the outer appearances.
> Essence and appearance are the same.
> Only ideas make them seem separate.
> Mystified?
> Tao is mystery.
> This is the gateway to understanding.'

One of the recurring images in the *Tao Te Ching* is water, a potent symbol for the ever-changing Tao. Without water, all life would cease:

> 'Great goodness is like water.
> It flows everywhere, filling everything.
> It is life-giving, by its very nature.
> It humbly settles in the lowest places,

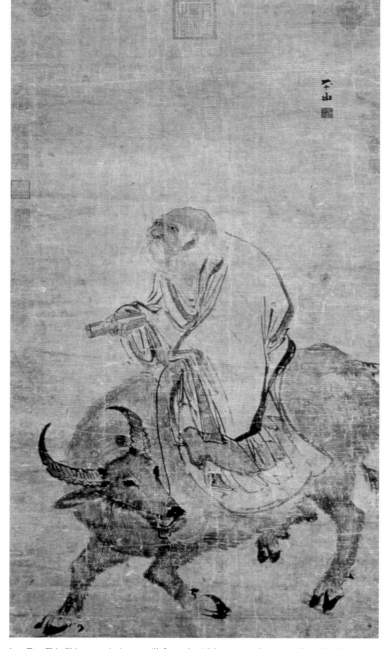

Lao Tzu *This Chinese painting on silk from the 16th century shows Lao Tzu riding his water buffalo to the far west of China before his disappearance.*

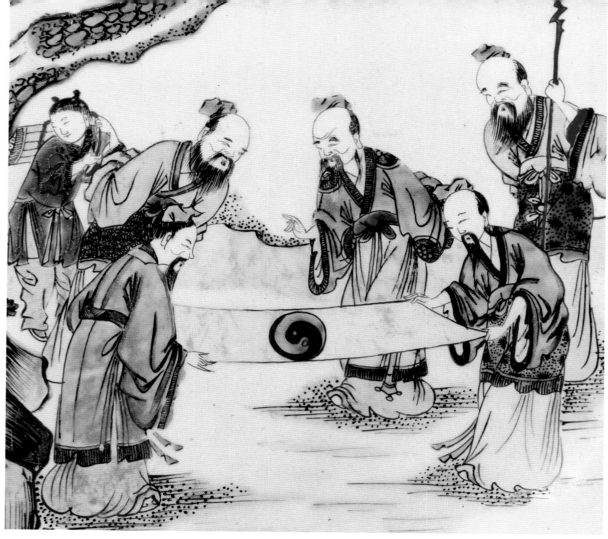

Yin/yang *This painted ceramic from the Kang Hsi Period (1661–1722) depicts sages gathered around a yin/yang symbol.*

Like someone who follows Tao.
Make your heart like a lake,
With a calm, still surface,
And great depths of kindness.
Nurture your true nature.
Make love your gift to others.
Only talk the truth.
Flow around obstacles, don't confront them.
Don't struggle to succeed.
Wait for the right moment.
No need for strife – no need for blame.'

The *Chuang Tzu*

According to Taoist tradition, Chuang Tzu was a revered Taoist master who lived in the 4th century BCE. Whereas the *Tao Te Ching* honours the virtues of acceptance and surrender, the *Chuang Tzu* celebrates qualities of intelligence and insight. Chuang Tzu teaches with a piercing philosophical acuity:

'Chuang Tzu and Huizi were strolling along the dam of the Hao Waterfall when Chuang Tzu said, "See how the minnows come out and dart around where they please! That's what fish really enjoy!"

Huizi said, "You're not a fish – how do you know what fish enjoy?"

Chuang Tzu said, "You're not I, so how do you know I don't know what fish enjoy?"

Huizi said, "I'm not you, so I certainly don't know what you know. On the other hand, you're certainly not a fish – so that still proves you don't know what fish enjoy!"

Chuang Tzu said, "Let's go back to your original question, please. You asked me how I know what fish enjoy – so you already knew I knew it when you asked the question. I know it by standing here beside the Hao."'

Although the tone of the *Tao Te Ching* and the *Chuang Tzu* could not be more different, they are both fundamentally concerned with the same issue – directing the seeker to the great mystery that is Tao. As in other Eastern traditions, attaining enlightenment is like waking up from a dream:

'Once I, Chuang Tzu, dreamed I was a butterfly and was happy as a butterfly. I was conscious that I was quite pleased with myself, but I did not know that I was Tzu. Suddenly I awoke, and there was I, visibly Tzu. I do not know whether it was Tzu dreaming that he was a butterfly or the butterfly dreaming that he was Tzu.'

CONFUCIANISM

If you are interested in **Confucianism**, you may also like to read about:
- **Taoism**, pages 216–217
- **I Ching**, pages 70–71

Confucianism is the name given to the religious and spiritual tradition associated with the Chinese sage **Confucius**. Its most important sacred texts are the *Five Classics*, which include the well-known oracle, the *I Ching*, and the Confucian Canon.

Confucius

Confucius, meaning 'Master of Merit', is believed to have been born in the State of Lu (now the Shandung Province) in 551 BCE. It is widely held that he developed his highly evolved system of personal and social virtue in response to the great social and political turmoil that he lived through. It was his purported aim to bring peace and prosperity to the troubled Chinese Empire.

Confucius *Confucius's writing comprises some of the widest-known philosophical teachings in the world. This Chinese illustration depicts him with some students.*

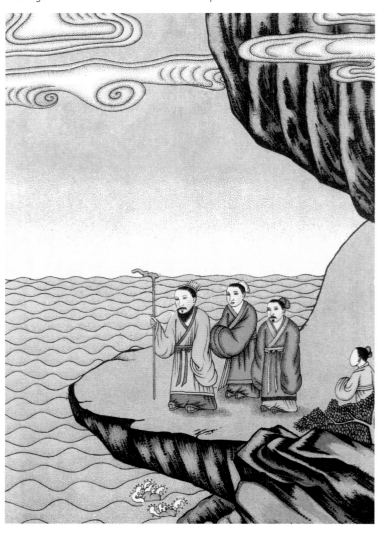

Confucianism has much in common with Taoism, with its clear emphasis on contemplation and compassion. Where it differs is in its unwavering focus on matters of right and wrong, which for Taoists largely disappears when one lives in harmony with the Tao. Confucius believed in the importance of cultivating virtue above all else:

> '*To be able under all circumstances to practise five things constitutes perfect virtue; these five things are gravity, generosity of soul, sincerity, earnestness and kindness.*'

Confucius taught extensively on the subject of good conduct in relation to others, stressing the rewards that befall both individuals and society as a whole when people cultivate courteous and caring relationships: 'Virtue is not left to stand alone. He who practises it will have neighbours.'

It is believed that the followers of Confucius faithfully recorded his extensive teachings after his death in 479 BCE, and so created a body of work known as the Confucian Canon. This work includes a wealth of timeless sayings that communicate deep spiritual insights with striking clarity, simplicity and force, such as the following examples:

> '*Ignorance is the night of the mind, but a night without moon and star.*'
> '*Men's natures are alike; it is their habits that carry them far apart.*'
> '*Before you embark on a journey of revenge, dig two graves.*'
> '*Wherever you go, go with all your heart.*'

The sayings of Confucius became firmly integrated into ancient Chinese culture, and were for many centuries considered essential in the education of all governmental officials.

The *Five Classics*

According to tradition, Confucius also wrote a great work of literature, now known as the *Five Classics*. The Five Classics in question were: the *Classic of Poetry*, the *Classic of Rites*, the *Classic of History*, the *Spring and Autumn Annals* and the *Book of Changes*.

The *Classic of Poetry* consists of poems, songs, hymns and eulogies to be read or performed at social gatherings and public ceremonies. The *Classic of Rites* was lost in the 3rd century BCE. The *Classic of History* is a collection of important historical documents and speeches given by ancient Chinese rulers. The *Spring and Autumn Annals* is a record of the history of the State of Lu, where Confucius was born. The *Book of Changes* is a collection of oracles and a profound in-depth commentary. It is known in the West as the *I Ching*.

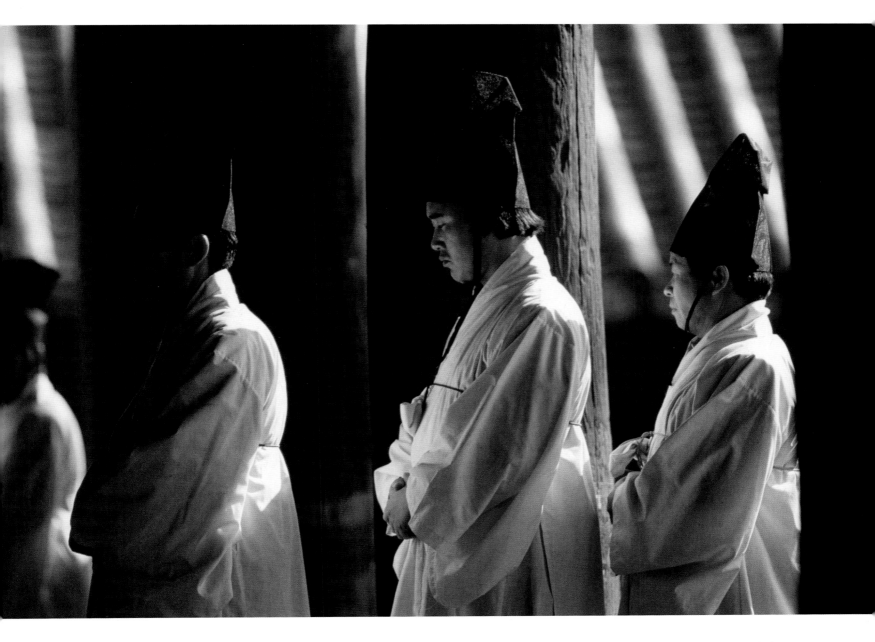

I Ching

This is a unique collection of oracles, with guidance on how they can be used as a system of divination. Taken together, the oracles, in the form of hexagrams and commentaries, give a complete yet concise introduction to all the major themes in Confucianism: virtue and the superior man, the inevitability of change, the balance of opposites and the importance of kindness and compassion.

For example, the hexagram known as Chun, which may be translated as 'sprouting', is associated with difficulty in beginning. In the *I Ching* the commentary on Chun includes guidance on how to move forward in life:

> *'Times of growth are beset with difficulties. They resemble a first birth. But these difficulties arise from the abundance of all that is struggling to arise. Everything is in flux: therefore if one perseveres there is a prospect of great success, in spite of the existing danger.'*

Confucianism *This picture shows participants in a traditional Confucian rite called Sokchonje, a celebration of Confucius's birthday.*

Confucianism as a religion

There is some debate as to whether Confucianism actually qualifies as a religion. As opposed to many other traditions, Confucianism does not recognize an afterlife, deities seem less important in human affairs and concerns such as the nature of the soul, which is a focus in most religions, is given little attention.

However, Confucius's strong emphasis on ethics and morality in daily life, his concept of perfect virtue, his strong regard for the family and his advocacy of the principle 'Do not do to others what you do not want done to yourself' have ensured that Confucianism remains central to the spiritual practice of millions of people around the world today.

JAINISM

Jainism is the ancient Indian religion of the **Jains**, having much in common with Hinduism and Buddhism. The spiritual aim of Jainism is to attain *moksha*, meaning 'liberation from the cycle of rebirth', which may be achieved by combining study and ritual prayer with observance of the **five vows**.

If you are interested in **Jainism**, you may also like to read about:
- **Buddhism**, pages 208–209
- **Hinduism**, pages 204–205
- **Buddhist Sacred Texts**, pages 210–211

The Jains

Jains are followers of Jinas, spiritually elevated beings who have achieved the state of *moksha*. According to Jain tradition, there have so far been 24 Tirthankaras, a special type of Jina who has chosen to teach the path of liberation to others. The last Tirthankara acknowledged by Jains was Shri Mahavir (599–527 BCE).

The 24 Tirthankaras are greatly revered, and their recorded teachings are viewed as holy scripture. Practising Jains say the following prayer every morning, taken from the Namaskara Sutra:

> *'I bow down to those who have achieved* moksha *and teach the path to liberation.*
>
> *I bow down to those who have attained perfect knowledge and liberated their souls.*
>
> *I bow down to those who have experienced self-realization through self-control and self-sacrifice.*
>
> *I bow down to those who understand the true nature of the soul and teach the importance of the spiritual over the material.*
>
> *I bow down to those who strictly follow the five great vows of conduct and inspire us to live a virtuous life.*
>
> *To these five types of great souls I offer my praise.*
>
> *Such praise will help diminish my failings.*
>
> *Giving this praise will bring*
>
> *Happiness and bliss.'*

The five vows

Shri Mahavir taught that right faith, right knowledge and right conduct were the essential steps on the path to liberation. In order to ensure right conduct, he taught five vows:

1. Non-violence – not to cause harm to any living things
2. Truthfulness – to speak only the harmless truth
3. Not stealing – not to take anything not freely given
4. Chastity – not to be seduced by sensual pleasures
5. Non-attachment – not clinging to people, places or things.

Jain monks and nuns are expected to follow these vows scrupulously, and lay Jains to follow them as best they can. Most Jains take the vow of non-violence extremely seriously, believing that harming any living thing creates

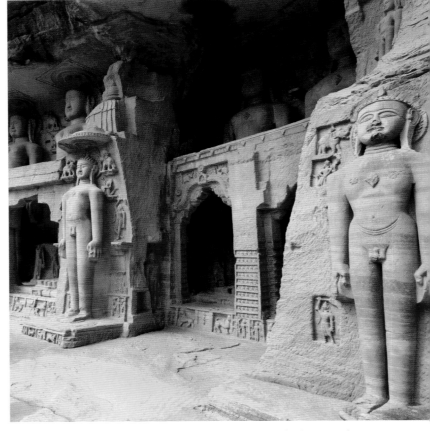

Jainism *These 7th-century Jain sculptures in a fort near the central Indian town of Gwalior depict the Tirthankaras, humans who achieve enlightenment.*

harmful karma (see page 204). As a consequence, the diet of some Jains often goes beyond vegetarianism, and even veganism, extending to not eating root vegetables, since tiny animals may be injured when they are pulled from the earth. Many Jains will not eat carrots, onions or garlic.

Mahatma Gandhi (1869–1948) was deeply influenced by the five vows of Jainism, having been tutored by a Jain in childhood. Gandhi took the vow of non-violence early in life, and this became a central tenet in his long-standing political campaign to liberate India from the rule of the British Empire. Gandhi was also a committed vegetarian.

SIKHISM

If you are interested in **Sikhism**, you may also like to read about:
- **Hinduism**, pages 204–205
- **Buddhism**, pages 208–209
- **Sufism**, pages 198–199
- **Jainism**, page 222

Founded by Sri Guru **Nanak** Dev Ji, Sikhism shares many of the values of Hinduism, Buddhism, Sufism and Jainism. However, at the same time, Sikhism promotes its own unique **spiritual beliefs** and **practices**. Most of the world's 20 million-plus Sikhs live in the Punjab states of India and Pakistan.

Nanak

Nanak was born in 1469 CE in a village close to what is now Lahore, Pakistan. It is said that he was an extraordinarily gifted child, blessed with strange powers and profound spiritual insights. As an adult he travelled throughout India and beyond, sharing his wisdom with all who sought it. Before his death he acquired the title Guru, which for Sikhs means much more than teacher, referring instead to Nanak's status as a divine messenger. Just before his passing, in 1539, Nanak appointed Baba Lehna Ji as his successor, and thus began a holy lineage of ten Sikh Gurus, culminating in Gobind Singh (1666–1708). Guru Singh proclaimed that he was the last human Guru, and that henceforth the text known as Adi Granth, which was first composed by Guru Arjan Dev (1563–1606), would be the final Guru of the Sikhs, thus establishing it as holy scripture.

Spiritual beliefs

In keeping with many mystical traditions, Sikhs do not think of God as an abstract being to be worshipped from afar, but rather as the divine presence in everything. According to Guru Arjan Dev: 'God is beyond colour and form, yet God's presence is clearly visible.'

Sikhs believe that the spiritual purpose of life is to progress from being self-centred to being God-centred. This involves acquiring the qualities of selflessness, devoting one's life to the service of others and following the teachings of the Gurus. The greatest obstacle to becoming God-centred is *maya* – referring to illusory or false values – which distracts us from our spiritual purpose. Sikhism lists five particular evils – ego, anger, greed, attachment and lust – which are capable of separating us from God.

Spiritual practices

Guru Nanak dismissed pilgrimages and other religious rites as pathways to God, instead stressing the importance of inner devotion and dedicated spiritual practice, including deep meditation and prayer: 'Realization of Truth is higher than all else. Higher still is truthful living.'

One of the most important spiritual practices in Sikhism is to meditate on *nam* (the divine name), or on *shabad* (the divine word). If an individual follows this practice with true devotion in his or her heart, they can, in Nanak's words, 'grow towards and into God', the ultimate goal for all Sikhs.

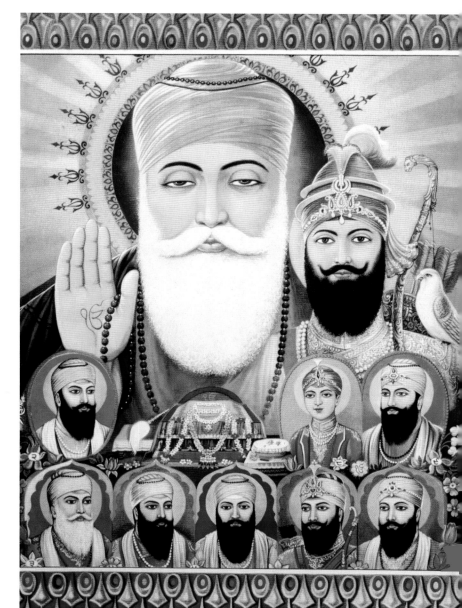

Sikh Gurus *This painting depicts Guru Nanak and the other nine Sikh Gurus, together with the final Guru, Granth Sahib (the text which was previously referred to as Adi Granth).*

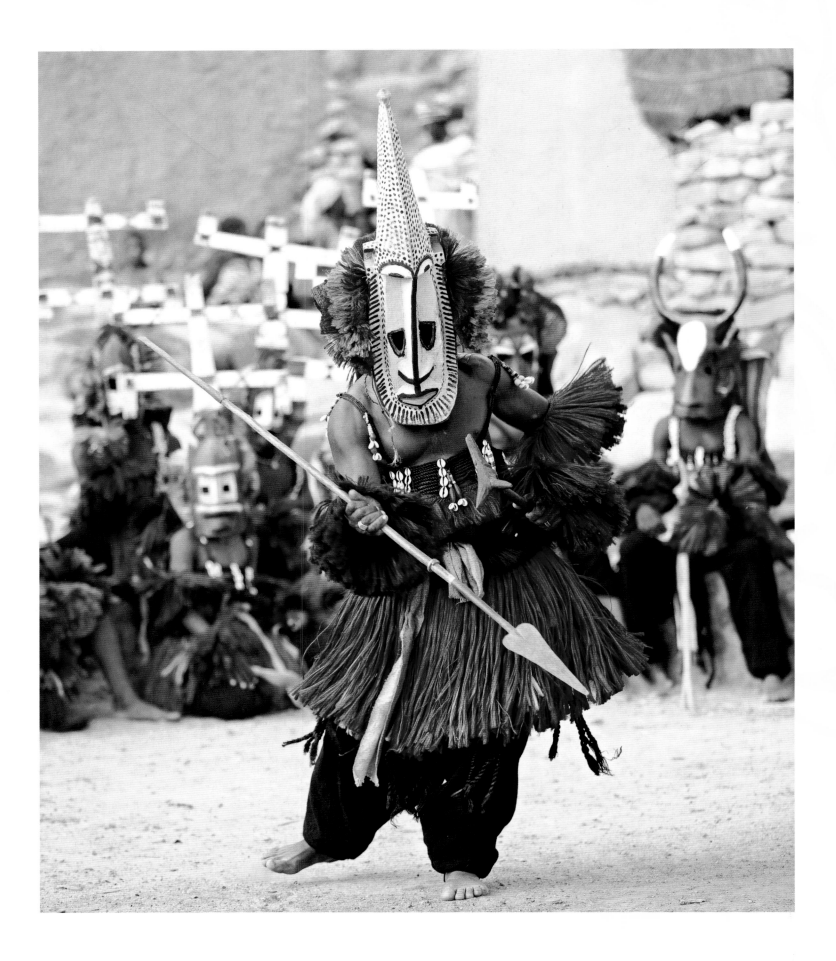

TRIBAL, SHAMANIC AND ANIMIST TRADITIONS

 Among indigenous and tribal peoples around the globe, spiritual practice and ritual was and still is as diverse as their mythology, mostly due to geographical need and cultural necessity. But what they have in common is the worship of and veneration for an array of gods and goddesses (polytheism), and a view that nature itself is imbued with 'cosmic breath'. Many indigenous peoples upheld this ancient belief to reflect and maintain the community's harmonious relationship with nature and the supernatural world. Tribal communities in many parts of the world would use a tribal medicine man or woman, priest or priestess or shaman to lead rituals, make sacrifices, recount the myths of the people as well as perform healing rituals directly informed by the spirits they invoked.

The universal animation of nature

'Animism', in the spiritual sense, was coined by German physicist G. E. Stahl (1660–1734) and introduced by English anthropologist Sir Edward Burnett Tylor (1832–1917) in 1871 in his theory of the universal animation of nature. The word comes from the Latin *animus* or *anima*, which is rooted in the Indo-European word for 'breath'. Thus the animistic spiritual belief is that every thing is permeated by spirit, soul or the breath of life, also known as prana in Hinduism and chi in Taoist philosophy. In Western language, animism can also be defined as a world-view that experiences God in everything.

Tylor argued that the general belief in the spirit or soul in everything was the most primitive principle of all religion. Animism can also refer to a specific belief in the relationship between humans and the non-human spirits that live around us. For example, the head-shrinking practice of the Jivaroan and Urarina peoples of Peru is based on the belief that the spirits of their enemies must be trapped in the head to prevent them escaping and taking revenge by inhabiting the spirit of a predatory animal. The Aboriginal peoples of Australia believe the spiritual essence of Dreamtime is manifest not only in living things, but in the landscape itself, such as Ayers Rock.

Dogon *A Dogon folk dancer during a traditional dance ritual. The Dogon people of central Mali believe that they are descended from a man-god called Nommo.*

Diverse beliefs

Before organized religions such as Christianity, Judaism, Islam, Buddhism and Hinduism spread worldwide, small communities or tribes had their own myths about how the world began or why mankind existed. These were the sacred stories of each tribe or community, and this spiritual heritage would be sustained through oral tradition.

There are many examples of a belief in a supreme creator deity among ancient indigenous peoples, such as Amana, the creator goddess of the Calina of South America, and most based their spiritual practice on polytheism, with various gods and goddesses fulfilling minor roles, such as Thor, the Norse god of thunder, and Ixchel of Mayan mythological belief, the goddess of storms and floods. But many communities also combined these beliefs with the concept of an animistic spirit inhabiting everything from a rock to a hummingbird. In traditions as diverse as Native American Spirituality and Shinto, spirits in nature were worshipped along with the spirits of ancestors. North American native traditions reinforce the belief in both supreme creator forces, such as Wakan Tanka, 'The Great Mystery', and in the spirit power of animals and plants. The notion that all living things and people are descended from the gods was also a commonly held belief within tribal communities. For example, the Maori peoples of New Zealand believed that the god of the sea, Tangaroa, was the ancestor of all fish, and to the Dogon of Africa, Nommo was the ancestor of all Dogon people.

Shamanism and paganism

Other diverse but worldwide beliefs include shamanism – the practice of communicating with the spirit world – which is still widespread among many indigenous peoples today, who share the belief that the shaman is the mediator between the human and spiritual realms. The shaman is a community ambassador who can enter the supernatural world to find out answers to human or local questions.

Modern paganism, particularly in the West, embraces the revival of a range of polytheistic, pantheistic and animistic beliefs and practices. These include, among many others, Wicca, Druidism, Viking Age pagans, heathenry and Goddess Spirituality.

SHAMANISM

Shamanism is the belief in and the actual practice of communicating or interacting with the supernatural world. 'Shaman' was the Mongolian or North Asian word for 'he or she who knows', and people 'who know' are now generically termed shamans among various indigenous peoples **worldwide**. As a healer, the shaman's **work** is usually undertaken alone rather than within an organized religious group, although some form elite groups within isolated communities. Having undergone **initiation and transformation**, shamans usually enter into a trance-induced state to invoke revelations and visions. So-called **New Age shamanism** constitutes a modern-day revival of shamanistic practice.

If you are interested in **Shamanism**, you may also like to read about:
- **Mystical and Transcendent States**, pages 34–35
- **Channelling**, pages 42–43
- **Meditation**, pages 78–79
- **Spiritual Healing and Therapeutic Touch**, pages 176–177

The work of the shaman

Although diverse in their methods depending on geography and cultural needs, each shaman shares the common belief that so-called 'reality' is filled with invisible forces such as spirits and demons, which influence the living in both positive and negative ways. These spirits play a key role in the society or culture in question. Shamans can leave their mortal body to engage in this spiritual world, and can communicate with spirit guides, often animals.

Besides curing illnesses, shamans may also undertake specific roles in the community, such as predicting events, preserving traditional mythology, leading sacrificial rituals and mediating between the community and the spirit world. The shaman is frequently a retriever of lost souls, particularly those of animals that are for hunting purposes, as in the rainforest Tucano people of South America.

Shamans often have specific symbols, objects, totems and codes to identify them from the rest of the group. The shaman's 'lore' expresses the beliefs and mythology of the community through ritual, storytelling, art, dance, taboos, amulets and sacred talismans. These beliefs are frequently symbolized on the shaman's clothing or in painted skin codes and in their choice of musical instrument, which indicates the particular helping spirits that are being employed. Totems such as rocks or stones are commonly used, these items often possessing their own spirit and magic powers. Some shamans claim to have learned the healing powers of plants directly from the plant's spirit.

Initiation and transformation

There are several ways of becoming a shaman in the community. There may be sudden awakenings or a crisis, such as coming through a serious illness. American mythologist Joseph Campbell (1904–1987) wrote: 'the shaman is one who, as a consequence of personal psychological crisis, has gained a certain power of his own'. Rites of passage into shamanism include disturbing or confusing psychological behaviour. This is sometimes induced by hallucinogenic tisanes such as *ayahuasca*, a tea drunk by the Urarina shamans of Amazonian Peru as a ritualistic way to determine shamanistic powers. Many New Age neo-shaman seekers still travel to Peru to work with these peoples.

Some shamans, as among the South American Tapirape peoples, are called in their dreams. Cultural imagery plays a part in the initiation process, as religious historian Mircea Eliade (1907–1986) suggested: 'meeting a spirit guide, transcending the world, and being transformed so as to interact between the visible and invisible worlds or traversing the "axis mundi"'. Once transformed, the shaman is implanted with magical talismans. To travel in this spirit world, the shaman must first enter a trance-like state, which may be induced by a variety of different means including self-hypnosis; tobacco; drugs such as psychedelic mushrooms, *Datura* or deadly nightshade; rapid drumming; sweat lodges; and vision quests (see page 233).

Shamanism worldwide

In Europe, due to the historical dominance of monotheism, indigenous shamans are now rare, apart from those found among some of the Uralic peoples of Russia and Siberia. In Asia, shamanism is still practised in South Korea and within the Bon religion of central Asia, and shamans can be found in small communities in Tibet, Nepal, Vietnam and Taiwan. Shamanism is more widespread among the Inuit peoples of North America and Canada, and is still practised in Africa by the Dogon peoples and in southern African tribal peoples such as the Zulus, who refer to a shaman as a *sangoma* (see page 234). In fact, in most areas of the world where people live close to nature and unaffected by industry and technology, shamanism survives.

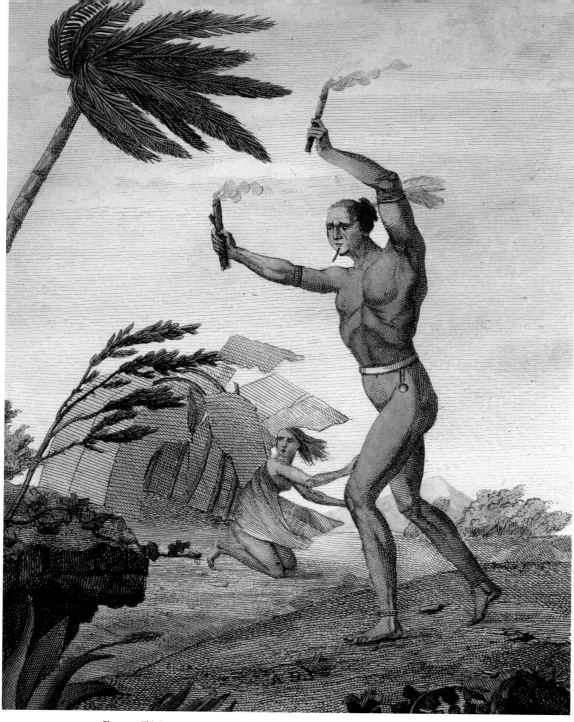

Shaman *This Paraguayan coloured engraving from 1811 depicts a Payaguas shaman attempting to ward off a hurricane with the powerful shamanic mastery of fire energy.*

There are also many shamans in South America, particularly in the Amazonian regions, such as those called *curanderos* of the Peruvian Amazon Basin and the *ayahuasqueros* of the Uravina peoples. In Australia shamans are known as 'clever men or women', or *kadji*. In Papua New Guinea shamans are known to exorcize *masalai*, or dark spirits.

New Age shamanism

There is currently much controversy over New Age shamanism. American anthropologist Michael Harner synthesized a set of beliefs gathered from traditional worldwide shamanistic practices to create what he called 'core shamanism', and established the Foundation for Shamanic Studies in 1985. The practice of this universal type of shamanism has since been popularized. Most contemporary shamans prefer to call themselves shamanic practitioners or neo-shamanists to differentiate themselves from traditional indigenous shamans. The modern methods of inducing a trance-like state include rapid drumming, ritualistic dance and spinning, vision quests, vigils, various entheogens (plant-derived psychoactive substances) and communication with what are often called 'power animals'.

AUSTRALIAN ABORIGINAL SPIRITUALITY

If you are interested in **Australian Aboriginal Spirituality**, you may also like to read about:

● Sacred Geometry, pages 250–251
● Megaliths and Earthworks, pages 252–253
● Landscape Lines, pages 258–259
● Native American Spirituality, pages 232–233

The earliest indigenous peoples of Australia arguably date from the Ice Age of 50,000 years ago, or in some accounts as far back as 125,000 years. These Aboriginal peoples, encompassing a diversity of social groups and languages, lived in small communities throughout the continent. Yet the consistent belief of all these peoples was that spiritual essence is manifest in the landscape and that all life is sacred. They based their spirituality on the **Dreamtime** or **Dreaming**, together with **songlines and sacred sites** – a labyrinth of mystical pathways and footprints left in the landscape by their ancestors.

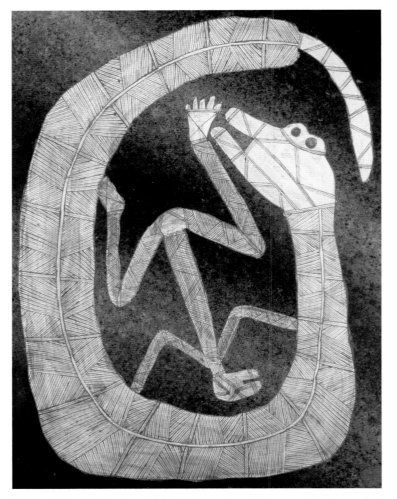

Rainbow Snake *The tale of Ngalyod, or the Rainbow Snake, is central to many Australian Aboriginal creation myths and the concept of Dreamtime.*

Dreamtime

Considered to be the beginning of creation, a time when ancestral spirits gave form to the land, Dreamtime is also an infinite spiritual dimension that includes present-day reality. In a sense, the individual is eternally in existence in the Dreamtime, before, during and after life.

During the time of creation or Dreamtime, creator spirits travelled the land. These included major ancestral spirits and totemic spirits such as the Rainbow Snake, the Djanggawul (two sisters and a brother creator gods) and Marindi (the wild dog), thought to be the spirit of the sacred Ayers Rock. Gods of Dreamtime were known by different names in different communities; for example, Altjira was also known as Arrernte and Pitjantjatjara. The Dreamtime mythology itself is diverse within each group or community. This knowledge includes creation stories, sacred sites, law and customs based on spiritual belief that were passed on via oral tradition.

The Rainbow Snake is an important image in Aboriginal spirituality, variously named Julunggul, Kunmanggur, Ngalyod, Ungar and Yurlunggur, and either male or female, depending on the community. In one account the snake emerged from a waterhole during the Dreaming; in others it came down from the sky. But in most accounts, as it slithered across the continent its movement created valleys, mountains and waterways of the sacred ancestral landscape. In some stories the snake was the creator and preserver of life as well as of water and fertility.

The Worora and Ungarinjin peoples of north and north-western Australia believed that the Wondjina – shape-changers that took the form of humans, hawks, owls and songbirds – were rain spirits who created the world. They painted images of the birds on the rocks where they basked in the sun at a ceremony every year so that the Wondjina would remember to send rain.

To the people of central Australia, the Wati-Kutjara were supernatural twins in the Dreamtime, also known as Kurukadi (white iguana) and Mumba (black iguana). Long before creation they slept under the Earth, and when they awoke, they wandered the Earth creating animals, rocks, waterholes, valleys and plants wherever they travelled.

The Dreaming

This also refers to a specific spiritual belief held by an individual or group. Dreaming was usually associated with an animal that was a manifestation of an ancestral spirit and must never be killed, but always protected as a spirit guide, and so individuals would talk about, for example, Kangaroo Dreaming or Serpent Dreaming. Native Cat Dreaming spirits, for instance, crossed the Simpson Desert and wherever they went left trails and sacred marks on the landscape like a map. The people who followed this Dreaming learned to navigate these trails by singing songs and telling stories about specific markers such as rocks or wells en route.

Songlines and sacred sites

Throughout Australia a huge web of invisible pathways and sacred sites known as songlines or dreaming tracks connects the entire continent, and are believed to reveal the existence of souls or ancestral spirits. These can be likened to the ley lines of Western Europe, the *naga* or serpent lines in India and dragon lines in China. Songlines are sometimes only a few miles long; others traverse deserts and many different groups and languages. The spirit would often transform into part of the landscape, and every rock or hollow had a totem spirit or *djang*. The most well-known and sacred *djang* location is Uluru, also known as Ayers Rock. The spiritual being of the Djabugay people of Queensland, Damarri, was held to have become a mountain range, lying on his back above the Baron River Gorge in north-eastern Australia, while the Noongar peoples in Perth believe that the Darling Scarp was once the serpent Wagyl.

If a group of people followed the exact rituals accorded to the sacred place or site, they would also be able to commune directly with the spirits. By reciting the myths associated with these sacred places, the people entered Dreamtime themselves.

There are few identifiable Aboriginal sacred monuments left in Australia due to the loss of valuable information during the 'Stolen Generation' of 1869–1969 when the Australian government policy dessimated indigenous aboriginal culture. But sites such as Biame's Cave (the place of a creator god situated near Lake Macquarie in New South Wales) are still fiercely guarded, as is the Dampier Rock Art site, the only surviving archipelago of the Yaburara people. This site, one of the world's largest collection of rock carvings, is currently under threat from industrialization.

Uluru *The world-famous sandstone rock formation in Australia's Northern Territory – Uluru, or Ayers Rock – reveals at sunset the blood of Marindi, killed in the Dreamtime.*

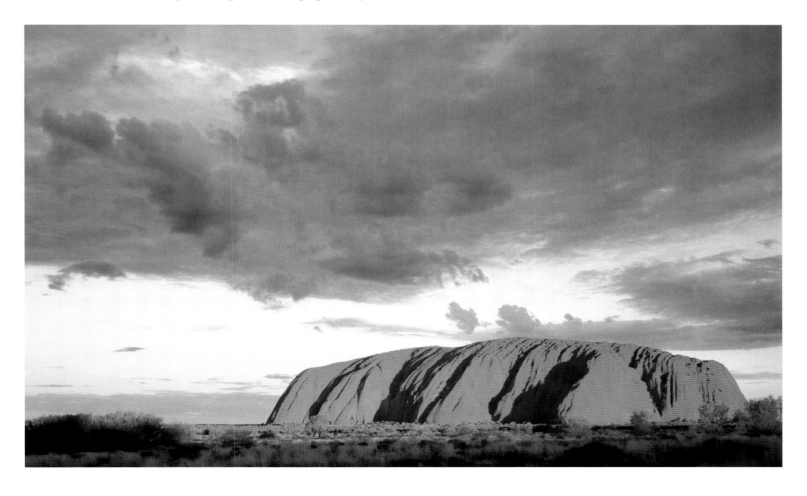

OCEANIA

If you are interested in Oceania, you may also like to read about:
- Mayan Prophecy, page 285
- Australian Aboriginal Spirituality, pages 228–229
- Megaliths and Earthworks, pages 252–253
- Hinduism, pages 204–205

Comprising Indonesia, Melanesia, Polynesia and Micronesia, this region has a geography that is often as desolate as it is sparse in population. Yet among its small, scattered communities there is a surprising degree of spiritual unity that adapted well to the introduction of Christian, Hindu and Muslim faiths. Key elements survived: the belief in **creator gods**, the concept of *mana* and **ancestral and animist traditions**, depending on their local weather, geographical or cultural conditions, with the **Philippines and Java** having a particularly **diverse spiritual culture**.

Creator gods

Beliefs in creator gods, such as the Polynesian gods Rangi and Papa, travelled across Oceania through oral tradition. After the arrival of the Portuguese explorer Magellan in the 16th century, many myths and traditions were recorded by Europeans with apparent distortion or embellishment of the region's cultural identity. Recently, however, the peoples of Oceania have recognized a need to reassert their culture by recreating and upholding their traditional spirituality through ritual and the written word.

Other popular gods in this region include Tangaroa, the god of the sea and fishing, and trickster gods like Maui. In Micronesia the Nauru indigenous peoples believe in a sole goddess creator called Eijebong who existed on a fantasy island of spirits called Buitani; the sky and earth were then created by the spider Areop-Enap. To the Balinese, creation began with a world snake, Antaboga, who meditated and created the world turtle, Bednang. Above the world are layers of skies: floating sky, dark blue sky and perfumed sky. The ancestors live above the perfumed heaven in a flaming sky, and above them live the gods.

Mana

The universal archetype of *mana* – a spiritual essence or power – is a core element of the Polynesian, Melanesian and Micronesian traditions. Certain people and objects are believed to be filled with this power. For example, in Hawaiian and Maori tradition it is a supernatural force that is acquired either by birthright or warfare. In Melanesian culture it is a sacred force associated with success and luck, and can be induced by wearing magic charms and talismans.

Ancestral and animistic traditions

The Maori belief, which spread across most of Polynesia, is that all things are connected through a genetic or genealogical link. Ancestry, or *whakapapa*, is

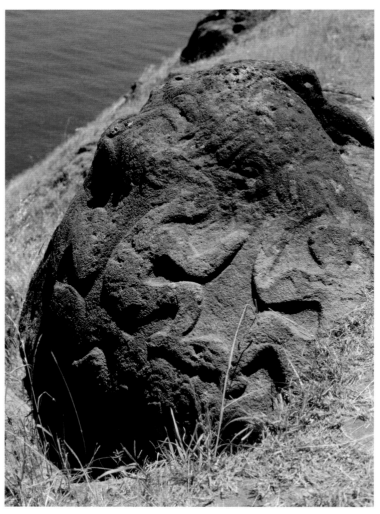

Easter Island *In the rock caves of Orongo, Easter Island, there are many sacred carvings of the gods, especially of Makemake and the birdman.*

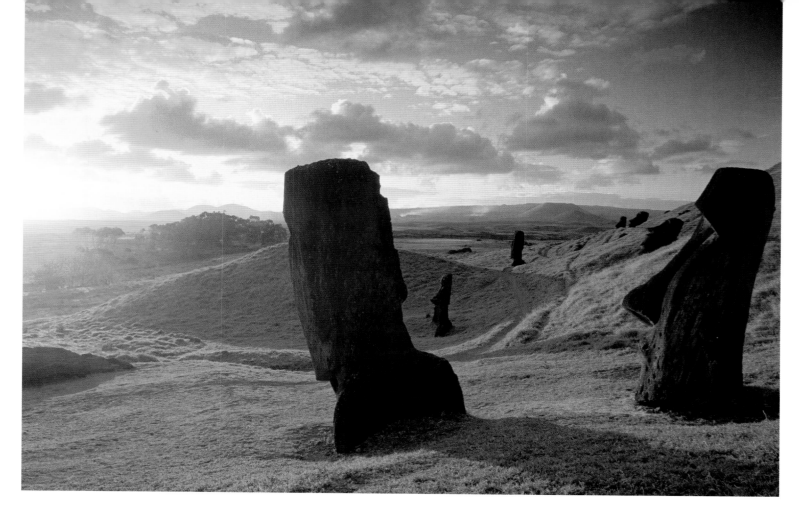

Moai *The enigmatic large stone head figures on Easter Island, known as Moai, have been subject to widespread speculation and debate.*

essential to their culture, and means that all things on earth, whether rocks, animals or people, are descended from the gods, the most widespread being Tangaroa, the god of the sea, ancestor of fish; Tane, the god of the forests, ancestor of birds; and Rongo, the ancestor of cultivation and agriculture.

Indigenous Maoris still believe in the sacredness of a place, animal or person. *Tapu* means sacred, and whether it is a private or public place or person, it must not be approached or touched. For example, a tribal chief and his house or possessions were considered *tapu*. Sacred places such as clearings, groups of trees and cleared land were called Marae and building on these sites was forbidden.

Easter Island (Rapu Nui) is world-famous for its Moai, large stone monolithic statues of the ancestors, such as the group at Rano Raraku, which is believed to date from 1250 CE. As with most of Oceania, the peoples of Rapu Nui believed in the ancestral link to the gods. They developed their own unique sacred race to collect the first sooty tern egg of the season, involving dangerous climbs up and down high cliffs and swimming in shark-infested seas, known as *Tangata manu*, the 'cult of the birdman'. Contestants were revealed in dreams by *ivi-attuas* (clairvoyants), and the winner was the sole harvester of the eggs for that season.

The diverse spiritual culture of the Philippines and Java

Mythological and spiritual traditions varied according to local community needs. Some ancient tribes believed in a supreme being; others in numerous tree and forest deities called *divatas*. To the Tagalog peoples, Bathala was the supreme creator god, Apalake the protector of the sun and Mayari the moon goddess. Various communities also believed in the Aswang, a vampire or ghoul spirit, and the Dila (Tongue), a spirit who rose up through the floor and licked its victims to death.

The Cebuano peoples believed in Gaba or Gabaa, a non-divine energy of negative karma that asserts an evil influence on wrongdoers. For the peoples of the islands of Siquijor, Talalora and Western Samar, a belief in magic was part of their spiritual culture. Kulam was a magic spell and a *mangkukulam* a magician who recited spells and was usually feared by the community. To prevent or cure the influence of bad magic, the community would turn to a shamanic healer, originally known as a *babaylan*, who was a miracle worker, seer and healer. In the pre-Hispanic era most of these healers were women.

One Javanese traditional belief was based on *kebatinan*, a spiritual search for harmony and wisdom inside oneself as a connection to the universal divine being. Via meditational techniques, such as hanging from a tree or fasting, the individual would contact a supreme power that determines all destiny and would thus be both informed and enlightened. Other pathways to induce divine contact include the avoidance of light and fire, fasting and eating saltless food.

NATIVE AMERICAN SPIRITUALITY

If you are interested in **Native American Spirituality**, you may also like to read about:

● Shamanism, pages 226–227
● Oceania, pages 230–231
● Sacred Geometry, pages 250–251
● Australian Aboriginal Spirituality, pages 228–229

Before contact with European settlers there were over a thousand tribal groups scattered across North America. They focused on **nature** and the land to provide spiritual meaning. The sacredness of all life, referred to by many of the communities as **Wakan Tanka**, was at the core of their tradition, and **rituals and totems** were key elements.

The spirit of nature

In contrast to the Judaeo-Christian traditions, where people are considered nearer to God than to animals, most Native American indigenous communities gave animals, plants, the elements and the landscape equal respect, believing in a connection between all living things, as well as the rocks, sand, sea and earth. Each local tribe or community adapted their beliefs according to their geographical needs. For example, the Native Americans of

Totem pole *This totem pole of a halibut spirit guide merging with a man stands in Nimpkish Burial Grounds, British Columbia, Canada.*

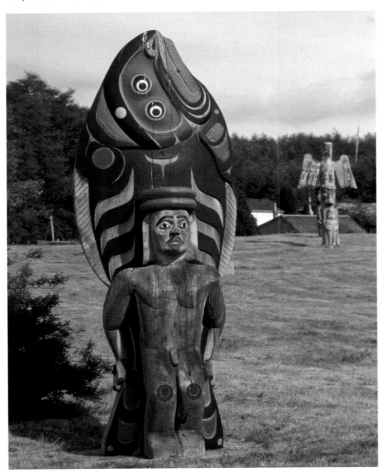

the Great Plains practised daily rituals to worship the sun and the great sky, while those who cultivated the land worshipped agricultural deities such as the Corn Woman of the Creek peoples of the south-east. According to Native American writer Professor John Mohawk (1945–2006): 'nature informs us and it is our obligation to read nature as you would a book, to feel nature as you would a poem, to touch nature as you would yourself, to be part of that'.

Wakan Tanka

For Native American indigenous peoples, the world and everything in it is imbued with spirit. This animistic belief in the sacredness of all things is known as Wakan Tanka or Wakanda. This all-pervading spiritual force is at the heart of their mythology too. Wakan Tanka is often referred to as the 'Great Spirit' but to the Sioux and Omaha peoples, it literally translates as the 'Great Mystery'. This sacred spirit is in everything from a grain of sand to a rock or tree. To the Dakota people of the Great Plains, Wakan Tanka was a creator god who divided himself up, which is why everything in the universe is part of Wakan Tanka. Every myth or story that was told in these oral traditions was also a way of working out this 'Great Mystery', and animals played a significant part, with many tribes believing that specific animals embodied spirit power. To the Sioux peoples, for example, the animal coyote was also the trickster god Coyote, a messenger between the real and supernatural worlds; to the Nez Perce people of the north-west, Wishpoosh was a monster beaver who ruled the primeval lake.

Rituals and totems

There were as many different rituals for connecting to the spirit world and maintaining the harmony in nature as there were tribal groups. For example, the Cherokee invoked spirits known as 'thunder beings' at their annual Green Corn Ceremony to ensure rain for a successful crop, while the Pawnee of Nebraska studied the stars and had sophisticated knowledge of Venus. Their creator god was Tirawa and they built lodges that represented the universe in detail, where they celebrated the creation of the universe with either Morning Star or Evening Star (Venus) ceremonies. The Navajos maintained harmony with the spirits through sand-painting rituals. Within the Blackfoot and Creek peoples, the symbolic totems and talismans of the 'Four Directions' or cardinal points were used to keep the universe in balance.

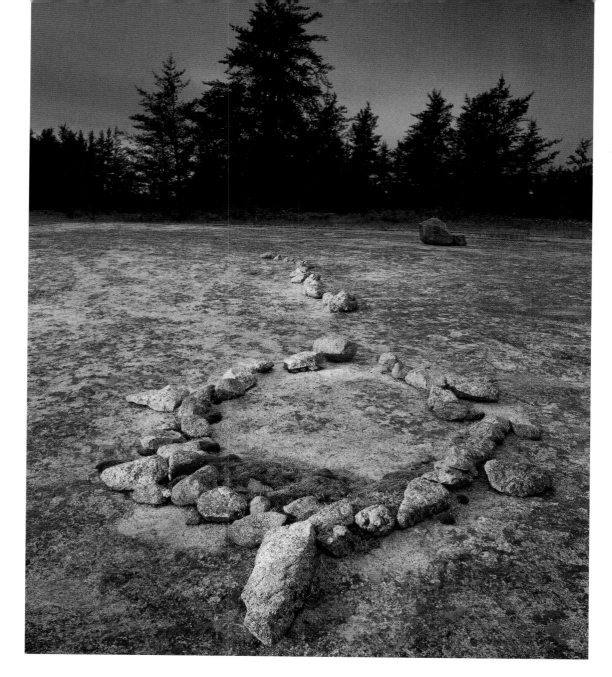

Petroform *A petroform or boulder outline in the shape of a turtle in Whiteshell Provincial Park, Manitoba, Canada. Such outlines were made by Native Americans for sacred and healing rituals.*

The sweat lodge

This was a hut constructed from tightly woven saplings with a small opening. In the middle was a pit containing hot rocks doused regularly with water to keep the interior as steamy and hot as a sauna. Groups would gather to meditate, pray, smoke or sing sacred songs to purify themselves and also to commune with the spirits.

Vision quests

After spending some time in a sweat lodge, a young man would travel into the wilderness to commune with a spirit guide for wisdom and power, and also to determine whether he was to be a hunter, herder or chief. Facing many natural dangers and without food or water, he would spend days or even weeks alone until a spirit guide would appear in a vision or dream and advise him of his future direction.

Spirit guides and power animals

Many peoples honoured a specific animal that had great significance to the community and was likened to a guardian spirit. Each individual had their own spirit guide, who added to that person's power and would represent the qualities of the animal. To the Lakota people, for example, the beaver embodied hard work and domestic tranquillity.

Smudging

This involved burning small amounts of herbs or sweet-smelling grass to purify the mind and drive away negative thoughts or spirits from an individual. Smudge sticks were bundles of dried herbs tied together with strips of hide or coloured thread. The most common herbs used were sage to drive out negative energy and sweetgrass to attract positive energy. Smudging was a way of connecting the realms of the physical and supernatural.

AFRICAN TRADITIONS

If you are interested in **African Traditions**, you may also like to read about:
- **Native American Spirituality**, pages 232–233
- **Oceania**, pages 230–231
- **Shamanism**, pages 226–227

Apart from the ancient Egyptian religions, there were very few large organized belief systems in Africa, which extended over large geographical areas. The majority of spiritual traditions there today are animist and shamanic, and belong to local tribal and ethnic groupings. These traditions refer to the **life force**, **creator gods** and **spirits of the ancestors**. Two of the most notable are the *orisha* **tradition of the Yoruba** and **Dogon spiritual beliefs**.

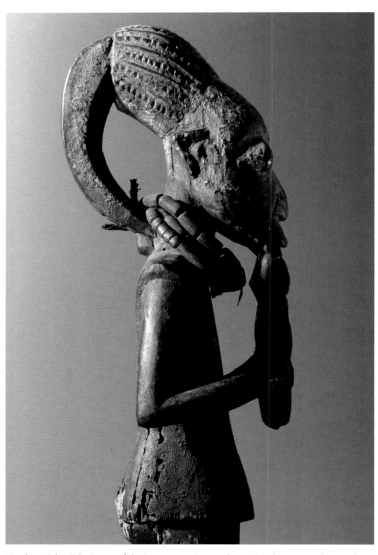

Yoruba *orisha* *Eshu is one of the important minor gods or spirits known as* oshiras, *who play a major part in the Yoruba people's daily life.*

The life force

Among the Shilluk peoples of southern Sudan, Juok was a formless creator who was present in everything. The word Juok, along with aliases Jok, Jwok and Joagh, was also used to signify the divine spirit itself in all Nilotic (pertaining to the Nile) languages, who was both good and evil and determined the fate of humans and animals accordingly. The Yoruba peoples of Nigeria call this life force *ase*.

Creator gods

In Zulu mythology the supreme creator god was Unkulunkulu and other important deities included Mamma, the goddess of rivers, and Unwaba, a chameleon messenger god who was sent down to Earth to give humans immortality; he was so slow that people began to die before he got there. When the chameleon changes his colour from green to brown, he is thought to be recalling Unwaba's misfortunate slothfulness.

Other indigenous groups recognized dualistic creator gods. For the Maasai, the supreme god was Enkai, his dual nature being Enkai Narok (Black God), who was benevolent, and Enkai Nanyokie (Red God), malevolent. The Ewe peoples of Ghana also worshipped a dual god called Mawu-Lisa.

Ancestral spirits

Among the Zulu and Swazi peoples of southern Africa, belief in ancestral spirits is widespread. *Sangomas* are shamans or healers who perform acts of healing through rituals and channelling ancestral spirits. They are usually called to heal after an initiation through a difficult illness themselves, and are most commonly women. They work in a sacred healing hut where the ancestral spirit resides and offer believers guidance, cure and relief through trance possession, bone throwing and the interpretation of dreams.

The *orisha* tradition of the Yoruba

The Yoruba believe that all humans are destined to become one with Olorun, sometimes known as Olodumare, the supreme creator god. This tradition also influenced many Afro-American beliefs when the Nigerian peoples were taken across the Atlantic in the slave trade.

There are scores of different *orishas* (spirits or minor gods) that reflect the many manifestations of Olorun, and spiritual growth and destiny are reinforced through contact and communion with an *orisha*. They also venerate the spirits of their ancestors, called Engungen. Believers often consult a *babalawo* for divinational advice, known as the practice of Ifa.

Dogon spiritual belief

Although highly complex, at its basic level this constitutes the worship of ancestors and their spirits. It is believed that the Dogon peoples of central Mali may have originally come from ancient Egypt. The following are their four main cults:

The Awa

This is a ritualistic dance originally performed to establish order in the universe after the spiritual forces were disturbed by the death of Nommo, a mythical ancestor of crucial importance. These rituals are commonly practised at funerals to lead the souls safely to join their ancestors, using over 70 different masks, all with symbolic decorative messages.

Lebe

Lebe is the earth god, and most Dogon communities have a Lebe shrine, devoted to the fertility of the earth. The chief priest or village leader is called a Hogon. Lebe is believed to visit the Hogons at night in the form of a serpent and nurture them with the beneficial life force by licking their skin.

Binu

This is a totemic practice and sacred places are used for ancestral worship and spirit communication. The Binu belief is associated with Nommo, and Binu shrines are imbued with the spirits and gods of pre-humanity. Most are painted with mystical symbols, and rituals include the sacrifice of blood and millet at sowing time to ensure a good crop. Binu diviners draw specific questions in the sand for the sacred fox to answer during the night. The next day the diviner interprets the fox's footprints left in the sand.

Nommo

When part of Nommo, the self-dividing first being, rebelled, the creator god Amma scattered another part of him into the universe to purify the cosmos. The Dogon also believe that Nommo gave them the sophisticated knowledge of the dog star, Sirius. For the ancient Egyptians the star was an important celestial marker for times when the River Nile was liable to flood just before the summer solstice, and it is possible that the Dogon inherited this knowledge from their ancient Egyptian roots. But American author Robert Temple's book *The Sirius Mystery* startled the world in 1976 with the revelation that the Dogon priests seemed to know about Sirius B even before this companion star or white dwarf was discovered in the 20th century. Dogons claimed that the Nommos had come from the Sirius system in a space ship with the secret knowledge. The Dogon calendar is based on the orbit of Sirius B around Sirius A, a cycle of 50–60 years. They believe that the Sirius star system is the axis of the universe, and maintain that they have known for thousands of years that Jupiter has moons, Saturn has rings and that the Earth orbits the sun.

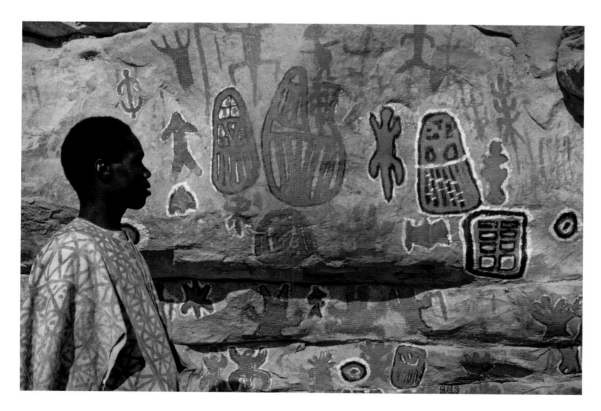

Rock painting *One of the Dogon people of Mali paints a symbol onto a rock. A new painting is added each time a young male undergoes the circumcision ritual.*

SHINTO

Shinto is both an animist and polytheistic tradition with ancient roots in Japan. It involves the worship and belief in *kami*, or spirits, and attempts to mediate and create harmony between the world of the spirit and the profane world of nature and man. Among other practices, it features a ritual dance of shamanic origin known as the **Kagura**, which is said to imply 'the site where the *kami* is received'. There are no sacred texts, but there are numerous **different styles of Shinto**.

If you are interested in **Shinto**, you may also like to read about:
- Buddhism, pages 208–209
- Taoism, pages 216–217
- Bahai, pages 200–201
- Hinduism, pages 204–205
- Shiatsu, pages 124–125

Kami

Native Shinto pre-dates the influences of Buddhism, which merged with Shinto belief in the 6th century. The basis of Shinto is that all things are animated by *kami*, or spirit. Anything from a rock to the Moon, even an abstract concept such as 'knowing', is permeated with *kami*. There is also a *kami* for collective groups, for example for all horses as well as for an individual horse.

The *kami* were long associated with deities such as Amaterasu, the goddess of the sun. Her myth concerning Susano lies at the heart of Shinto worship and the political and social dynastic rule of Japan; the imperial family of Japan believed themselves to be direct-line descendants of the sun goddess herself.

Amaterasu

Worshipped since ancient times as the Great Heaven Shining Deity, Amaterasu is the most deified of the *kami*. Her symbols of power as the sun goddess are a necklace made of light, the Milky Way and the first clothes ever made, sewn with fabulous jewels and the golden light of the sun itself. Every 20 years her simple thatched shrine at Ise on Honshu is renewed in her honour, but there are many other shrines dotted around Japan, sometimes empty except for a mirror. This symbolizes that everything in the mirror (the reflected world) is the embodiment of every *kami* including Amaterasu.

Amaterasu *This woodblock print from 1860 by artist Utugawa Kunisada depicts the Japanese goddess Amaterasu emerging from the Earth.*

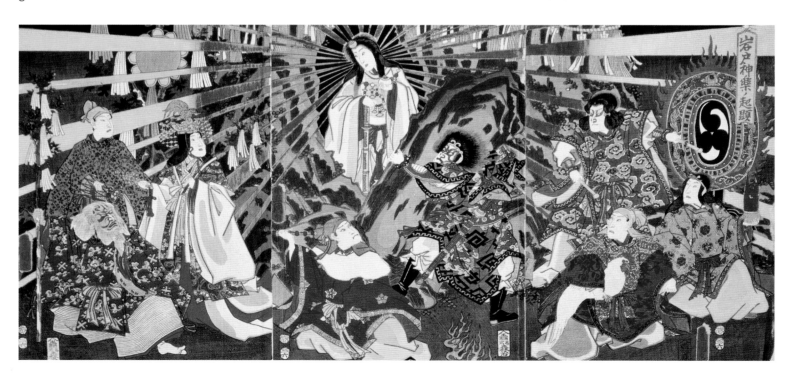

Susano

A key Shinto deity, Susano was Amaterasu's brother, who forced Amaterasu to hide in a cave for fear of his wrath. Later Shinto priests embellished one of his myths by adding that Susano also discovered a magic sword and gave it to Amaterasu, who later gave it to her grandson, Ninigi, when she sent him to rule the Earth. This sword was handed down from generation to generation and became one of the most sacred objects in the Imperial family, another proof that they were descended from the gods.

Hachiman

The Shinto god of war, Hachiman, was also the divine protector of Japan. Originally he was a multi-tasking god of fertility, agriculture and fishing. Many Shinto shrines are devoted to Hachiman, whose main cult following is centred on the temple at Kamakura. Young men still celebrate their rite of passage into adulthood at Hachiman temples.

Kagura and other practices

The origin of this dance is the myth of Uzume's (goddess of magic) trick to lure Amaterasu out of the cave and restore light to the world. The dance invites the *kami* to bring blessings and is accompanied by sacred songs and drumming. Kagura is also performed as a rite of passage for the spirits of the departed. Rites of purification called *asobi* and *chinkon* were also performed, initially only for the Emperors of Japan.

The most ancient Kagura was known as Miko Kagura. The ancient *miko* were female shamans, and their dance was a means of channelling oracles and prophecies from the gods and spirits. Another type of Kagura is the Izumo Kagura, involving participants wearing exotic masks in a dramatic performance based on mythological tales. The Yamabushi Kagura of northeast Japan has retained its ritualistic tradition; authentic practitioners wear lionheads and dance as if possessed by the *kami*.

Many purification rites are still practised to placate *kami*, for example if a shrine has to be moved to a new location. New buildings are still blessed by Shinto priests, and water purification remains the most popular method.

Ema is a small wooden plaque on which a Shinto worshipper writes prayers or wishes and is hung in the appropriate shrine where the *kami* can read it. The usual image that accompanies the *ema* is a horse. Real horses were once given as offerings by wealthy merchants in exchange for blessings.

Different styles of Shinto

Shrine Shinto is the most commonly practised form of Shinto today. Ko Shinto, on the other hand, emphasizes the traditional values of ritualistic pre-Buddhist influence. Sect Shinto was developed in the 19th century, and various sects evolved that worship mountains such as Mount Fuji or are concerned with faith healing or purification. Minzoku-Shinto is folk Shinto based on the most ancient, yet fragmented local beliefs. The practice includes divination, spirit possession, shamanic healing and sometimes Buddhist elements. Shinto has inspired many new Shinto sects and religions in contemporary Japan.

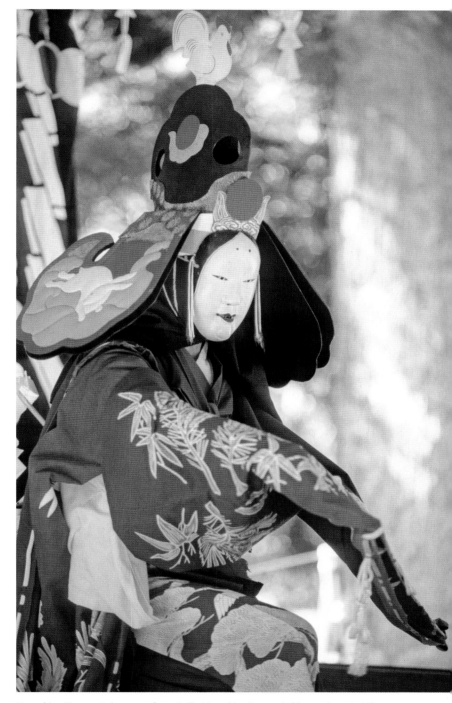

Hayachine Kagura *A dancer performs in the Hayachine Kagura, held every August at the Hayachine Jinja Shrine, Iwate, Japan. This fast-paced dance ritual is believed to have been started by followers of the nearby mountain religion of Sangaku Shinko.*

Since Shinto's interaction with Buddhism over a thousand years ago, the peoples of Japan often practise Shinto in their daily lives, but elect to have Buddhist ceremonies for more important occasions. The four most important affirmations of Shinto are the preservation of the traditional role of the family, respect for nature, cleanliness and sustaining and attending the festivals dedicated to various *kami*.

PAGANISM

If you are interested in **Paganism**, you may also like to read about:
- **Shinto**, pages 236–237
- **Druidry**, pages 242–243
- **Wicca**, pages 240–241
- **Runes**, pages 64–65
- **Western Astrology**, pages 56–57

'Pagan' comes from the latin *paganus*, meaning 'country dweller', and paganism is an umbrella term for a diverse group of spiritual approaches that occur worldwide, usually active among small groups, and that focus on ancient local traditions and practices. It can be divided into **three cateogies**: paleopaganism, such as the **Celtic belief system**, mesopaganism and neo-paganism, including **Goddess Spirituality** among many other revival movements. **Pagan beliefs** usually focus on the divine or spiritual essence in nature, including an array of deities.

The three categories of paganism

In the late 1970s, influential American Druid priest and pagan leader Isaac Bonewits classified paganism into the following main categories:

Paleopaganism

This category encompasses traditional animist and polytheistic beliefs of indigenous peoples that have not been disrupted or influenced by other religions. Examples include the oldest form of Shinto, Dogon (see page 235) and the Celtic belief system.

Mesopaganism

These are pagan belief movements, both organized and non-organized, that sought to revive the original beliefs of their heritage, but were influenced by other religious ideology, while still remaining independent of them. These revivals usually occurred before the 20th century, such as African Voudoun, Odinism and Druidism.

Neo-paganism

This category refers to the 20th-century revival of pagan beliefs and is a generic term for the many groups of animistic, pantheistic and polytheistic beliefs. It also includes the revival of nature worship and 'folk' religions of indigenous peoples worldwide, such as Wicca, Sacred Ecologists, Theodism, German Pagan Reconstructionism and, further afield, the revival of Mayan paganism in Guatemala, shamanism in Siberia and Korea, Greek polytheism in both Greece and the USA, as well as other diverse practices such as Goddess Spirituality and Kemetism, the ancient Egyptian belief system.

Pagan beliefs

Neo-paganism has absorbed many influences from around the world, but most pagans specialize in a specific tradition. For example, the Heathen 'path' follows ancient Germanic, Scandinavian and Anglo-Saxon beliefs, Greek paganism follows early Greek polytheistic traditions, and so on.

Most pagans believe that the divine is both immanent (internal) and transcendent (external). They also simultaneously, or alternatively, believe that the natural world is divine, everything is filled with the life force or spirit, everything that exists is part of the whole and that gods and goddesses are everywhere. The well-known American feminist practitioner of Goddess Spirituality, Starhawk, states: 'the Goddess is another way of saying the great creative forces of life'.

The Celtic belief system

The Celts ('fighters') were a huge group of peoples spread across Europe. Comprising many tribes and settlements, and renowned for their guerrilla warfare, they appeared in Eastern Europe in the 2nd millennium BCE and moved west and south, dominating European culture in Northern Europe. One of the few civilizations to revolt against Roman rule, their mythology is diverse and their belief system remained intact, although it went underground with the rise of Christianity. Celtic paganism is animistic and also polytheistic. Shrines and monuments were placed in various landscapes to honour trees, rocks, clearings, rivers and streams, as well as sacred altars and festivals to honour various deities such as the sun god Lugh, in Irish myth, the horned god Cernunnos and the god of thunder, Taranis.

Heathenry, Norse and Viking Age paganism

The Vikings travelled the world around the 8–11th centuries CE mostly in search of trade, conquering places along the way, and their beliefs remained secularized and undiminished despite the Christianization of Europe. A considerable amount of Norse poems and prose also appeared in Iceland between the 11th and 14th centuries, known as the Eddas, Skalds and Sagas. Most neo-paganists who follow these beliefs honour a vast array of deities

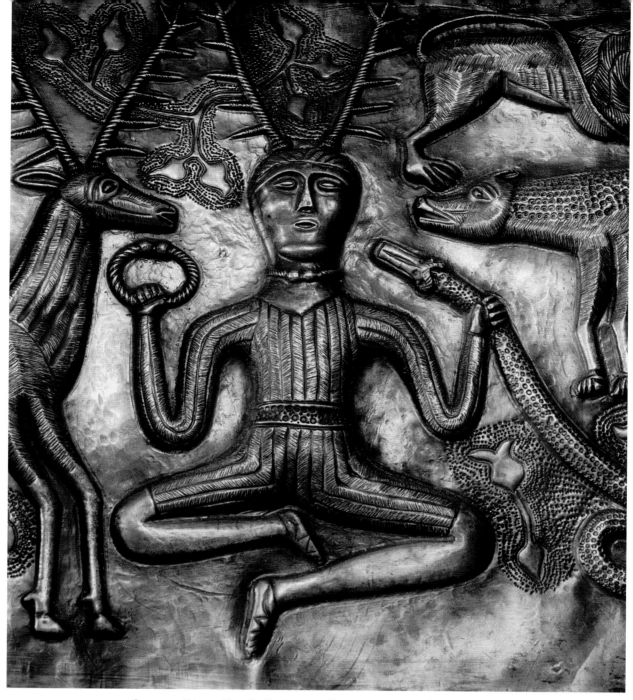

Cernunnos *This panel from the Gundestrup cauldron shows an image of the god Cernunnos surrounded by beasts. Thought to be Celtic in origin and to date to the 1st century BC, it was discovered in a Danish peat bog and is now in Copenhagen.*

and spirits, sometimes called wights. Priests are known as *godhis* within small groups and communities. Wyrd is an important concept in Heathenry, basically meaning 'that which has become'. It is the moment of turning, making choices and accepting the consequence of one's choice and action, similar to karma (see page 204).

Once a sacrificial ceremony, the Blot is now a feast of offerings of mead and food, in which a place is usually laid for the god, wight or ancestral spirit who is being propitiated. Symbel is a drinking ceremony where a drinking horn is passed around the group and the gods and ancestors are toasted.

Goddess Spirituality

Bronze and Stone Age figurines and carvings throughout Europe constitute strong evidence of the existence of the 'Great Goddess' religion before the patriarchal civilizations with their own pantheon of deities took over Europe. Goddess Spirituality has been an important revival of ancient traditional goddess worship, mainly for women both in Europe and the USA. A goddess temple has recently been set up in Glastonbury, England, to celebrate the divine feminine. Goddess worship there includes Brigit, the Celtic triad of goddesses, and Domnu, the goddess of the sea.

WICCA

Wicca is a neo-pagan nature-based mystery religion founded by **Gerald Gardner**, with its origins debatably lying in a pre-Christian witch cult. Although there are different forms of Wicca, most Wiccans **worship the God and Goddess** and believe in the sanctity of nature. Wicca has nothing to do with Satanism; spells and **magic rituals** are performed for the good of the whole. 'An it harm one, do what ye will' is the most fundamental philosophy of Wiccan practice, along with the Law of Threefold Return – a belief that whatever action one performs, benevolent or malevolent, it will return three times greater.

If you are interested in Wicca, you may also like to read about:
- **Paganism**, pages 238–239
- **The Tarot**, pages 62–63
- **Alchemy**, pages 296–297
- **Mythical Creatures**, pages 286–287

Gerald Gardner

In the early 1950s, Gerald Brousseau Gardner (1884–1964) claimed to have been initiated into an ancient secret coven of witches of the New Forest in southern England. Originally Gardner called the initiates in the coven 'the wica', and simply called the practice 'witchcraft', but it became an inspiration for the worldwide development of Wicca after the publication of his books *Witchcraft Today* (1954) and *The Meaning of Witchcraft* (1959).

What came to be known as Gardnerian Wicca, or British Traditional Wicca in the USA, was centred around an ancient witch-cult initiation system of the coven whereby 'only a witch can make another witch'. However, many sceptics, such as author and Gardnerian Wiccan Aidan Kelly, believe that Gardner invented the rituals he apparently discovered in the New Forest, which were very similar to ideas and practices that had already been noted in the writings of occultist Aleister Crowley (1875–1947) and anthropologist Sir James Frazer (1854–1941).

In Gardnerian Wicca there are three levels or degrees of initiation. The highest or third degree is the status of High Priestess or Priest, able to initiate both the first-level initiates and the second-level, who can become high-level priests and priestesses themselves and thus continue the Wicca lineage by creating new covens. The common belief is that 13 is an appropriate number for a coven. The initiation usually lasts for a year and a day and includes taking part in a dedication ceremony.

Other forms of Wicca

Alexandrian Wicca, founded by Alex Sanders (1926–1988) in 1960, is based on Gardner's rituals and initiation ceremonies, but also includes elements of the Kabbalah, an ancient Jewish mystical pathway, and Enochian magic, based on the apocryphal Book of Enoch, great-grandfather of Noah. It became highly popular in the USA and more recently in Canada. Ritual nudity, or appearing 'skyclad', is optional.

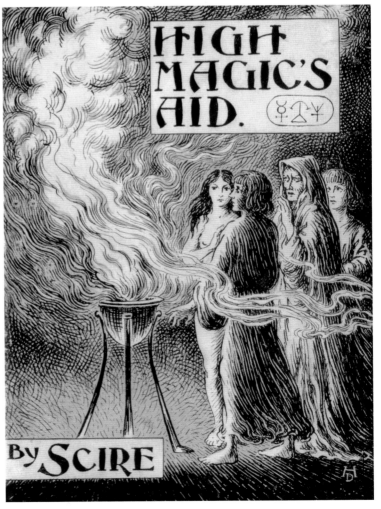

High Magic's Aid *Written under the pseudonym of 'Scire' this is the first published book of Gerald Gardner and is sometimes credited as beginning the popular revival of Wicca.*

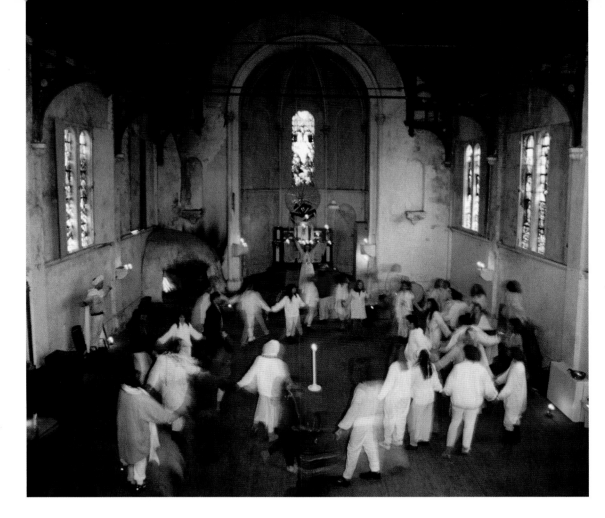

Wicca *A group of Wiccans dance in an old church's nave during a ceremony near Amsterdam, Holland.*

Eclectic Wicca maintains Gardnerian Wicca's essential elements of ritual, belief and practice, but there is no insistence on initiation or lineage, although it can be part of the practice. Eclectic Wiccans far outnumber the traditional lineage Wiccans.

Many other traditions and branches of Wicca have developed their own distinct magic or secret cults. Some are solitary practitioners, but also gather in small groups or communities to perform spell casting, rituals and worship, or for celebrations such as *sabbats* and *esbats*. Dianic Wicca, founded by American feminist writer Zsuzsanna Budapest, combines elements of Gardnerian Wicca with feminist values and is usually practised only in women's groups where the male god is no longer worshipped. It draws on ritual and Italian folk magic. Founded in California in 1975, the Covenant of the Goddess is now an international Wiccan organization with over 100 covens and many solitary members.

Worship of the God and Goddess

Some Wiccans believe that the gods and goddesses are all aspects of the God/Goddess duality (pantheism), but many worship separate gods and goddesses in their own right (polytheism). It is also believed that the God or Goddess can manifest through the bodies of the High Priest or Priestess via rituals such as the 'drawing down' of the sun or moon.

The gods most commonly worshipped are the Horned God, usually known as Cernunnos, Pan, the Green Man, the Sun God and the Oak King. The Goddess is usually the Triple Goddess, conceiving and containing all as Maiden, Mother and Crone.

Magic rituals and ceremonies

Most Wiccans celebrate a cycle of festivals throughout the year, four concerned with the sun's cycle at the equinoxes and solstices, another with the cycle of fertility and the remainder with the yearly cycle of growth, death and rebirth, referred to by different names, but perhaps most often as Samhain, Yule, Imbolc, Ostara, Beltane, Midsummer or Summer Solstice, Lughnasadh and Mabon.

The most common symbol in Wicca is the pentagram, which represents the five elements of Wiccan belief – fire, air, earth, water and spirit or quintessence. It symbolizes the human as a microcosm of the universe reflected in this elemental balance.

The usual ritual begins with the coven or solitary practitioner entering a protective magic circle, followed by invocation of the guardians of the cardinal points represented by the pentagram. Seasonal rituals, spell working and worship of the God/Goddess may or may not be included. Many Wiccans use magical tools such as the chalice, wand, crystals, pentacle and, sometimes, a besom (broomstick). Most have a 'book of shadows' containing the coven's sacred text of magic spells, core beliefs and practices, kept by initiates and only accessible to that coven. Solitary Wiccans may also keep their own book of spells.

DRUIDRY

If you are interested in **Druidry**, you may also like to read about:

● **Western Mystery Traditions**, pages 184–185
● **Wicca**, pages 240–241
● **Paganism**, pages 238–239
● **Megaliths and Earthworks**, pages 252–253

Among the ancient Celtic tribes of Britain and Western Europe the Druids were once magicians, priests, ambassadors, advisors to kings, teachers and judges who worshipped the natural world. Suppressed by the Romans around the 2nd century CE, there is, however, little surviving evidence of **original Druidry**. But its **revival** over the past few hundred years and renewed interest in its **beliefs and practice** have resulted in the establishment of a great many **Druid orders** worldwide.

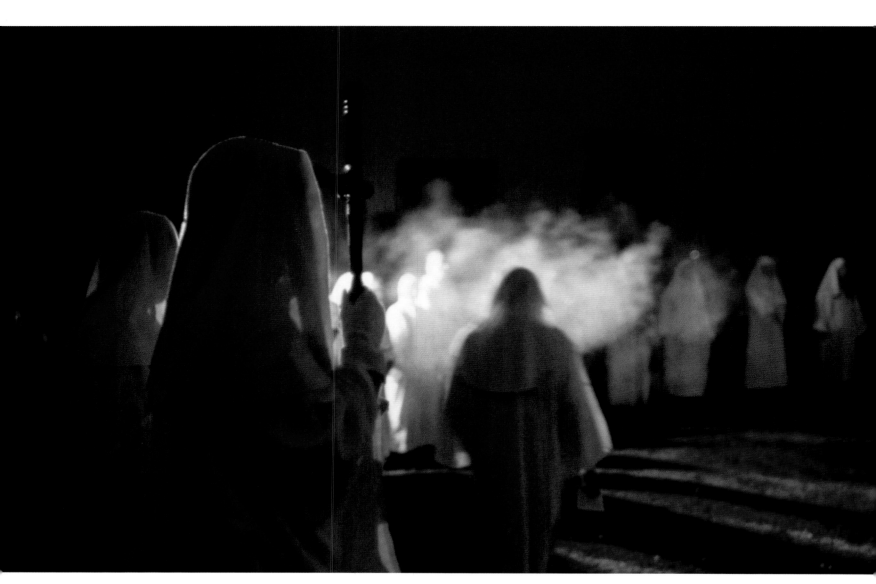

Druids *Druids gather in the inner ring of Stonehenge for the summer solstice. The World Heritage site was constructed over a period of 1,500 years, beginning in around 3000 BC.*

Original Druidry

It is thought that the original druids were both polytheistic and animistic, and revered the natural world. In Greek mythology the Dryades were oak nymphs (the Greek word *drys* meaning 'oak') associated with the priestesses of Artemis. In pre-patriarchal Europe the cult of Artemis was a mystery religion restricted to women. According to the Greek geographer Strabo (c. 64 BCE–24 CE), followers practised rites in oak or hazel groves throughout northern Europe, 'similar to the orgies of the Samothrace'. Eventually, male priests were admitted. In Celtic Europe this developed into a class of bardic soothsayers, who memorized orally transmitted material that later became the basis of medieval stories and ballads. Lewis Spence (1874–1955) in his book *The History and Origins of Druidism* (1949) believed that the knowledge that had been transmitted 'arose in the Veda-like sacred hymns which formed the depository of the learning professed by the body of the druidical teachers and diviners and taught orally in the druidic school'. It seems that most of this was never recorded but, like myth, was passed on in the form of spoken poetry and prose from generation to generation.

References to Druids are found throughout Irish mythology, particularly those myths from medieval sources. For example, in the Irish Ulster Cycle, Cathbad was the chief Druid at the King of Ulster's court of Conchobar. In the epic *Tain Bo Cuailnge*, Medb, the Queen of Connacht, consulted her Druid before setting off to war, thus delaying the battle for several weeks while waiting for an auspicious omen. Dalgn, the High King of Ireland's Druid, took a whole year to find the king's wife, Etain, who eloped with her former god consort, Midir.

The revival of Druidry

The 17th century onwards saw a renewed interest in Druids when John Aubrey (1626–1697) developed ideas connecting megalithic sites such as Stonehenge with the Druids. However, it was John Toland (1670–1722) who established the Ancient Druid Order in 1717, using Aubrey's unpublished ideas, without giving him any credit. The Ancient Druid Order finally split into two groups in 1964.

Beliefs and practice

The core belief among all Druid orders is that nature is sacred. Many contemporary Druids are also pantheistic, but it is not known if this was ever part of Celtic polytheism. Druids also venerate their ancestors as well as preserving cultural and local heritage.

Ceremonies are usually performed in a circle around a fire or altar. According to the Council of British Druid Orders, these rituals are usually concerned with the solar cycle and its associated festivals, and Druids believe that 'all that we do, we do in the eye of the sun and before and in the presence of the assembled congregation'. In other words, these festivals are open to public observation. Like many other pagan groups, Druids usually celebrate the equinoxes and solstices as well as four lunar-cycle celebrations. Unlike the ceremonies of many other pagan religions, these practices are performed in public places.

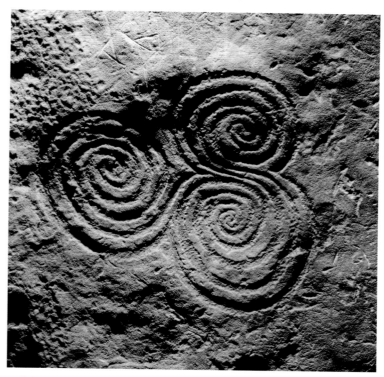

Triskelion *This triple spiral motif is carved into the rock walls of the central chamber of the Newgrange prehistoric mound in County Meath, Ireland.*

Group meetings are often called 'groves', and favoured places are among groves and copses, or in the presence of pre-Celtic megaliths such as Stonehenge in Wiltshire, England. Glastonbury in Somerset, England, is also favoured because of its sacred associations. Druids usually wear ceremonial robes to indicate the order to which they belong. One of their important symbols is the triskelion, a Celtic symbol for the cycle of life. An example lies at the entrance of the Newgrange monument in County Meath, Ireland.

Druid orders

There are many different orders of Druid. Some work with the local landscape, while others are more concerned with national heritage; some teach, while others prefer the divinational or ritualistic side of Druidry. The Order of Bards, Ovates and Druids, founded in 1964, is the largest body of organized Druids in the world with over 10,000 members. Meanwhile, the Ancient Order of Druids in the USA was revived by John Michael Greer in the 1990s and is believed to have its roots in Freemasonry. There are three basic 'levels' of Druid. At the first level is the Bardic grade, made up of Druids concerned with music, art, literature and intellectual skills. The next is the Ovate grade, where Druids are concerned with magic, healing, astrology and divination. The last group is called the Druid grade, with these Druids performing public rituals and ceremonies, and promoting the ethical beliefs of Druidry. The Bardic grade is responsible for passing on their knowledge, the Ovate grade for using that knowledge for the good of the planet and the Druid grade for supporting this belief and showing the external world how to be responsible for the preservation of the planet and all life.

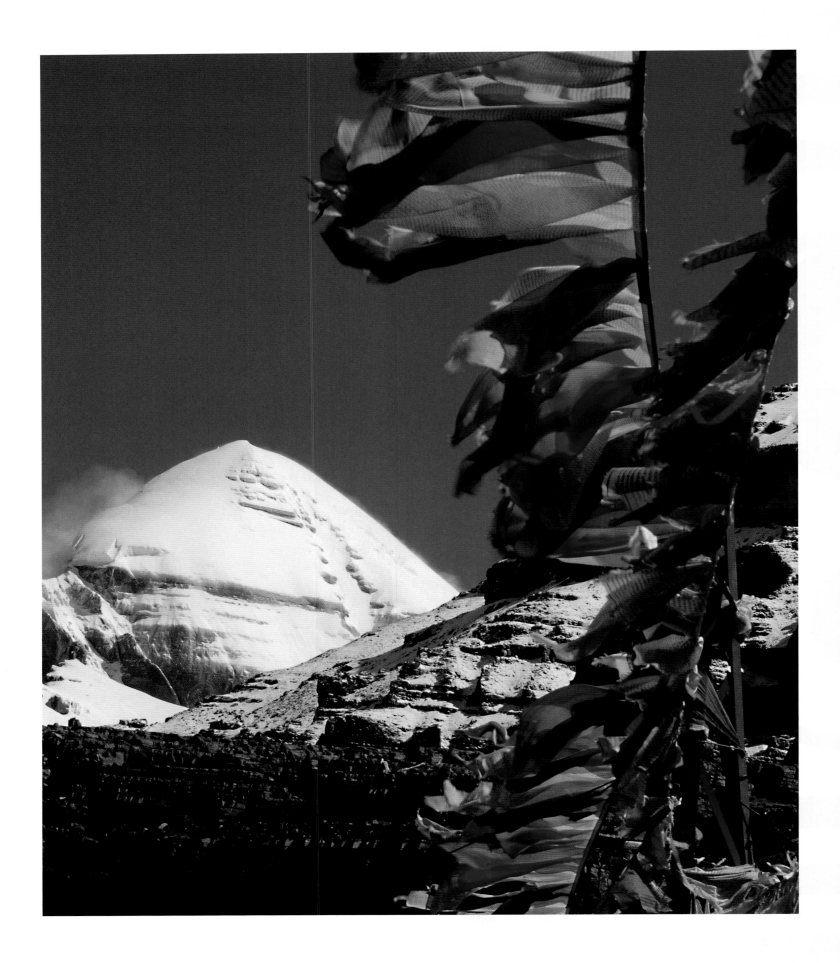

EARTH MYSTERIES

We live within an increasingly circumscribed and urbanized world. Most of us only occasionally come into direct contact with raw nature, more often seeing simply a flash of countryside out of our car, train or aircraft windows, or watching nature at a remove on our TV screens. Our spiritual compasses are awry, and the facts, figures and explanations of our scientists squeeze the mystery out of being in the world. Time is measured in ever-shorter units, and many of us feel buffeted by the winds of rapid social and technological change. In consequence, it is no wonder that two, somewhat opposed, reactions are increasingly occurring in response to such spiritual suffocation. One is an escapist tendency to enter into an alternative cyber reality where antidote can all too readily turn into addiction, and the other is an urge to journey to rural and even wild and remote places in order to experience ancient sacred monuments that speak of mystery and a depth of time our souls crave.

The origins of Earth Mysteries

Earth Mysteries is a curious hybrid of such spiritual succour and simultaneously a kind of escapism. Essentially, it is a successor to the Romantic movement in Europe and Britain, which began in the 18th century as a reaction to the Enlightenment, the dawn of scientific thinking. Its remit encompassed a fascination with antiquity, exemplified by the re-invention of Druidry, which still continues; the rise of occult interest, as exemplified by the Golden Dawn and Theosophy, and a general yearning to re-enchant nature, the land. In effect, it reflected a homesickness for Eden, for the Golden Age.

The term 'Earth Mysteries' covers a broadly based area of interest rather than a single subject. Its focus is on ancient sacred sites and lost knowledge, and it encompasses archeology, anthropology, ancient astronomy, enigmatic landscape lines (ley lines and Nazca lines), sacred geometry, earth energies,

Mount Kailash *Kailash, which means 'crystal' in Sanskrit, is an important sacred place in four of the world's great religions: Buddhism, Hinduism, Jainism and the ancient Tibetan religion of Bön Po. For many pilgrims the journey to Kailash is the fulfilment of a lifetime's ambition.*

green spirituality, shamanism, feng shui, UFOs, Atlantis and more. This umbrella term was coined in 1974 by *The Whole Earth Catalog* to give a simple journalistic handle to this disparate collection of topics that had actually started to coalesce during the previous decade.

In the psychedelic-tinted social ferment of the 1960s, various factors merged to create an unprecedented wave of popular interest in the ancient past. A key one was the idea of 'ancient astronauts', largely due to Erich von Däniken's *Chariots of the Gods?* (1968), though there had been other writers on the same theme before him. This entered the mix along with interest in 'flying saucers' (UFOs), Atlantis, speculations about earth energies, a renewed interest in ritual magic and the neo-pagan Wicca (introduced in the 1950s by Gerald Gardner).

Over the same period, radiocarbon dating techniques in archeology revealed Stone Age monuments to be older than had previously been thought and at the same time new understandings about ancient astronomy ('archeoastronomy') indicated that prehistoric people had been cleverer than had hitherto been acknowledged. Everything went into the same pot, and the magical mystery soup that was to be dubbed 'Earth Mysteries' began to be cooked up.

The early writings of John Michell (especially *The View Over Atlantis*, 1969) and of Janet and Colin Bord (notably *Mysterious Britain*, 1972), among others, were influential in focusing and shaping Earth Mysteries into a more integrated subject area, superficially at least.

Earth Mysteries today

Earth Mysteries has now fragmented to some degree into separately designated, yet still generally interrelated areas, such as neo-paganism, 'ancient mysteries' and even scholarly, researched-based work. In general, it continues to acknowledge the mysteries of the natural world; an attitude that grows more valid as environmental awareness and concerns press more strongly on our consciousness. But misinformation and wishful thinking needs to be guarded against, as the role Earth Mysteries can play in the authentic re-enchantment of our perceptions of our environment and our human heritage is too valuable to misuse.

SACRED LAND

If you are interested in **Sacred Land**, you may also like to read about:
- **Australian Aboriginal Spirituality**, pages 228–229
- **Native American Spirituality**, pages 232–233
- **Buddhist Sacred Texts**, pages 210–211

The first human societies were animistic, considering spirit and spirits to be present throughout the natural environment. In some indigenous cultures this sensibility eventually developed into two broad aspects: **landscapes imbued with meaning**, in which a mindscape was effectively superimposed on the physical topography, and the identification of certain landscape forms and features as **sacred places**.

Landscapes imbued with meaning

A well-known case of this is the Australian Aboriginals' 'Dreamtime'. This term was actually coined by Europeans in 1927, though the Aborigines felt it well enough described the *tjukuba*, one of their many names for the timeless time still cloaking the land. According to this concept, the present topography was formed in the Dreamtime, when the country was flat and uninhabited, and giant totemic, creator beings emerged from under the ground. Everything they did left a mark – a rock outcrop is still the head of a Dreamtime being, certain boulders remain the droppings of a totemic creature, and so on. The inner, living mythic world of the Aborigines and the physical environment were inextricably fused. As the anthropologist Lucien Lévy-Bruhl (1857–1939) put it, for Aborigines 'legend is captured in the very outlines of the landscape'.

This has been equally true of other cultures. For instance, Buddhists in the Himalayan region make pilgrimages to places whose topographical forms present the accidental likenesses – the simulacra – of deities or religious figures. In La phyi in south-east Tibet, for example, the main sacred mountain is seen as the body of a goddess, Vajravarahi, with a rock outcrop known as Ras chen perceived as her head, the Seng khyams rock as her belly and a rock in front of the cave, known as bDud'dul, as her knee. Such places are considered to be where active spiritual forces reside. Similar ways of seeing sanctity in the landscape by means of simulacra also occurred with the Incas in the Andes, in pre-dynastic Egypt, in the Celtic lands and indeed with cultures throughout the ancient world.

In some societies, the land became a kind of sacred scripture – the landscape of the Kunisaki peninsula in Japan, as a classic example of this, is seen by Buddhists as the topographical embodiment of the Lotus Sutra (see page 210). Other cultures, such as the ancient Celts, embedded their tribe's mythology in the land by associating legends with places. For the Apaches of Arizona, the complex names of certain natural features constitute stories that can inform social behaviour. Every Apache knows the names of hundreds of such places, and if someone transgresses, an appropriate place name is used to point out diplomatically the person's error. The Apaches say that place names are 'arrows' and that the land 'stalks' the people. Even young Apaches who move to the cities say such places still guide them in their actions.

Because the native territory of a traditional society is like a collective mindscape, the removal of the people from it can cause a kind of cultural amnesia, leading to tribal disintegration. This is hard for the modern world to appreciate because we no longer have such a close relationship with the land.

Sacred places

The power of place is the other major aspect of seeing the land as sacred. Our modern-day familiarity with temples, churches, mosques and sacred monuments makes it easy to forget that originally there were no such things. The first holy places were venerated natural locations – certain hills and mountains, caves, springs and waterfalls and specific trees. Selected caves became the cathedrals in the Palaeolithic era, tens of thousands of years ago, with painted walls. In the later Stone Age, fragments of special places in the form of ceremonial hand-axes and other objects were circulated because of the *mana*, the supernatural power, they were thought to possess. In a similar way the relics of saints were circulated in medieval times.

It can be difficult to decipher all the reasons why particular places came to be venerated, but some are clear. Places that stood out as landmarks, such as Glastonbury Tor in Somerset, England, seemed to emanate an aura of sanctity, as did those that produced unusual sounds like echoes, ringing rocks or roaring waters, or where vegetable or mineral materials existed that could be prepared for ritual or ceremonial purposes. And some places simply had a haunting, numinous quality, where the spirit world seemed especially close.

Gradually, venerated natural places became marked by rock art, or by the building of subtle walls or boundaries, until mankind eventually started constructing artificial sacred places. At first these acknowledged their original, natural sacred features in the vicinity. Stone circles on Bodmin Moor in Cornwall, England, for instance, were positioned within sight of the moor's weirdly weathered rock outcroppings ('tors'), sometimes precisely at the extreme limits of visibility. And the Minoan palace-temples on Crete relate to sacred cleft-peak mountains. As just one example, Knossos faces out to Mount Juktas, where a summit fissure contained pre-Minoan votive offerings.

It was the land that stirred the idea of the holy in the human heart and mind, and our places of worship ultimately derive from that initial interaction.

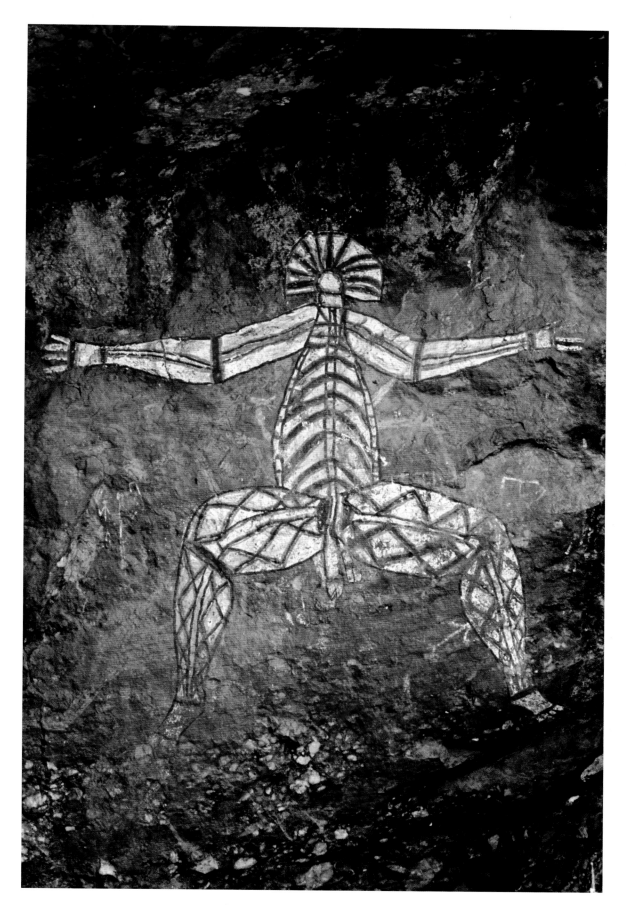

Aboriginal rock painting *This rock painting at Nourlangie Rock depicts Nabulwinjbulwinj, a dangerous spirit who kills women by striking them with a yam and then eats them.*

FENG SHUI

Feng shui ('wind-water') is a Chinese system of landscape divination that derives from ancestor worship practices requiring the specialized siting of family tombs. Feng shui aims to control a subtle force, **chi**, for the betterment of the living and the dead. There are two basic feng shui disciplines, the **Form School** and the **Compass School**. Popularized **modern feng shui** is a simplified version of these two schools, much as a newspaper horoscope is merely a snapshot of serious astrology.

If you are interested in **Feng Shui**, you may also like to read about:
- **I Ching**, pages 70–71
- **Chinese Astrology**, pages 58–59
- **Traditional Chinese Medicine**, pages 98–101
- **Taoism**, pages 216–217

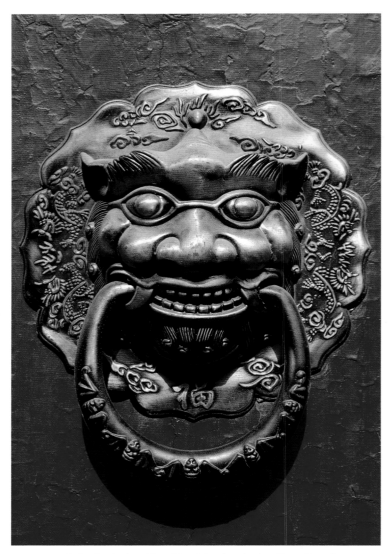

Doorway god *This detail of an old traditional door knocker in Beijing, China, shows an intimidating doorway god designed to ward off evil spirits.*

Chi

The concept of 'chi' is difficult for the Western mind: it is nowadays thought of as 'energy', but this is a rather crude equivalency. It is probably best understood as an overarching concept covering the dynamic forces expressed by breath, growth, motion, flow and so on, the converse being stagnant, unhealthy *sha* chi; in short, the qualities exhibited by wind and water.

The Form School

The archaic principles involved in the siting of tombs subsequently spread to locating homes and major buildings, and by the Han Dynasty (206 BCE–220 CE) feng shui as such began to be developed, becoming more or less fully fledged by the Sung Dynasty (960–1279 CE). Two basic styles of feng shui, the Form School and the Compass School, emerged.

The Form School is the oldest and is concerned directly with the lie of the land. The feng shui diviner (*hsien-sheng* or *kan-yu jia*), brought in to locate the most propitious site for a building, looks for a spot where a harmonious confluence of chi forces exists or can be engineered. The yang (masculine) element in the landscape is symbolized by the dragon; yin (feminine) by the tiger. Rugged places are excessively yang, where chi rushes like mountain streams; flat or swampy country has excessive yin and is imbued with sluggish *sha* chi. Straight landscape features such as roads, ridges and avenues are 'secret arrows' along which chi tends to hurtle dangerously. A secret arrow directed towards a dwelling, for example, would bring harmful influences. So the ideal location for a building is in undulating countryside with no harsh elements, and the building should be angled to the wind, sun and hillsides, and in a favourable relationship to water, as feng shui tenets dictate.

If the ideal spot cannot be found, the feng shui master can try to create a better balance of factors by, say, altering the slope of a hillside, modifying watercourses or planting trees. In unremittingly flat, excessively yin country, a hollow can be scooped out of the ground where chi would collect, or fountains or ponds installed (water can carry and attract chi). And sharp sounds such as the tinkling of wind chimes can add a dash of yang. If a

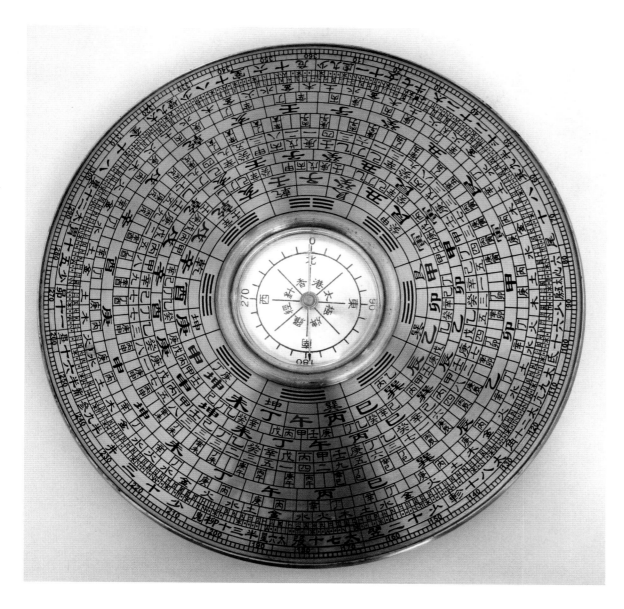

Luopan *The Compass School of feng shui uses a special compass, called a luopan, that is used to determine the flow of chi and subsequently determine the most advantageous orientation of buildings, rooms and furniture.*

straight feature points towards the entrance of a dwelling and cannot be diverted or masked, the doorway itself may be protected by sculptures or paintings of fearsome creatures – doorway gods – harking back to when feng shui related to the idea of spirits that could be scared away. Another ruse would be to deflect unwanted influences by placing a small mirror on or above a door, usually surrounded by an arrangement of the eight trigrams that form the basis of the *I Ching* (Book of Changes) divinatory method. Each trigram consists of arrangements of three lines, broken ones representing yin and unbroken ones yang.

The Compass School

This style of feng shui puts a greater emphasis on the eight trigrams and also involves five planets, the five elements (wood, fire, water, earth and metal), time, seasons, constellations, compass directions and astrological symbolism, as well as landscape forms. It employs the *Pa Kua* or *bagua*, an octagonal representation of the eight trigrams (as around the protective mirror), and

can be overlaid on the plan of a building, a city or even a room. As its name implies, the school also uses a special compass, the *luopan* or *lo'pan*. This consists of a square or circular tablet of lacquered wood, set into the centre of which is a magnetic compass. This is surrounded by concentric rings of symbols providing tiers of information that have to be brought into correspondence when the magnetic needle has oriented the compass.

Modern feng shui

Earth Mysteries pioneers became aware of feng shui in the 1960s, re-publishing books such as Ernest J. Eitel's *Feng Shui* (1873). Decades later feng shui has become a New Age staple, with articles regularly appearing in glossy magazines. However, feng shui is a complex subject and one that cannot always be simplified. Furthermore, it is a system that is not fully portable, as many of its rules relate specifically to Chinese conditions. As one example, a feng shui tenet states that a house with a narrow frontage brings good fortune, but this is because in old China taxes were levied on a house's width.

SACRED GEOMETRY

If you are interested in **Sacred Geometry**, you may also like to read about:
- **Megaliths and Earthworks**, pages 252–253
- **Archeoastronomy**, pages 254–255
- **Ancient Egyptian Wisdom**, pages 278–279

Sacred geometry, also referred to as canonical geometry, is not the invention of human beings, but is based on the **patterns** inherent in **nature**, such as growth spirals in organic forms, and their ratios, the most famous of which is **the golden proportion**. These ratios and proportions were then used by initiated builders to enhance the spirtual atmosphere of temples and **monuments**.

Patterns of nature

The term 'sacred geometry' describes the mathematical patterns that can be found in nature, ranging from the logarithmic structures of growth in plants and organisms to the vibrational patterns of atoms and molecules and the motion and proportions of planets, stars and galaxies.

The golden proportion

The nature of sacred geometry is such that only a straightedge and compass are required, since it is to do with ratios and not quantitative measure by number. Probably the best-known element of sacred geometry today is the golden proportion. In the diagram below, the rectangle ABFE is a golden rectangle because the ratio of its length to its width is 1.618, a ratio referred to by the Greek letter *phi* (ϕ). The famed golden section occurs on the line AE at D (AD:DE). Proportionally, the ratio works out at about 8 to 13 parts.

Monument architecture

A figure of sacred or canonical geometry, therefore, can be seen as a frozen moment in the process of becoming; a freeze-frame of the endless creative power of the universe or a thought cast from the Divine Mind. The ancient builders drew on this geometry of nature because they wanted to encode the ratios of creation in their temples and monuments. Two structures in particular provide an interesting illustration of the use of sacred geometry. They are very dissimilar to one another, yet both are derived from a very simple piece of geometry: two equal overlapping circles, the circumference of one passing through the centre of the other. The fish-shaped form created by the overlap is known as a *vesica piscis*. This was the mark of the early Christians in the catacombs of Rome because the fish was the symbol for Christ. It later became incorporated into ecclesiastical architecture. Architect Keith Critchlow detected this figure in the ground plan of the Neolithic stone

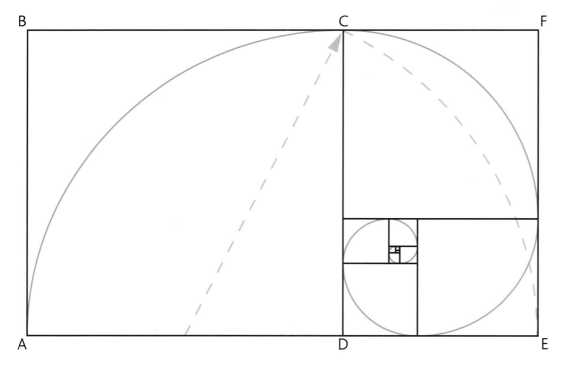

The golden rectangle and growth spiral

A square (ABCD in the diagram left) can be added to the longer side of a golden rectangle, or subtracted from a golden rectangle, to create a proportional progression growing larger or smaller respectively. As indicated in the diagram, a spiral can be generated from this progression, which is known as a logarithmic or growth spiral, such as is apparent in a conch shell. Pentagonal geometry can be derived from golden-section geometry, and this can be found in nature in the proportions of the human figure, in snowflakes and in some flowers. An example of the golden proportion exists in the Fibonacci series of numbers, where each number is the sum of the two preceding ones: 1, 2, 3, 5, 8, 13 and so on. A geometric example of Fibonacci progression can be seen in the distribution of seeds on the head of a sunflower.

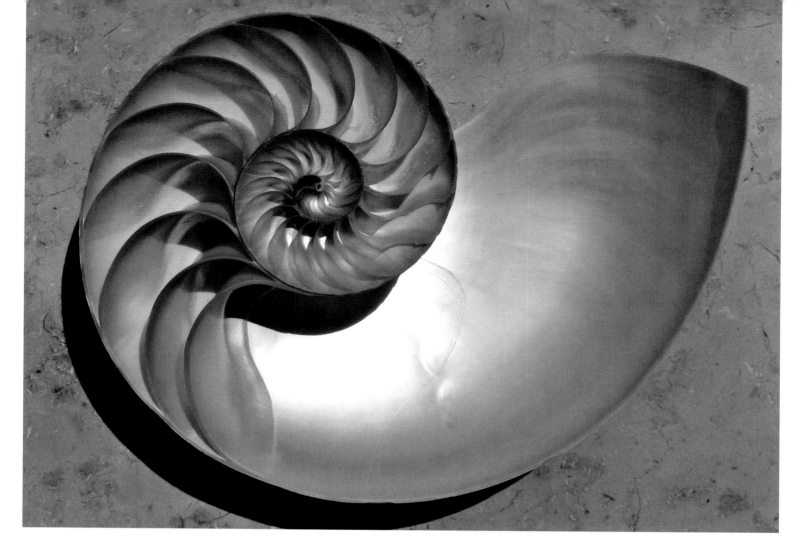

Nautilus shell *The structure of the nautilus shell conforms to the geometry of the golden-proportion growth spiral.*

circle of Castlerigg in the English Lake District, when he related the existing ground plan of the monument to the solar and lunar alignments incorporated into the ring of stones (see his 1979 book, *Time Stands Still*).

Earth Mysteries author and geometer John Michell considers the *vesica piscis* figure to be 'the matrix figure of sacred geometry', and has published some fascinating developments of it. For example, he has shown in his book *The View Over Atlantis* (1969) (revised edition *The New View Over Atlantis*, 1986) and later works how Egypt's Great Pyramid expresses *vesica piscis* geometry. At first glance, there seems to be no connection between the angular form of the pyramid and the curves of the fish-shaped *vesica*, but Michell shows how the proportions and angle of slope of the Pyramid can be reproduced using just a compass and straightedge from overlapping circles. The Great Pyramid also embodies *pi*, the constant ratio of the circumference of a circle to its diameter, and the golden section. Remarkably, a development of the Great Pyramid's geometry can create a figure that produces two circles which accurately display the ratios between the diameter of the Earth and that of the Moon. The ancients had their own ways of knowing, which defeat our modern logic.

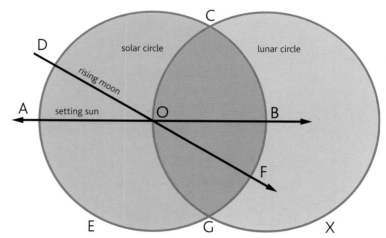

Castlerigg ground plan *The basic geometry underlying the ground plan of the Castlerigg stone circle. The axis AB is determined from the position of sunset on midsummer's day as observed from the stone circle. A 'solar' circle is drawn from centre O. The 'lunar' circle (centred at B) interlocks with it through O, creating points C and G on the circumference. An arc (EOBX) centred on G gives the point X on the lunar circle, which allows the axis (DOF) of the most southerly rising moon to be marked. This astronomically related geometry can be developed further to provide the precise 'flattened circle' ground plan defined by the stones at Castlerigg. (After Keith Critchlow)*

MEGALITHS AND EARTHWORKS

If you are interested in **Megaliths and Earthworks**, you may also like to read about:
- **Sacred Geometry**, pages 250–251
- **Archeoastronomy**, pages 254–255

Standing stones and other megalithic ('large stone') monuments, together with earthworks and structures built of both stone and earth, generally started to be constructed at locations around the world from around 6000 BCE, when settled agriculture began to supplant nomadic hunter-gatherer ways of life. The purpose and meaning of these monuments have been the subject of extensive research.

Standing stones

These were placed in circles or rows, or erected as solitary pillars – monoliths or menhirs – and occur in many locations worldwide. In Africa the Msoura site in Morocco comprises small stones surrounding a tall pillar stone; there are dozens of stone circles in Senegambia on the west coast; and hundreds of standing stones survive in Ethiopia, including sculpted menhirs and a monstrous 30 m (100 ft) tall monolith. In the Middle East the Yemen can boast rows and rings of standing stones, while in Israel there is a megalithic complex in Upper Galilee. Parts of the Himalayan region, Pakistan and India are scattered with standing stones. In Japan there is a set of concentric stone

Standing stones *The stones at Carnac, France, are at least 5,000 years old and represent one of the most concentrated collections of standing stones still visible today.*

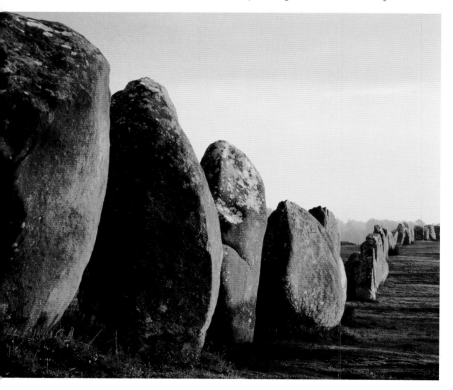

circles on the summit of the Tatetsuki Mound at Okayama. Generally, more recent standing stone sites occur in parts of South East Asia and Oceania – the Moai, the giant sculpted stones of Easter Island, being the most famous.

Megaliths as such are rare in the Americas, but one example is in the San Augustin region of Columbia, where sculpted stone uprights occur along with other megalithic structures. And in 2006, a ring of over 100 unhewn granite blocks was unexpectedly uncovered in the Brazilian Amazon.

Europe has probably the greatest concentration of extant standing stones. Over 5,000 are said to survive in Brittany alone, primarily in extensive stone rows. Scandinavia possesses standing stones laid out in boat-shaped settings as well as more recent monoliths emblazoned with runic engravings. Ireland and the UK have an exceptional megalithic heritage, with sites such as Stonehenge and Avebury in Wiltshire, England.

Stone and earth

Many megalithic monuments are composed of both stones and earth. A prime example is Newgrange in County Meath, Ireland, dating back to c. 3200 BCE. This giant earthen mound, over 100 m (328 ft) across and 13 m (43 ft) high, has carved kerbstones around its perimeter and a stone-lined passage 24 m (79 ft) long, leading inside to a stone chamber some 6 m (20 ft) high. At midwinter, the beams of the rising sun shine through an aperture known as the roof-box above the entrance to the passage and illuminate the chamber, making its stones glow like luminous gold. Neighbouring Newgrange are the equally great megalithic mounds of Knowth and Dowth. Ireland, the UK and northern France are peppered with smaller examples of similar structures, a classic being Gavrinis in Brittany.

Dolmens, which now appear as gaunt, table-like stone structures with uprights supporting a capstone, were once wholly or partially covered by earth or small rocks. They are found primarily in Europe, parts of the Middle East and India, as well as the Russian steppes.

Earthworks

Prehistoric earthen monuments occur throughout the world and are usually burial mounds, but there are some very mysterious ones too. In the UK, for instance, there are long earthen avenues, or 'cursuses', whose purpose is unknown, and Avebury's Silbury Hill, the largest artificial mound in prehistoric Europe at 40 m (130 ft) tall, has been probed for centuries, yet it still remains enigmatic. In the northern Midwest states of the USA thousands of effigy mounds survive. Most are geometrical forms, but there are also many in the shapes of animals and humans. Although usually not very high, effigy mounds can be large in plan. Man Mound, in Baraboo, Wisconsin, which depicts a human form with a headdress, is over 61 m (200 ft) long, and an earthen depiction of a bird in Madison in the same state has a wingspan of 213 m (700 ft). Not all effigy mounds contain human burials.

Monumental mysteries

Prehistoric monumental structures would have had varying purposes, some of which we can only guess at. Certain monoliths seem to have been used as waymarkers for hunters or pilgrims, while others delineated tribal boundaries, marked burial places or were associated with fertility rites, being generally phallic in shape. Yet others, especially shaped or engraved stones, represented ancestral figures or tribal symbols. The Scandinavian rune stones commemorated famous people or events in the Viking era. Numerous prehistoric sites, Stonehenge and Newgrange being famous cases in point, seem to have been built to mark astronomical events for ritual or calendrical purposes. Stonehenge is built on an axis aligned to the midsummer sunrise and possibly originally had a lunar axis before that.

Another puzzle is how megalithic sites were constructed. Speculations include exotic notions such as levitating stones or extra-terrestrial assistance, but the more likely answer is that they were built by human labour and ingenious human engineering. The prehistoric monuments around the world testify to enormous effort on the part of our remote ancestors in the service of beliefs and perhaps knowledge that we no longer possess.

Serpent Mound *Located in Adams County, Ohio, USA, the great Serpent Mound is the largest and most distinctive serpent-effigy mound in the world.*

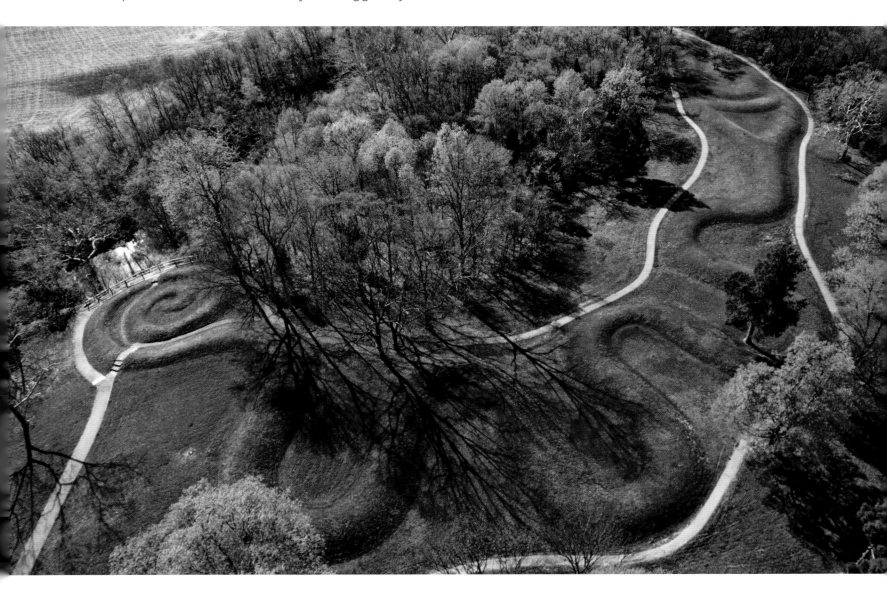

ARCHEOASTRONOMY

Archeoastronomy is the study of ancient astronomical knowledge. Its main origins date back to the turn of the 20th century, when scientist Sir Norman Lockyer found that Egyptian and Greek temples had solar and stellar orientations. **Stonehenge** and other **megalithic** monuments then took centre stage, followed by archeoastronomical research worldwide, including the astronomy of ancient **Chinese** and **Native American** cultures.

If you are interested in **Archeoastronomy**, you may also like to read about:

- **Megaliths and Earthworks**, pages 252–253
- **Sacred Geometry**, pages 250–251
- **Native American Spirituality**, pages 232–233
- **Mayan Prophecy**, page 285

The Stonehenge story

Although Lockyer (1836–1920) did some work at Stonehenge, it was not until the 1960s that archeoastronomy there began to mature. An amateur astronomer, C. A. Newham, found that the stones' positions, which mark out an almost perfect rectangular area within the monument, gave alignments to key solar and lunar rise and set positions. His further studies indicated that the builders of Stonehenge had used movable wooden poles for over a century to work out the skyline positions of the Moon in the course of its complex cycle of 18.61 years. It is now generally agreed that Stonehenge may indeed have been initially laid out on a lunar axis, which was later realigned to a solar one.

A little later in the decade, Smithsonian astronomer Gerald Hawkins (1928–2003) also studied the monument's astronomical possibilities, including the suggestion that the ring of 56 pits known as the Aubrey Holes surrounding the stones of Stonehenge was related to the 56-year lunar eclipse cycle. His bestselling book (in association with John B. White), *Stonehenge Decoded* (1965), made archeoastronomy much more accessible to an enthusiastic public.

Megalithic astronomy

In 1967 Scottish engineer Alexander Thom (1894–1985) published the findings resulting from his decades of accurately surveying many prehistoric megalithic monuments in the UK and calculating how they could have been used as Stone Age observatories. His work was so detailed that finally archeologists were reluctantly obliged to accept that astronomy was used in prehistory for ceremonial, ritual or calendrical purposes, even if not for scientific enquiry as we would understand it today.

Early Earth Mysteries enthusiasts willingly incorporated archeoastronomy into their range of interests, and one of their luminaries, John Michell, wrote a well-received book on the topic entitled *A Little History of Astro-Archaeology* (1977).

Archeoastronomy has now become a standard aspect of archeology because it has been realized that ancient astronomy was widespread, as the following selected examples illustrate.

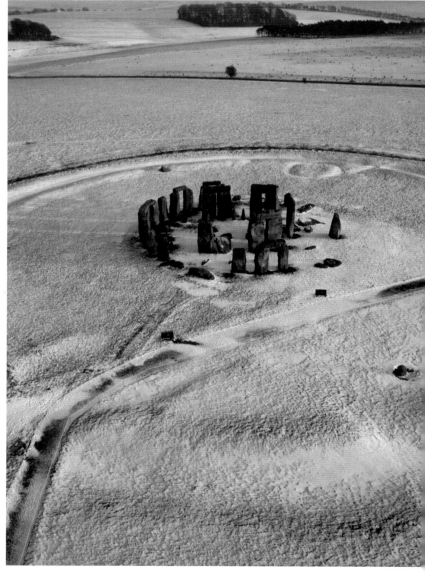

Stonehenge *The positioning of the standing stones at Stonehenge, Wiltshire, UK, clearly aligns with key solar and lunar rise and set positions.*

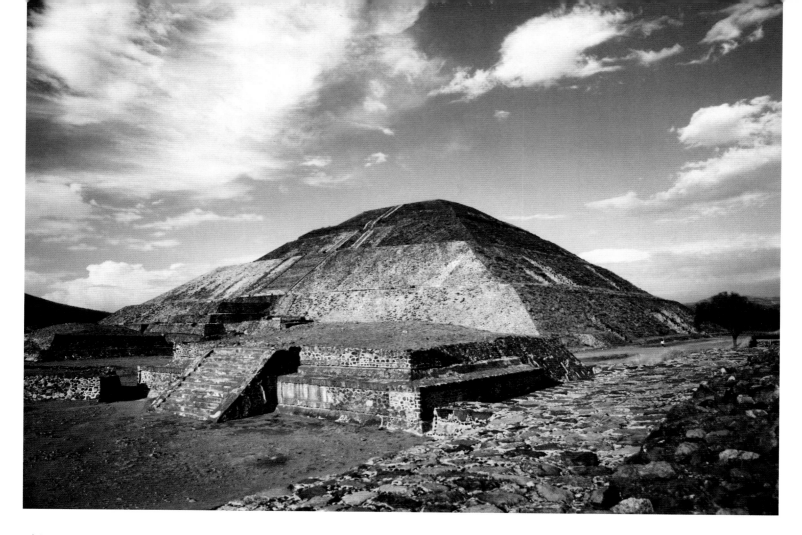

Chinese precision

In 8th-century CE China, pillars were erected along a north–south line over 2,000 miles (3,220 km) in extent, and their shadows, which varied in length on a given day according to latitude, were measured to enable the curvature of the Earth to be calculated. An even more 'high-tech' measuring device was built at Gao cheng zhen in the 13th century. This consists of a tall, pyramidal tower, from the north side of which a low wall extends for 37 m (120 ft). This was water-levelled using narrow troughs and calibrated. At noon on the summer solstice (21 June) the tip of the shadow cast by the tower was marked on the wall, and again when the sun was at its lowest, at midday on the winter solstice (21 December). Because of the height of the tower, the differences in the length of these shadows was considerable and could be precisely measured, allowing the exact length of the year to be determined.

Native American astronomy

In the Americas, most archeologists now regularly consider astronomical possibilities when working at specific sites. As one example, it was found that the Mississippian Indian city of Cahokia, Illinois, where the tallest prehistoric earthwork in North America – Monks Mound – still stands, had a ring of giant wooden posts (nicknamed 'Woodhenge') that was used for accurate observation of the solstices and equinoxes (21 March and September) a thousand years ago. In Arizona, as another example, the adobe ruin of Casa

Teotihuacan *The Pyramid of the Sun in the great ruined city in the Valley of Mexico was built around 150 CE on top of a cave that aligned to the setting point of the Pleiades constellation. This gave the orientation for the whole city grid of Teotihuacan.*

Grande, built by the Hohokam people around 800 years ago, has a square aperture that aligns to a key stage in the lunar cycle and a circular one that faces towards the summer-solstice sunset. In Mexico, the entire street grid of the vast, 2,000-year-old ruined city of Teotihuacan was discovered to have been laid out in relation to the setting point of the Pleiades star cluster, which had great significance for ancient Native America. And numerous Mayan and later Aztec temples have been found to align to the Sun, Venus and other culturally significant astronomical objects.

Archeoastronomers note that the ancient builders sometimes manipulated light from the Sun and Moon to create bravura performances of ceremonial showmanship. A classic case is that of the Castillo, a temple dedicated to the plumed serpent Kukulcan, situated on a stepped pyramid at the Mayan ceremonial city of Chichén Itzá, Mexico. At equinoctial sunrises, a serrated shadow of one of the pyramid's stepped corners is thrown on to the north balustrade, creating a pattern of light and dark triangles that moves as the sun rises, giving the effect of a diamond-backed serpent sliding down from the temple. This impression is enhanced by a carved stone serpent's head at the base of the balustrade.

EARTH ENERGIES

Ideas about 'earth energies' have always been prominent in Earth Mysteries. While there are ancient, **traditional beliefs** relating to subtle forces in nature, today's concepts of earth energies, typically promulgated by **energy dowsers**, are rather different. The only attempted scientific inquiry into earth-energy claims has been by the **Dragon Project**.

If you are interested in **Earth Energies**, you may also like to read about:
- Ayurveda, pages 94–97
- Landscape Lines, pages 258–259
- Traditional Chinese Medicine, pages 98–101
- Energy, pages 302–303

Traditional beliefs

The idea of an all-pervading, subtle force in nature is deeply embedded in the human psyche. There is the chi, *ki* and prana of oriental systems, the *kurunba* of Australian Aborigines, the *mana* of Pacific Islanders, the *maxpe*, *orenda*, *po-wa-ha* and many more names of Native American tribes, the *baraka* of northern African peoples, the *wouivre* of the pagan Druids and the *prima material* of the alchemists – the list is extensive. The idea was resurrected in a fictional context with 'The Force' in the *Star Wars* movies, in the late 1970s.

Energy dowsing

A more technological notion of magical energies began to gather strength in the 1960s with the arrival of the transistor radio and solid state electronics. This coincided with the rise of Earth Mysteries, and soon there were claims that 'ley lines' were lines of energy and could be dowsed. Theories proliferated in which the land became envisaged as being superimposed with a kind of printed circuit of subtle energies. Mother Earth became motherboard.

Traditional dowsing is a form of primary sensing using a rod, pendulum or other device for finding underground water, mineral veins and lost objects. While such targets are either found or not, Earth Mysteries 'energy dowsing' is different because it does not have such objectivity, being based only on the claims of individual dowsers. The practice derives from a conceptual amalgam that has three basic sources. One was the introduction of dowsing into 'ley hunting' by Arthur Lawton in 1938 – he believed that the positioning of ancient sites was related to a dowsable cosmic force. The second was the rise of interest in 'flying saucers' (UFOs) at roughly the same time as the advent of Earth Mysteries. A bestselling book, *Flying Saucers Have Landed* (1953), by Desmond Leslie and George Adamski, claimed there were 'magnetic paths' interpenetrating the planet that were used for navigation by extra-terrestrial craft. This idea found its way into early Earth Mysteries.

The third and main source of Earth Mysteries energy dowsing related to a specific development of dowsing, 'radiesthesia', conducted in Continental Europe. Radiesthetists claimed that natural radiations emerged from the ground, some saying that these fell into various kinds of grid patterns. This telluric radiation could be disturbed by subterranean water, mineral veins and other factors, causing it to mutate into dangerous or 'black' radiations and have negative effects on buildings and individuals situated above them. It was claimed that such 'black streams' can adversely affect the immune system and lead to chronic health conditions, now usually referred to collectively as 'geopathic stress'. The claimed clearing of such terrestrial radiations from a home or other environment has become very popular, with consultants offering specialized gadgets and techniques, sometimes borrowing traditional ceremonial purifying practices such as Native American smudging with smoke from smouldering sage.

Some British dowsers were influenced by the work of their Continental counterparts, one of them being Guy Underwood. His book, *The Pattern of the Past* (1969), included a look at the effect of underground streams at megalithic sites. Energy dowsing was firmly established in Earth Mysteries circles by Tom Graves' book *Dowsing* (1976).

The understanding of leys as energy lines has become a New Age doctrine and it remains highly influential despite its unproven nature.

The Dragon Project

The only attempt at a scientific investigation of earth-energies claims began in 1977. The Dragon Project was a shifting consortium of volunteers from various backgrounds, scientific and otherwise. It operated on a part-time basis with limited resources. It monitored megalithic sites – particularly its field headquarters, the Rollright Stones near Oxford, England – with electronic instrumentation, and also brought dowsers and psychics on site.

The dowsers were given the same working parameters, but did not produce matching results, and neither did the psychic work. The physical monitoring, though, did result in a few tantalizing findings. Magnetic anomalies were found at certain sites; some were permanent, being due to the geological composition of megaliths, but others were transitory and unexplained. Natural radiation anomalies also featured at some sites, ranging from dolmens in Cornwall, England, to the King's Chamber in Egypt's Great Pyramid. These anomalies were related to granite, which is radioactive. Some Dragon Project volunteers experienced vivid visionary episodes in such environments. Did the ancient builders know the effect granite could generate, perhaps explaining why the Egyptians brought Aswan granite hundreds of miles to clad the interior of the King's Chamber, for instance?

An overview of the Project's findings was published in Paul Devereux's *Places of Power* (1990, 2000).

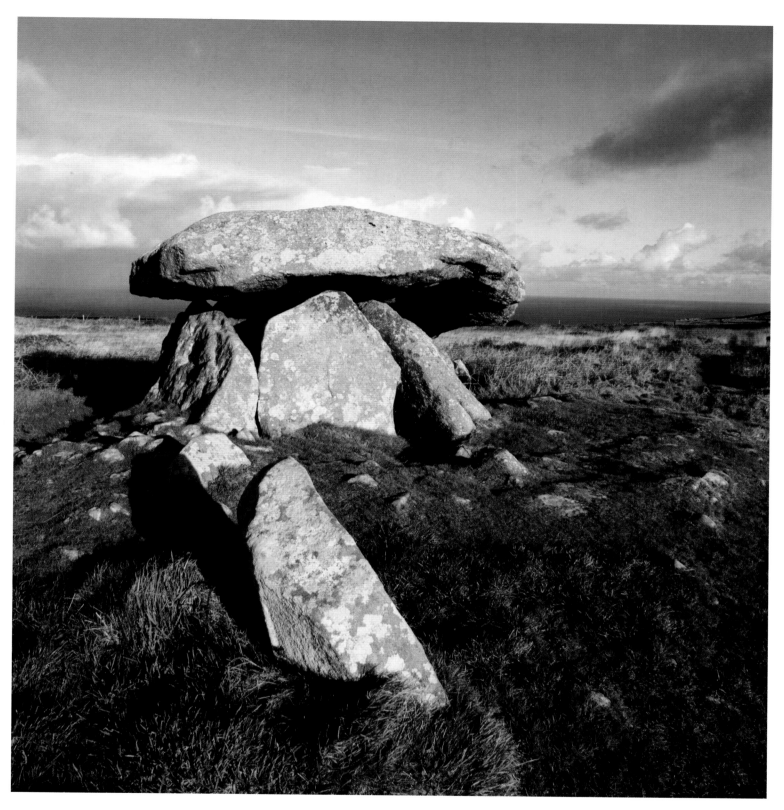

Dolmen *A number of Earth Mysteries experiments have been conducted at the 5,000-year-old monument of Chun Quoit in Cornwall, UK. In the 1980s, the Dragon Project measured heightened natural radiation inside the structure – the same level as inside the King's Chamber in the Great Pyramid, in fact. Also, at nightfall, dull flickering lights on the underside of the capstone were reported by project volunteers.*

LANDSCAPE LINES

Unexplained ancient landscape lines such as alignments of sites, stone rows, earthen avenues and desert markings have always been a key interest within Earth Mysteries circles. In particular, **ley lines** and the **Nazca lines** of Peru have long been a focus of attention. It is the **straightness** of many landscape lines that is the real puzzle.

If you are interested in **Landscape Lines**, you may also like to read about:
- **Earth Energies**, pages 256–257
- **Native American Spirituality**, pages 232–233
- **Shamanism**, pages 226–227

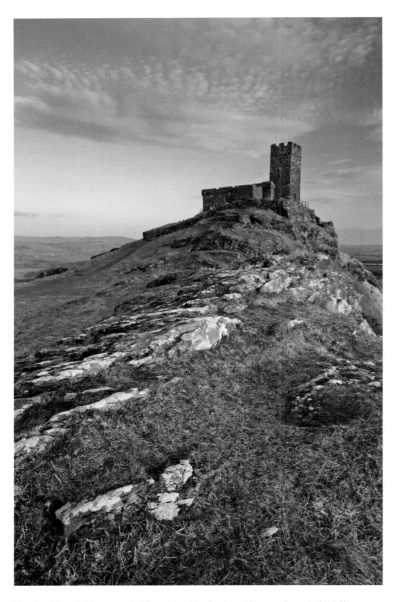

Brentor Church *The purported 'St Michael ley line' is said to run through this hilltop church in Devon. It is a point on a contentious alignment across southern England that was first suggested as a map line by John Michell, but was later claimed as a complex 'energy line' by some dowsers.*

Leys and ley lines

These were first understood as being the remnants of old straight tracks by the British businessman and photographer Alfred Watkins (1855–1935), whose main work was *The Old Straight Track* (1925). He believed that they had been laid out in prehistory as traders' routes using line-of-sight surveying methods (hence their straightness), and that the vestiges of these survived mainly as alignments of various kinds of ancient sites. It was these alignments that he dubbed 'leys'. After Watkins's death this modest observation became endowed with various accretions so that leys became interpreted as being, variously, lines of supernatural force, an idea initiated in a 1936 novel, *The Goat-Foot God*, by the occultist Dion Fortune; or magnetic lines in the ground used by UFOs, a belief originated in *Skyways and Landmarks* (1961) by ex-RAF pilot Tony Wedd; or dowsable lines of unspecified energies, a claim first spawned by Arthur Lawton in his pamphlet *Mysteries of Ancient Man* (1939) and built upon by many self-proclaimed energy dowsers up to the present day.

Much that is now written in the popular literature about leys (or 'ley lines' as they came to be called) is usually dubious hearsay, and most people remain unaware that there has never been such an archeological entity as a ley or ley line. For many years, most 'ley hunting' was accomplished by drawing straight lines on maps to connect symbols representing ancient sites such as stone circles, earthworks and even old churches. In the 1970s, there was intense debate about the statistics associated with such methods, and it was found that chance played a larger part than had been assumed, especially as ley hunters tended to include indiscriminately sites of many different periods as 'ley marker points'.

The original interest in leys has now resulted in two contrasting outcomes: a broadly popularized New Age notion of ley lines as energy lines, and a much smaller but scholarly based research strand interested in actual, yet unexplained archeological and historical linear features and tracks. Among these are the Nazca lines.

Nazca lines

On the desert tableland (*pampa*) between Nazca and Palpa, Peru, there is a complex pattern of ruler-straight lines of varying widths and with lengths of up to 6 miles (10 km) thought to date back to c. 600 CE. Scattered among them are probably older, giant images of creatures and abstract designs. All these ground markings, lines and images alike, were created by the removal of the oxidized, darkened desert surface to reveal bright-yellow subsoil.

The purpose of the lines remains uncertain. Suggestions have included that they map burial spots or underground water sources on the *pampa*, or that they point to distant sacred mountains, but these ideas do not explain the complexity of the lines or their strict straightness. Of course, the best-known 'theory' concerning the Nazca lines is writer Erich von Däniken's claim that they were the landing strips for the 'chariots' of extra-terrestrial 'gods' in his book *Chariots of the Gods?* (1968). The real answer seems most likely to lie with the spiritual life of ancient Native America.

The Kogi Indians of Columbia have ancient paved paths on their territory that they say the Earth Mother has instructed them to walk as a religious practice. Kogi *mamas* (shamans) claim that these pathways are the material traces of paths in the spirit world, which often continue where the physical ones end. Close examination of the Nazca lines reveals that they contain deep furrows made by countless feet walking them, Kogi-like, seemingly from and to nowhere in this world. In Bolivia there are longer straight lines than at Nazca, and even today some Indians proceed 'Indian file' along them on religious occasions. Prehistoric straight paths or roads occur at numerous places throughout the Americas – great straight roads left by the lost Anasazi people radiate from Chaco Canyon in New Mexico, and similar straight roads were made by the shamanistic Hopewell peoples in Ohio; in the Mayan lands of Central America, straight causeways – *sacbes* – link ceremonial cities, and the Maya still talk about invisible *sacbes*; straight lines are etched into the Atacama desert of Chile, and straight ways are even now being discovered deep within the Amazon rainforest.

Mysterious straightness

It seems that straightness had some spiritual connotation for ancient American Indians, and current research by archeologists and ethnobotanists, as well as research-based ley hunters, indicates that this at least partially had to do with the effects of mind-altering plant substances ingested by most ancient American Indian societies, and may possibly link to the sensation of flying out of the body that such drugs typically produce. The enigmatic ground markings of the Americas, at least, form shamanic landscapes – the visible signs of a sacred geography that lived within the American Indian soul.

Nazca lines *The condor is one of hundreds of images of animals, humans, flowers and geometric shapes at Nazca, Peru, which are only properly visible from the air. They are thought to have been drawn by the Nazca civilization in 200–600 CE.*

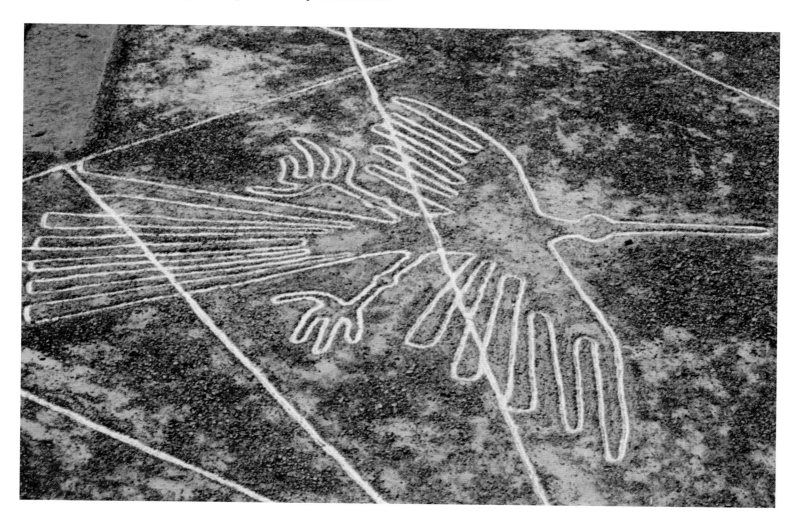

GREEN SPIRITUALITY

If you are interested in **Green Spirituality**, you may also like to read about:
- **Sacred Land**, pages 246–247
- **Paganism**, pages 238–239
- **Wicca**, pages 240–241
- **Fairies**, pages 292–293
- **The Goddess**, pages 294–295

In 1969, James Lovelock presented his **Gaia Hypothesis**, which showed how the Earth acts like a living, self-regulating organism. There was a strong **spiritual response** to this concept, resulting in areas like eco-paganism and **ecopsychology** emerging, along with **New Age notions** such as 'earth acupuncture' and 'earth chakras'.

The Gaia Hypothesis

In 1957 British scientist James Lovelock invented an incredibly sensitive device consisting of a gas chromatograph fitted with an electron-capture detector. This detector could register minute traces of chemicals in the atmosphere and was arguably the trigger for the environmental movement, in providing the data that enabled Rachel Carson to write her seminal book *Silent Spring* (1962), which warned of global poisoning by chemicals like DDT. Lovelock's findings with the instrument showed him that the world was far more environmentally interconnected than had previously been thought. Further research convinced him that the Earth was dynamic – its atmosphere and temperature range could be maintained because the planet acts like a self-regulating organism, a 'tightly coupled system' comprising the totality of its life (the biosphere) and its environment, including the oceans, the atmosphere and the surface rocks. Lovelock saw that the biosphere creates, regulates and maintains the environment that best suits it. This system has 'emergent properties', he argued, that make it greater than the sum of its parts, and the whole planet is, in a certain sense, alive.

It was the novelist William Golding, author of the famous *Lord of the Flies*, a neighbour of Lovelock's, who suggested that the system be named 'Gaia' after the ancient Greeks' Earth goddess. Lovelock put forward his tentative Gaia Hypothesis in a 1969 lecture at Princeton University, USA. No one took much notice except for life scientist Lynn Margulis, who became Lovelock's principal collaborator on the development of a fully fledged theory.

Spiritual response

Lovelock found that two-thirds of the letters he received from readers of his first book, *Gaia – A New Look at Life on Earth* (1979), were framed in religious terms. He suspected that the import of the theory had been supercharged by the then relatively novel imagery of Earth from space, which aroused much emotion in people everywhere. A generalized notion of our planet as a living being took hold, as if it were the modern rediscovery of the Earth Mother Goddess known to the ancients. This was expressed particularly strongly by an emergent neo-paganism, which reveres nature. Neo-paganism has now grown into a major movement with various denominations, including eco-paganism where pagan sensibilities merge with environmental and political activism. It is one form of a broader green spirituality ethic that has been summed up as 'soil, soul and society'.

New Age notions

The emergence of the Gaia Hypothesis coincided with the rise of Earth Mysteries. The people involved – some of them neo-pagans – readily accepted a 'living Earth' philosophy, equating it with ancient world-views, but it perhaps created some questionable hybrid notions within Earth Mysteries in which refined and ancient oriental body-energy systems were mixed with a simplistic concept of the Earth's 'body'. For instance, standing stones

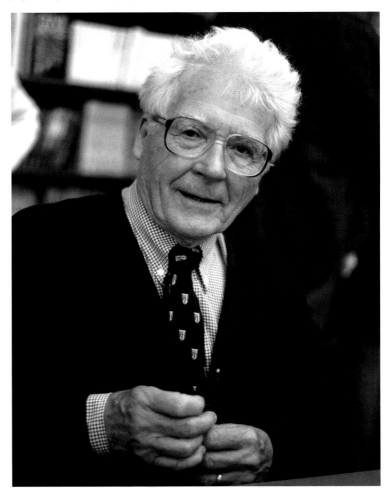

James Lovelock *The invention of James Lovelock's detector and his subsequent research played a key role in developing environmental awareness.*

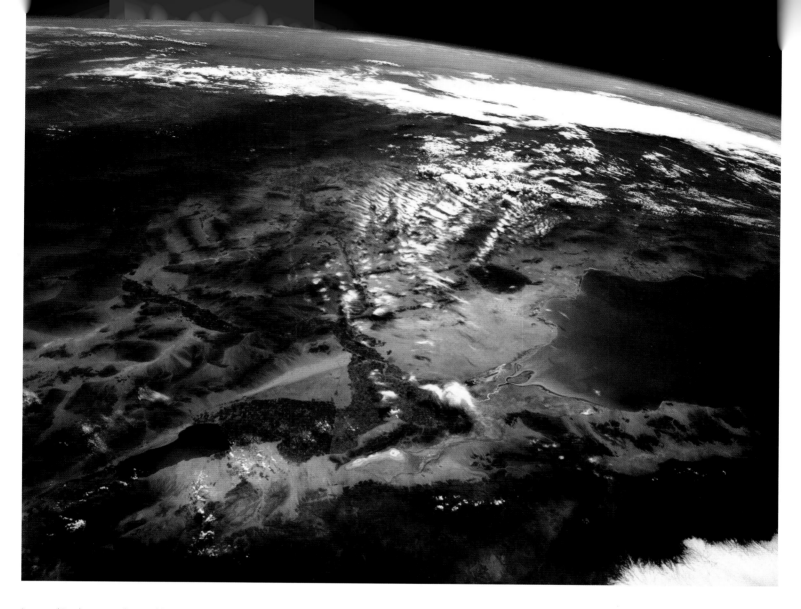

inserted in the ground were likened to acupuncture needles. This was seemingly first suggested by Earth Mysteries author John Michell, but it was Tom Graves's *Needles of Stone* (1978) that really cemented the image. Graves now privately states that he was being metaphorical, playing with ideas, but if so it was nevertheless taken literally by many readers. Another example is the appropriation of the Hindu system of chakras – energy centres in specific parts of the human body – for use in claims about 'earth chakras'. These are selected sacred sites or landscape features forming points in supposed national or global subtle-energy systems. Identification of earth chakras varies considerably from one claimant to another, and in all cases involves but a tiny selection from a vast number of other equally valid sites; it also probably reflects the knowledge level of the claimant.

Ecopsychology

There were also other, more formal ways in which an Earth-based spiritual impulse manifested. In 1972 Norwegian philosopher Arne Naess (1912–2009) complained to a Future Research conference in Bucharest, Romania, that the environmental movement was too shallow and materialistic, and

Earth *The Apollo programme, which captured pictures of the Earth from space during the 1960s and 1970s, revolutionized the public's perception of our planet. It created fertile soil for the timely Gaia Hypothesis to take root.*

was still promoting the view that humans were somehow separate from, and superior to, nature. This resulted a few years later in the emergence of the Deep Ecology movement, in which the concept of 'self' was to be expanded to include the natural world beyond the skin – an ecological self.

Some environmentalists disapproved of this apparent intrusion of psychology into ecology, but Naess saw ecology as being based on 'how we experience the world', that world-views *are* psychology. A full ecopsychology eventually developed in which a deep, almost poetical relationship with nature is felt to be necessary for mental health. Rather than trying to heal the Earth, the idea is for the Earth to heal us.

The broad thrust of ecospirituality actively seeks and builds upon any traditional faith approach that appreciates and honours landscape. It draws on animist and shamanic traditions that particularly reverence the natural world, but also Buddhism, Hinduism and Taoism.

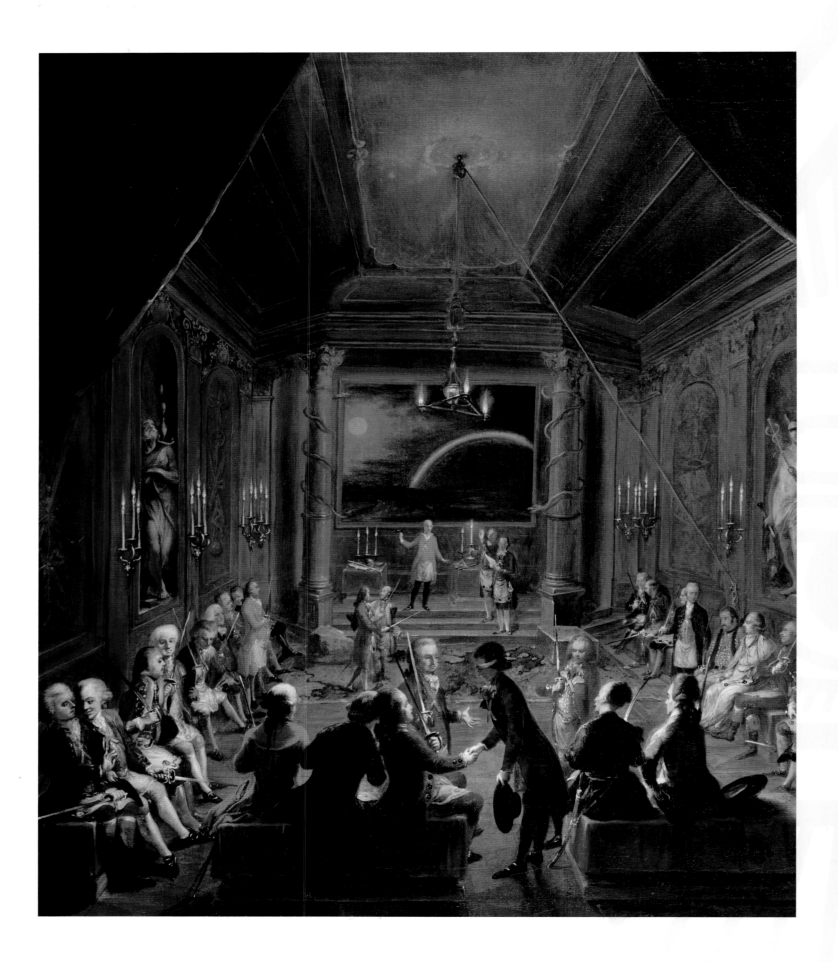

SPIRITUAL, SECRET AND OCCULT SOCIETIES

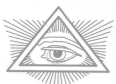

In recent times secret societies, including the Knights Templar and the Freemasons, have captured the public imagination. Novels such as *The Da Vinci Code* (2003) and the non-fiction work that informed it, *The Holy Blood and the Holy Grail* (1982), have introduced millions of people around the world to organizations that appear exotic, exciting and possibly dangerous. Yet such societies were, by and large, founded with the most spiritual of aims and over the centuries have inspired and guided many in the quest for enlightenment. Some, such as the Theosophists in the 19th century, were responsible for popularizing faith traditions, including Hinduism and Buddhism, for a Western audience; others, such as Rudolf Steiner's Anthroposophy, which emerged in the early 20th century, continue to provide inspiration to educationalists and healers today. This section explores the truth behind the fiction surrounding such organizations and tries to capture the ideals that prompted their formation.

Defining characteristics

Clearly not all spiritual societies are secret, and not all secret societies are spiritual; some, for example, are political or criminal. Here we look at spiritual societies that had heterodox – out of the ordinary – beliefs and practices or, in the case of the Knights Templar, are popularly believed to have had them.

Since there has been much ignorance and prejudice surrounding unorthodox approaches to religion and spirituality, it is important to look at what the related terms actually mean. 'Occult' comes from the Latin for 'hidden'; it is used in astronomy to mean 'eclipsed', without any other connotations. In the context of mind, body and spirit, occult means hidden in the sense of spiritual and secret. The word 'esoteric' is less contentious, meaning 'inner' or 'within', and applies to something taught to, or understood by, only the initiated rather than by everyone.

A defining characteristic of esoteric spiritual movements is that they encourage a personal quest for spiritual understanding and an individual

Masonic lodge *This detail from an 18th-century painting shows an initiation ceremony in a Viennese Masonic lodge during the reign of Joseph II, with Mozart seated on the left.*

relationship with the divine, in contrast to – as in mainstream orthodox religions – being told what you must believe by a specialist priesthood.

The enduring influence of the Golden Dawn

A number of societies evolved from earlier organizations. The Hermetic Order of the Golden Dawn, for example, was founded in London in 1888 by the leaders of an existing Rosicrucian Order within Freemasonry. Unusually, women could join as well as men; the only prerequisite was an enquiring mind. The Golden Dawn drew together and distilled Western esoteric teachings dating back to the Rosicrucians and earlier, to the Hermetic philosophers, the alchemists, astrologers and Kabbalists of the 16th and 17th centuries. It drew particularly on the teachings of French esoteric societies of the 19th century, and authorities such as Eliphas Lévi (1810–1875), who published the influential *Dogme et Rituel de la Haute Magie* in 1855–1856.

In its Outer Order the Golden Dawn taught the theory of magic based on four factors: the power of the will, the astral medium, correspondences, and directed imagination. Correspondences include the symbolic significance of Hebrew letters and numbers, together with astrological signs and their properties; gods and angels; the traditional four elements; plants; animals; parts of the body; colours; scents; precious stones; musical notes; and much more. In a magical ritual, practised in the Inner Order, all of these would be carefully selected to work together to bring about the desired result.

Members of the Golden Dawn included the poet W. B. Yeats (1865–1939), the actress Florence Farr (1860–1917) and, for just one year until he was expelled, the well-known occultist Aleister Crowley (1875–1947).

As a result of internal tensions and external pressures, the Golden Dawn fragmented at the turn of the century; the group that continued its magical teaching was called Stella Matutina. Although the Golden Dawn only lasted about 15 years, its influence on later 20th- and 21st-century esoteric societies is incalculable in terms of the focus on the tarot, Kabbalah and ritual magic, for instance. It remains an excellent example of the enduring power of spiritual societies to maintain an influential presence beneath the surface of mainstream society, adapting and evolving, yet continuing to act as transmitters of secret knowledge and faith.

KNIGHTS TEMPLAR

If you are interested in the **Knights Templar**, you may also like to read about:
- **Christianity**, pages 190–191
- **Freemasonry**, pages 268–269
- **The Holy Grail**, pages 282–283

Founded in the 12th century, the Knights Templar was an **order of warrior monks**, whose influence and great wealth ultimately led to its **downfall** at the turn of the 13th century. The Templars have long been the subject of colourful **myths**, and in recent years there has been much speculation concerning their connection to **Freemasonry** and other occult societies.

Order of warrior monks

The Knights Templar, or the Order of the Poor Knights of Christ and the Temple of Solomon, was founded around 1119 by Hugues de Payen, a noble from Champagne in France, with eight other knights, mostly of noble families. They took their name from their original quarters on Temple Mount in Jerusalem, which were supposedly built over the ruins of Solomon's Temple.

The Knights Templar took the monastic vows of poverty, chastity and obedience common to other religious orders. However, it was remarkable for being a Christian religious order whose members dedicated their lives not to prayer, contemplation and study, but to fighting. Their purpose was to protect Christian pilgrims going to Jerusalem, which had been captured by Crusader knights and established as a Christian kingdom in 1099. Their numbers quickly grew; by 1130 there were around 300 knights in Palestine.

These were well-trained, disciplined fighting men: an elite force that would fight to the death rather than surrender. Each knight had two or three horses, a mounted sergeant and a number of foot soldiers. It has been estimated that for every knight there were ten other men, including infirmary brothers, priests, cooks and labourers; at their height the order had some 15,000 men, 1,500 of these being knights.

From almost their beginning the Templars were in high favour with the Catholic Church. Their Rule was written by the influential abbot Bernard of Clairvaux and they were formally established as an order at the Council of Troyes in 1129. In 1139 Pope Innocent II granted them independence of all secular or religious authority, save that of the pope himself. In 1161 Pope Alexander III granted them exemption from paying tithes and allowed them to receive tithes themselves. They could also have their own chaplains as well as their own burial grounds, and so were completely outside the ecclesiastical structure of the Church.

The downfall

As the Templars grew in size, they also grew in influence and prestige. Kings and nobles gave them castles, land and the rents from land. With their wealth the Templars became 'the bankers of Europe'. They loaned money to kings and nobles, and this eventually led to their downfall.

King Philip IV of France was massively in debt to the Templars, and decided to cancel his debts by destroying the order – and in so doing seize their wealth. He arrested all the Templars in France, accusing them of conspiring with the Saracens, the enemies of Christianity in the Holy Land; of homosexual acts; of spitting on the Cross; of blaspheming against Christ; and of worshipping the head of an idol called Baphomet. Although Philip had no authority over the Templars, he used torture to extract confessions from some of the knights.

Templar myths

Most scholars today accept that there was little or no truth to any of the accusations, but some speculative historians claim that the Templars were secret believers in a cult of John the Baptist rather than Jesus, and venerated Mary Magdalene. There is absolutely no evidence for these claims, or that the Knights Templar supported the Cathars, a 12th-century Gnostic religion, or held the secret of where Jesus or the Magdalene were buried, or possessed the Holy Grail. Neither is there any evidence that in their early years in Jerusalem the Templars dug under Temple Mount and came across either great treasure or an heretical secret, or that after the dissolution of the order they escaped with their treasure to Scotland and fought for Robert the Bruce at the battle of Bannockburn in 1314, or that they discovered America a century before Columbus. All of these are modern fantasies imposed on a group of dedicated Christian knights.

The Templars and Freemasonry

But the idea that the Templars influenced Freemasonry and other esoteric societies is somewhat older. In 1736 a Freemason, the Chevalier Andrew Ramsay (c. 1681–1743), wrote his famous *Oration* in which he stated that knights returning from the Crusades met in lodges for the symbolic study of architecture, and so brought brotherhood, symbolism and secret signs into Freemasonry. In the 18th and 19th centuries a number of Masonic orders invented histories of the surviving Knights Templar to add a romantic tradition to their ritual histories. All these stories were allegorical accounts of Freemasonry's origins and were never intended to be taken as literal history.

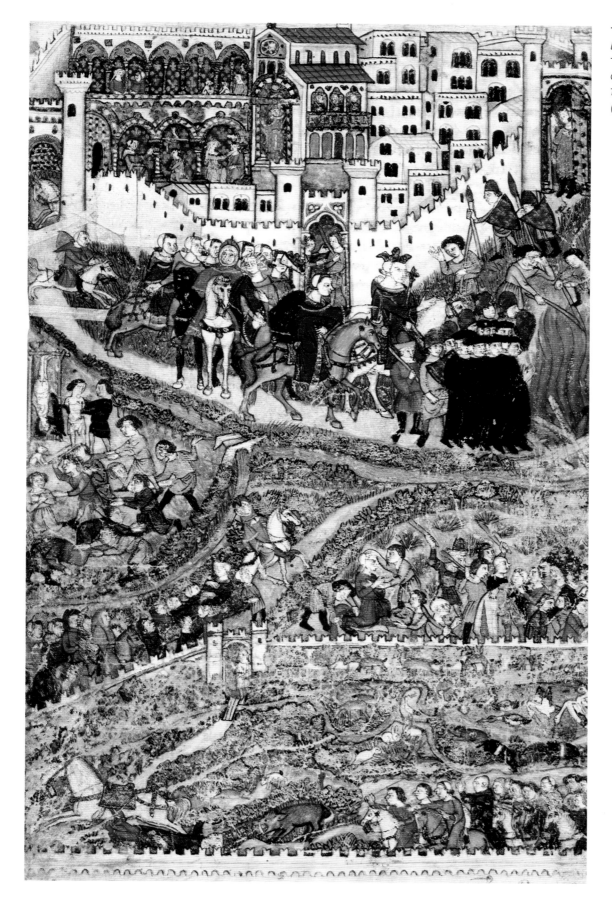

The destruction of the Templars *This late 14th-century illustration from the Treatise of the Vices by Cocharelli of Genoa shows the destruction of the Templars and the death of King Philip IV (1268–1314) of France.*

ROSICRUCIANISM

Rosicrucianism is a form of esoteric Christianity that first emerged in the 17th century. It was based on **three manifestos**, which described a secret brotherhood founded by Christian Rosenkreuz, and has left behind a **lasting legacy** in its influence on other esoteric societies and the establishment of modern-day Rosicrucianism orders.

If you are interested in **Rosicrucianism**, you may also like to read about:
● **Western Mystery Traditions**, pages 184–185
● **Freemasonry**, pages 268–269
● **Alchemy**, pages 296–297
● **The Kabbalah**, pages 188–189

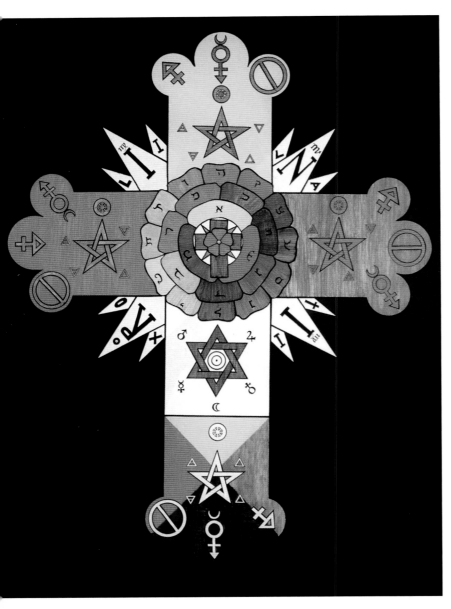

The Rose Cross *A classic late-19th-century interpretation of the rose-cross imagery from the Hermetic Order of the Golden Dawn: co-founder William Wynn Westcott's lamen, or the Rose Cross lamen. A lamen is a magical pendant worn on the chest.*

The three manifestos

The *Fama Fraternitatis*, published in 1614, told the story of how the tomb of Christian Rosenkreuz (Rosy Cross) was discovered in 1604, 120 years after his death at the age of 106. Rosenkreuz, it was claimed, had gained great esoteric learning while travelling in Europe and the Middle East, and established the Brotherhood of the Rosy Cross as an Invisible College of enlightened men.

The *Confessio Fraternitatis*, published in 1615, explained that the Brotherhood were learned men skilled in medicine, and through their personal spirituality they quietly brought good to the world. People of like mind were invited to join them. *The Chemical Wedding of Christian Rosenkreuz*, published in 1616, was a very different document. This was a spiritual fable, in a similar way to John Bunyan's famous *Pilgrim's Progress* over 60 years later, in which Rosenkreuz was invited to a wedding between a king and queen, and over a period of seven days had to overcome a series of obstacles in order to progress from one stage to the next. It is an allegorical romance of a personal spiritual journey, and can be interpreted in many ways, including as a veiled description of the alchemical process.

The Rosicrucians had never been heard of before the publication of these anonymous documents. In fact the Rosicrucian Brotherhood of the manifestos did not exist. But the ideas were not new; throughout Europe there were many 'natural philosophers' (sometimes called Hermetic philosophers), the scientists of their day, whose studies seamlessly interwove mathematics, astronomy, medicine, biology, botany, herbalism, alchemy, astrology, Kabbalism, neo-Platonism, forms of Gnosticism and much more in the search for truth about God and his creation.

Lasting legacy

In its emphasis on the importance of the individual's path to reaching spiritual enlightenment and its interest in esoteric traditions including alchemy, Rosicrucianism has proved highly influential in the development of other esoteric societies. For example, Freemasonry shared many of the ideals of Rosicrucianism, while the Hermetic Order of the Golden Dawn (see page 263) incorporated a number of Rosicrucian ideas. Rudolf Steiner (1861–1925), founder of Anthroposophy, lectured on the importance of Rosenkreuz's life as an example for humanity. Today there are many Rosicrucian orders worldwide claiming inspiration from the manifestos.

THE ILLUMINATI

The Bavarian Illuminati was a short-lived 18th-century society with both **political and spiritual aims**. Despite its members' ultra-radical aims, the many **claims by conspiracy theorists** that they were the secret rulers of the world, responsible for wars and revolutions, and the hidden power behind all business and finance, remain unfounded.

If you are interested in **The Illuminati**, you may also like to read about:
- **Western Mystery Traditions**, pages 184–185
- **Rosicrucianism**, page 266
- **Freemasonry**, pages 268–269

Political and spiritual aims

In May 1776 Adam Weishaupt (1748–1830), a young Professor of Natural and Canon Law at the University of Ingolstadt in Bavaria, founded the Illuminati or the Ancient Illuminated Seers of Bavaria. As with the Rosicrucians, his aim was to perfect the individual, and hence society, but his aspirations were as much political as spiritual and were extremely radical. The world could be perfected, he believed, if nations, monarchies, religions and other such artificial social structures were abolished.

But Weishaupt was not anti-spiritual; he was fascinated by the ancient pagan mystery religions and the work of the ancient Greek mathematician Pythagoras, and by the ancient wisdom teachings, the secret doctrines that underlay Rosicrucianism and Freemasonry, which he believed the Christian Churches had lost.

By 1784 the Illuminati had 650 members in lodges around Germany, and in Austria, Hungary, Bohemia, Switzerland and northern Italy. But in that same year the Elector of Bavaria banned all secret societies, and in 1785 the Illuminati was specifically named as a seditious group. Weishaupt lost his university position and was banished from Bavaria. Less than a decade after their formation, the Illuminati ceased to exist.

Conspiracy theorists' claims

Were it not for the hidden agendas and poor research of two writers, the Illuminati would have been no more than a curious footnote in history books. But in 1797 the Freemason John Robison (1739–1805), Professor of Natural Philosophy at the University of Edinburgh, wrote a book entitled *Proofs of a Conspiracy Against All the Religions and Governments of Europe*, and in 1797 and 1798 Abbé Augustin de Barruel (1741–1820), a former Jesuit, wrote the four-volume *Mémoires pour servir à l'histoire du Jacobinisme*. Both books were full of factual errors and both cited the Illuminati as a dangerous organization that was behind the French Revolution.

As a result of these books, 200 years later the internet abounds with conspiracy theorists asserting with false evidence and faulty logic that the Illuminati secretly rule the world in what is often called 'the Jewish-Masonic conspiracy'. They are said to have gone underground, resurfacing today as, amongst others, the Freemasons. Almost any organization containing wealthy, powerful or influential people is claimed to be a front for them.

But if the Illuminati are so all-powerful, why have they been so ineffectual at controlling the world? If they are so secretive, why is it so easy for conspiracy theorists to uncover their supposed members, aims and plans? If the Secret Rulers of the World are so inept, perhaps we don't need to worry too much about them.

Adam Weishaupt *The founder of the Bavarian Illuminati ended his days living in Gotha, Saxony, and teaching philosophy at the University of Göttingen.*

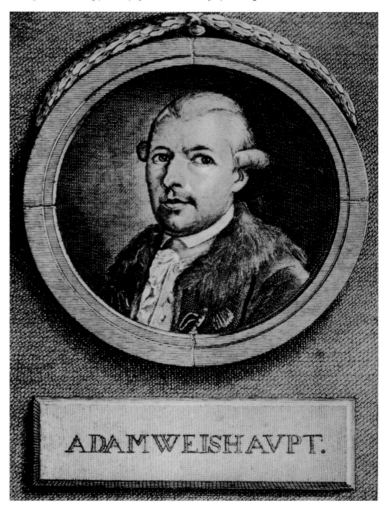

ADAMWEISHAVPT.

FREEMASONRY

If you are interested in **Freemasonry**, you may also like to read about:
- Christianity, pages 190–191
- Knights Templar, pages 264–265
- Rosicrucianism, page 266

Freemasonry has millions of members around the world, but is surrounded by a great deal of misinformation and even mistrust. While its **origins** are cloaked in mystery, the **orders, degrees and rituals** associated with modern Freemasonry are becoming more widely understood and appreciated, including the concept of its **mystical heart**.

Origins

Claims by early Masonic historians that the origins of Freemasonry date back to the Druids, to Moses or even to Adam may easily be seen as 'foundation myths', but even official Masonic historians cannot agree on the actual details of how Freemasonry began.

It is known that in June 1717 four London lodges met in a public house in St Paul's Churchyard in London, agreeing to set up a Grand Lodge as a regulatory body. Over the next few years lodges all over England joined the Grand Lodge, and new ones were founded; by 1730 there were over a hundred.

The earliest reference to lodges in England was in the 1646 diary of the antiquary and alchemical scholar Elias Ashmole (1617–1692), founder of the Ashmolean Museum in Oxford, noting that he was initiated into a lodge in Warrington. Many authorities believe that Freemasonry has Scottish rather than English origins, and some historians now suggest that the formation of the Grand Lodge in 1717, just two years after the first Jacobite Rebellion, was a deliberate move by the newly formed (and London-based) Hanoverian establishment to wrest any claim to Freemasonry from the Scots.

There are three main theories as to the origins of Freemasonry: from the Knights Templar, Rosicrucians or stonemasons. Despite the Chevalier Ramsay's *Oration* (see page 264), there is no evidence that returning Crusaders originated Freemasonry. There have been several Legends of Perpetuation, claiming that the last Grand Master of the Knights Templar passed the leadership and the 'secrets' of the order to one or another successor. In 1754 Baron Gotthelf von Hund founded the Order of the Strict Observance, claiming it to be a direct successor to the Templars, but this, like all similar claims, was no more than a romantic fantasy.

There is some evidence that the ideas and ideals of Rosicrucianism passed into Freemasonry, and certainly some of the scholars and scientists who came under the loose umbrella of Rosicrucianism were among the early Freemasons. There does not, however, appear to have been any direct linear progression from one movement to the other.

The earliest known reference to 'ffremasons', dating to 1376, refers to stonemasons, skilled craftsmen who carved 'freestone'. These were the men who designed and built the great cathedrals of Europe between 1050 and 1350, and who lived, did some of their finer stone carving and discussed their work in lodges – temporary buildings against the cathedral walls. Like many other craftsmen, the stonemasons had guilds to preserve high standards, protect the secrets of their trade and look after the welfare of their members.

Why should these guilds resurface in the early 18th century for people who were not stonemasons? One theory is that the rebuilding of London after the Great Fire of 1666, including St Paul's Cathedral, many other churches and public buildings and thousands of new houses, brought a great number of skilled masons to London. The work was largely complete by 1717 and many masons subsequently left London, so in order to survive, their lodges had to recruit 'gentlemen' members not only to maintain numbers but for their fees, which were twice those of craftsmen.

Orders, degrees and rituals

The aim of Freemasonry, like that of the Rosicrucians, is spiritual and moral improvement, and in consequence the improvement of society. The rituals, especially at each level of initiation, are effectively short mystery plays, teaching stories laden with symbolic meaning, but they are not intended to be taken as literal history.

Essentially, Freemasonry consists of three degrees – Entered Apprentice, Fellow Craft and Master Mason. In all three degrees initiates are taught hand grips and signs of recognition, and are given secret words, most of which come from the Old Testament; for example, two are the names of the pillars of Solomon's Temple, Boaz and Jachin. Beyond the three degrees of Craft Freemasonry there are many other orders, including the Holy Royal Arch, considered to be the fulfilment of the Master Mason degree; Mark Masonry, based on the identifying marks that stonemasons would often use to 'sign' their work; and the Ancient and Accepted Rite often known as Rose Croix.

The mystical heart of Freemasonry

For many Masons the rituals associated with the society serve to bond and organize members and dramatically express certain moral ideas. For others, progress through the orders and degrees represents allegorically the journey to mystical union with the divine. This was described by Freemason Joseph Fort Newton in *The Builders,* published in 1914:

> *'Here lies the great secret of Masonry – that it makes a man aware of that divinity within him, wherefrom his whole life takes its beauty and meaning, and inspires him to follow and obey it.'*

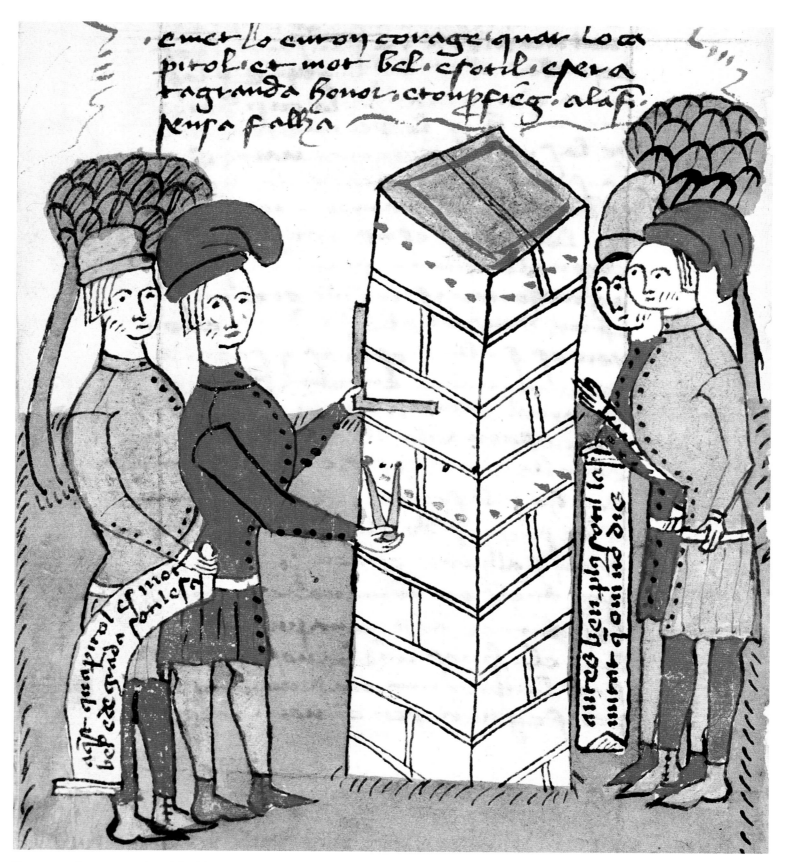

Stonemasons *Freemasons may have their origins in stonemasonry. This illustration is taken from* Traité d'Arpentage (Treatise on Surveying) *by Arnaud de Villeneuve (c. 1240–1312).*

THEOSOPHY

If you are interested in **Theosophy**, you may also like to read about:

- **Chakras and the Aura**, pages 172–173
- **Spiritualism**, pages 194–195
- **Hinduism**, pages 204–205
- **Buddhism**, pages 208–209
- **Rudolf Steiner and Anthroposophy**, pages 272–273
- **Atlantis**, pages 276–277
- **Spiritual Leaders**, pages 300–301

The Theosophical Society, founded in 1875 by **Madame Blavatsky**, has had a major role in introducing Eastern spiritual traditions to the West. Its central aims were to form a universal brotherhood of man; to study the ancient religions, philosophies and sciences; and, by studying the laws of nature, to reveal and develop the psychic powers latent in human beings. Subsequently, under **Annie Besant's stewardship**, Theosophy explored the nature of physical matter through psychic research and discovered spiritual teacher Jiddu Krishnamurti. Theosophy's **influence** can still be seen today in the New Age movement.

Madame Blavatsky

Born in Russia, Madame Helena Petrovna Blavatsky (1831–1891) was a colourful and often controversial figure. Throughout her life she claimed to have gained her spiritual insights from two teachers, Mahatma Morya, a spiritual initiate from Rajput, and Tibetan Master Koot Hoomi, whom she met in the Himalayas during what she herself called the 'veiled periods' of her life, 1848–1858 and 1863–1870. Whether her two teachers were actual physical people cannot be known, but they are now accepted as ascended masters by movements stemming from Theosophy.

Madame Blavatsky's biographical details up to the 1860s are somewhat confused, but what is known is that she moved to New York in 1873, where she impressed many with her psychic abilities and mediumship. In 1874 she met lawyer and journalist Henry Steel Olcott (1832–1907), who shared her interest in Spiritualism, and in 1875, in part as a result of illness that led to a personal awakening, she founded the Theosophical Society with Olcott and William Q. Judge (1851–1896), a mystic and occultist. In 1877 she published her first book, *Isis Unveiled*, subtitled 'A master key to the mysteries of ancient and modern science and theology', which painted a picture of a perennial philosophy underpinning every religion, often obscured by the outer forms of that belief system.

The following year she and Olcott moved the society's headquarters to Adyar, near Madras. Here they met A. P. Sinnett (1840–1921), a writer and journalist who became of major importance in disseminating Theosophy's key ideas. Sinnett was placed in contact with Blavatsky's spiritual masters Morya and Koot Hoomi, and this formed the basis of many Theosophical books and teachings. In 1880 Blavatsky and Olcott became Buddhists. By 1888 Blavatksy had returned to London where she published her second book, *The Secret Doctrine*, which set out the teachings of Theosophy.

Theosophy was rooted in its time: as well as its concentration on psychic abilities, it was heavily influenced by the newly fashionable theory of

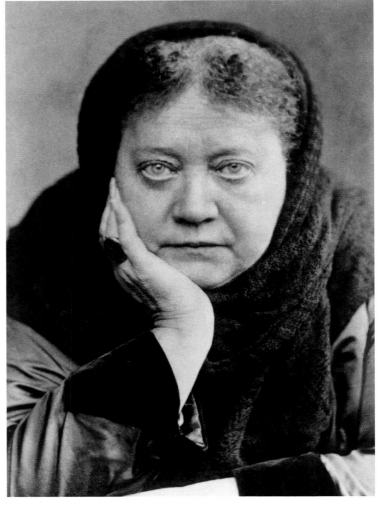

Madame Helena Petrovna Blavatsky *Author and founder of the Theosophical Society, she was a great intellect, but was criticized for faking her mediumship powers.*

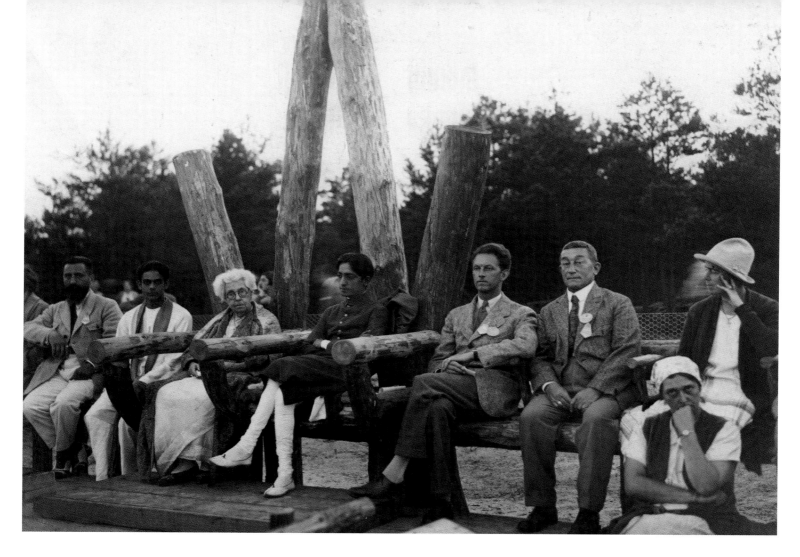

evolution – Charles Darwin's *The Origin of Species* was published in 1859. But instead of looking at evolution in the past up to the present day, Theosophy focused on the future evolution of the human race, both collectively and individually, believing that every person, progressing from life to life, and evolving to a higher state, can eventually become masters themselves.

Annie Besant's stewardship

Following her death in 1891, Madame Blavatsky was succeeded by Annie Besant (1847–1933), a freethinker and political radical, member of the left-wing Fabian Society and an early feminist campaigner. Besant was also prominent in Co-Masonry, a version of Freemasonry open to women, but she is perhaps best known for her involvement in Indian politics: she founded the Indian Home Rule League and became president of the Indian National Congress. She also founded what is now the University of Benares.

Together with Charles W. Leadbeater (1854–1934), Besant embarked on a number of occult experiments between 1895 and 1932 exploring the nature of physical matter. Some of their results, it is claimed, anticipated by many years scientific discoveries concerning the nature of subatomic particles. They also turned the emphasis of Theosophy away from esoteric Buddhism towards esoteric Christianity. Leadbeater became a bishop in the newly formed Liberal Catholic Church (an offshoot of the Old Catholic Church),

Annie Besant *This photograph shows Theosophist Annie Besant (centre left) at an assembly of the Order of the Star in the East with Jiddu Krishnamurti (centre).*

which became in some ways the formal religious wing of the Theosophical Society. Its teachings include reincarnation.

Leadbeater discovered the 14-year-old Jiddu Krishnamurti (1895–1986) and, along with Besant, believed him to be the prophesied new World Teacher, the embodiment of the Maitreya. In 1911 they set up a new Order of the Star in the East, with Krishnamurti at its head. However, he finally rejected their proposition and in 1929 disbanded the order. Krishnamurti refused to be the head of any new religion or spiritual organization, though he became a well-respected spiritual teacher.

Theosophy's influence

The ideas in Theosophy, particularly the concept of the Great White Brotherhood of Secret Masters, influenced both the New Age and other new religious movements, such as the 'I AM' movement, the Church Universal and Triumphant, Eckankar and the Aetherius Society. Theosophists were also responsible for the promulgation of many key ideas embraced by the New Age movement today, including the concepts of chakras and auras, the Akashic Record and karma and reincarnation.

RUDOLF STEINER AND ANTHROPOSOPHY

Rudolf Steiner was one of the most respected spiritual teachers of the early 20th century. **Founder of the Anthroposophical Society**, he also had a wider **influence** on the leaders of numerous other esoteric organizations. His **innovations in education, agriculture and architecture** are still highly regarded nearly a century after his death.

If you are interested in **Rudolf Steiner and Anthroposophy**, you may also like to read about:
- **Homeopathy**, pages 160–161
- **Colour Therapy**, page 162
- **Western Mystery Traditions**, pages 184–185
- **Christianity**, pages 190–191
- **Rosicrucianism**, page 266

Founding the Anthroposophical Society

Rudolf Steiner (1861–1925) combined a search for esoteric wisdom with a deep urge for social reform. His remarkable intelligence was recognized early; at the age of just 22 he was asked to be the scientific editor of a new standard edition of the works of German writer and philosopher Johann Wolfgang von Goethe (1749–1832).

Rudolf Steiner *This illustration shows Steiner at work in his studio near the Goetheanum in 1914 sculpting his great statue of Christ, which he called* The Representative of Man.

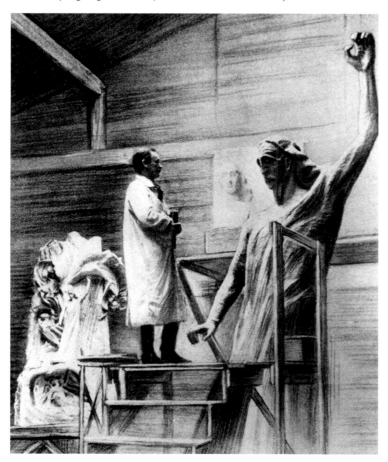

Steiner joined the Theosophical Society around 1900, and became its German leader in 1902. But in 1912–1913 he fell out with the society's president, Annie Besant, partly because she overturned his decision over expelling a member, and partly over her championing of Krishnamurti as the new World Teacher. Steiner left, taking many German Theosophists with him, and set up his own Anthroposophical Society. Theosophy translates from the Greek as 'god wisdom'; Anthroposophy translates as 'man wisdom'.

Theosophy had taught that humans were evolving towards higher powers; Steiner taught instead that humans used to have godlike powers, but had lost them. In Steiner's view, there are spiritual secrets buried deep within us and through study and meditation we can achieve spiritual growth on four levels: the senses, imagination, inspiration and intuition. With Christ's help we may regain the higher spiritual levels that mankind once knew. Steiner believed that these deeper truths were held in what he described as the Akashic Chronicle – the record of all events and experiences that could be read or directly perceived by a trained and sincere clairvoyant, first described by the Theosophists. Steiner emphasized mystical awareness; he himself had well-developed psychic powers.

Innovations in education, agriculture and architecture

Anthroposophy, like Theosophy, aimed to unite religion and science, and Steiner developed innovative ideas in many areas, particularly in education, agriculture and architecture. In education he pioneered a teaching method in which teachers support and keep awake the natural spiritual essence of each child, rather than force-feeding the same facts into several children simultaneously. His ideas, such as guided movement to music, work particularly well with children who have learning difficulties. Today there are nearly one thousand Steiner Schools, sometimes called Waldorf Schools, around the world. He also established what are now called Camphill Communities, designed to meet the needs of the disabled, in whom he took a particular interest.

In agriculture Steiner pioneered 'biodynamic' farming methods, an organic approach that emphasizes nature's rhythms, such as the seasons, for sowing and harvesting. He also championed homeopathic remedies.

In Steiner-inspired buildings, door and window frames are often made of naturally curving branches, rather than artificially straight planks of wood. His Goetheanum, built near Basel in Switzerland between 1913 and 1919, had two interlocking domes, the larger one bigger than the dome of St Peter's Basilica in Rome. It featured pillars of different woods, and colours based on Goethe's interpretation of the 'moral' qualities of colours. The roofs of the 'wings' from the intersection of the two domes were curved like a turtle shell. The original having been destroyed by fire in 1922, Steiner designed a second Goetheanum in Dornach, Switzerland, which was completed after his death and is the Anthroposophical Society's headquarters.

Steiner's wider influence

Steiner had never been happy with the Hindu and Buddhist foundations of Theosophy, nor with the Tibetan Secret Masters such as Koot Hoomi from whom Madame Blavatsky claimed to have received her teachings. Always more closely wedded to mystical Christianity, he helped found a new Christian denomination known as the Christian Community. It has no fixed theology, but lays great emphasis on the symbolism of the sacraments. It has around 15,000 members worldwide, 10,000 of them in Germany.

Steiner had connections with several influential individuals and organizations in the esoteric community. In 1906 he was made an officer of a quasi-masonic Order, the Rite of Memphis and Misraim, by Theodor Reuss, founder of the Ordo Templi Orientis (OTO). There is no evidence that Steiner was ever a member of the OTO, and he ended all association with Reuss in 1914. He had a strong influence on Max Heindel (1865–1919), whom he met in 1907, and who went on to write *The Rosicrucian Cosmo-Conception* (1909) and found the Rosicrucian Fellowship. Around 1910 Steiner met Dr Robert Felkin (1853–1926), leader of Stella Matutina, one of the successor organizations to the Hermetic Order of the Golden Dawn (see page 263). Greatly impressed by Steiner, Felkin sent one of his members to study under him; some of his teachings on meditation and homeopathy were incorporated into the teachings of the inner order of Stella Matutina.

Steiner published a large number of books, many of them based on the notes for the 6,000 lectures he gave over 25 years, on all areas of his interests, psychic, spiritual and practical.

Goetheanum *Built in Dornach in Switzerland, Steiner's Goetheanum is a classic example of his preference for using curves rather than straight lines.*

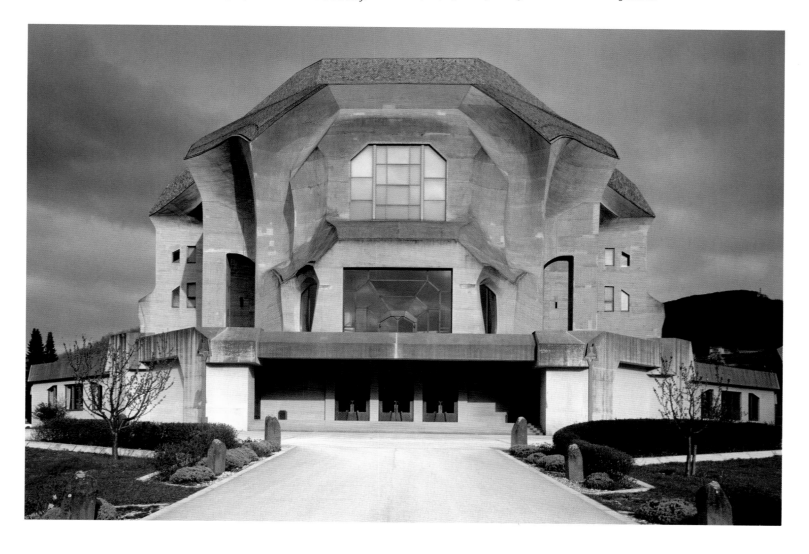

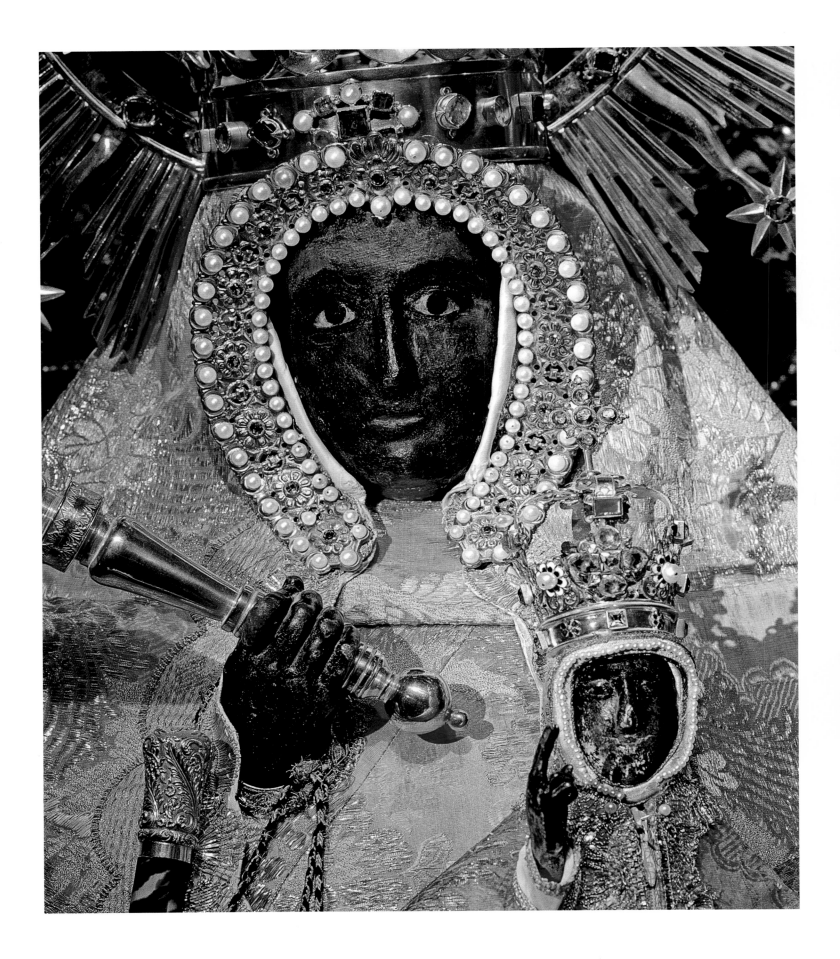

ANCIENT MYSTERIES

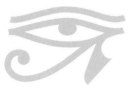

The immense diversity of contemporary global culture, married to the ever-extending frontiers of human experience and discovery, together present wonders and mysteries sufficient to occupy anyone for a lifetime. Yet amidst the clamour of the modern world, the mysteries with the deepest resonance and most enduring attraction often seem to be those that belong to the past.

Gathered together here under the rubric 'ancient mysteries' is a selection of these puzzles from the past. Included are some of the most famous historical mysteries and some less well-known ones. What makes these mysteries important? What, if anything, can be learned from them? Why should we care about the artefacts and beliefs of dead civilizations and extinct cultures? Why should we privilege ancient mysteries over modern?

Back to basics

There is a sense in which historical mysteries touch something more profound, more valuable than modern ones. Perhaps it is an atavistic urge, stirring primitive emotions, offering a way to access values and realities with which the modern world has lost touch. The human condition today is the result of long millennia of experience, but on the whole this experience is inaccessible. Many modern men and women are alienated from important aspects of their heritage: the roots of culture and community, and most of all the wellsprings of spirituality and mysticism. Though they may never be revealed, explained or resolved, the simple contemplation of ancient mysteries is a way to approach these wellsprings.

The power of the New Age

The prevalence and popularity of ancient mysteries owes much to two major developments in modern culture. The first is the growth of the New Age movement. Starting in the 1960s, but with its roots in 19th-century

Black Madonna *The Guadalupe Madonna from the Monasterio Real in Spain is a classic example of a Black Madonna, a statue of the Blessed Virgin Mary (and sometimes the Christ child as well) with black skin.*

movements like Theosophy, the New Age tied together disparate strands of ecological consciousness, personal development theories, freethinking and pagan religious thought, the occult and paranormal, mysticism and fringe science with enthusiasm for the wisdom of ancient cultures.

Ancient mysteries stand at the nexus of many of these fascinations. For instance, the venerable European tradition of the Black Madonnas, objects of local cults and folk veneration, was reinterpreted as a neo-pagan survival of pre-Christian fertility rituals and goddess worship, and recast as an act of spiritual and ideological opposition to the reactionary forces of the establishment. Another example is Atlantis. Made popular in the 19th century by an enthralling piece of pseudo-historical/anthropological detective work, for the New Age movement the lost continent became the *locus classicus* of many of its favourite tropes and concerns – psychic powers, reincarnation, channelling, crystal energies, occult technology, the dangers of empire and hubris. Atlantis was adopted both as the ultimate warning from history for corrupt and decadent modern civilization, and as an antediluvian utopia of spiritual self-actualization.

In these and many other instances, ancient mysteries become both a tool for modern agendas (feminism, anti-capitalism, eco-awareness) and a way to explore liminal phenomena and transcendent experience (magic, the paranormal, personal access to the divine, spiritual growth).

Mass media and popular culture

The other major cultural development has been entertainment and mass media. Ancient mysteries are cemented in the popular consciousness thanks to blockbusters such as the Indiana Jones films, the Dan Brown novels, the *X-Files*, Lara Croft and many other comics, books, games and films. Again this development can be traced back to the 19th century, when works such as Ignatius Donnelly's *Atlantis: The Antediluvian World* and Edward Bulwer-Lytton's *Vril: The Power of the Coming Race* reached huge audiences, and Orientalism triggered a vogue for all things ancient and Eastern.

The cultural success of ancient mysteries underlines the importance of their narrative content – in many ways they function as contemporary myths and legends, embodying archetypal quests for meaning and spiritual truth.

ATLANTIS

If you are interested in **Atlantis**, you may also like to read about:

● **Past Lives and Past-Life Therapy**, pages 50–51
● **Theosophy**, pages 270–271
● **Rudolf Steiner and Anthroposophy**, pages 272–273
● **Ancient Egyptian Wisdom**, pages 278–279
● **Channelling**, pages 42–43

The lost continent of Atlantis was first described in ancient times by the philosopher **Plato**, but it was not until the 19th-century theories of **Ignatius Donnelly** that the more familiar image of Atlantis as the Mother of Civilization emerged, a concept developed by a succession of mystics into the **New Age Atlantis**. In modern times scientists and explorers have sought **lost prehistoric civilizations** that may have inspired the legend.

Plato's Atlantis

In the *Dialogue of Timaeus* and the *Dialogue of Critias*, written c. 360 BCE, the ancient Greek philosopher Plato describes an island continent of mountains encircling a great central plain. Here, a mighty empire flourished before being destroyed in a natural disaster sent by the gods, which caused the land to sink beneath the sea.

Plato explained that the story of Atlantis had come down to him via Egyptian priests who had preserved knowledge of the lost civilization for 9,000 years, and went on to describe its geography, history, religion and constitution, and in particular the capital, with its concentric rings of canals

Plato *The ancient Greek philosopher Plato gave a famous early account of Atlantis. This mosaic found at Pompeii depicts him teaching a group of his students.*

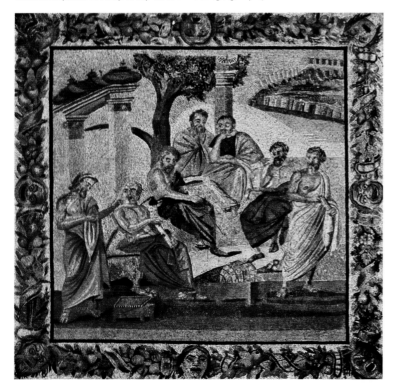

around a central citadel or acropolis. It was a high Bronze Age civilization, with great temples, dockyards and city walls. On top of the acropolis was a palace-temple complex sacred to Poseidon, the tutelary deity of Atlantis, and within this were lush gardens, hot baths, a giant statue of the god and a pillar of orichalcum (a copper-gold alloy), upon which were inscribed the laws of the land. Atlantis had been located, according to Plato, before the Pillars of Hercules – generally understood to be the Straits of Gibraltar, placing the continent in the Atlantic Ocean (continent and ocean derive their names from two different mythical figures named Atlas).

Plato's version included few of the features popularly associated with Atlantis today, with no pyramids, sun-worshipping, telepathy or flying vehicles. Most scholars think that Plato invented Atlantis as a moral fable – an example of an ideal state gone astray.

Ignatius Donnelly

Modern popular conceptions of Atlantis owe much to American politician, writer and eccentric Ignatius Donnelly. His 1882 bestseller *Atlantis: The Antediluvian World* highlighted similarities between the great civilizations of history, from ancient Egypt to the Aztecs, and argued that they had so much in common because they could all be traced back to one source – Atlantis, the ur-civilization, the original source of writing, metallurgy, architecture and other technologies.

Donnelly claimed that Atlantis had been a real continent and that refugees from its submergence had founded the known civilizations. Donnelly's evidence included the presence of pyramids and sun-worshipping on both sides of the Atlantic, and the prevalence of flood myths in cultures around the world. He claimed that the Azores and the newly discovered Mid-Atlantic Ridge were the last remnants of the lost continent.

New Age Atlantis

The 19th century was a ferment of new ideas about history, race and evolution. It was also a period of great fascination with the occult and mysticism, spiritualism and psychic powers. All of these concerns came together in Atlantis.

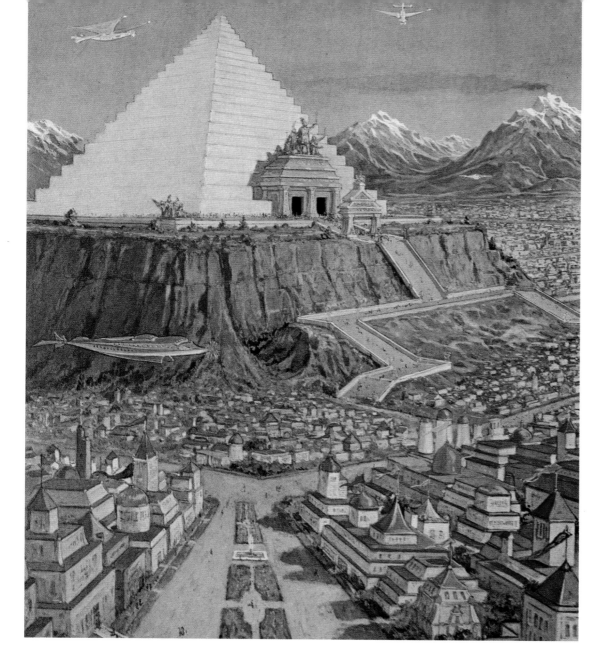

Atlantis *Fanciful representations of Atlantis have existed for centuries. J. Augustus Knapp's 1928 illustration of the city with a great Mystery Temple at its heart bears little resemblance to Plato's description.*

Madame Blavatsky was a charismatic spiritual explorer who invented a new discipline known as Theosophy, a beguiling blend of pseudoscience and the occult that offered a sweeping vision of millions of years of human history and evolution, in which Atlantis and other lost continents, such as Lemuria, played pivotal roles. Claiming to have clairvoyant access to occult records, Theosophist William Scott-Elliot revealed how the ancient Atlanteans had used psychic energy to power airships and other strange technologies, until their dark sorcery triggered the continent's destruction.

Subsequent figures such as Rudolf Steiner and Edgar Cayce also drew on psychic wisdom, such as the Akashic Record, to reveal more about Atlantis, developing a picture of spiritually evolved superbeings with access to godlike wisdom, technology and power. Cayce claimed that many people are reincarnated Atlanteans. Today this New Age conception of Atlantis continues to develop. Atlantis is seen as a pathway to Gnostic revelation; a parable of the dangers of unchecked technology, over-consumption, ecological peril or simple hubris; and a repository of spiritual wisdom that can be accessed if you have the right tools (such as channelling). People who study and write about Atlantis are known as Atlantologists.

Lost prehistoric civilizations

Advances in the understanding of geology and plate tectonics have shown that it is not possible for a continent to sink into the ocean, while mainstream archeological opinion is that the date that Plato gives for Atlantis (c. 9500 BCE) is deep in the Stone Age, before the earliest towns and cities. In other words, Plato's account cannot be literally true. Many Atlantologists believe, however, that Plato's Atlantis is a garbled recollection of a genuine lost prehistoric civilization, and that by following clues from his tale the 'real' Atlantis can be found. Candidates for the real Atlantis have been proposed on almost every continent, including Antarctica. One of the most popular is Thera in the Mediterranean.

ANCIENT EGYPTIAN WISDOM

If you are interested in **Ancient Egyptian Wisdom**, you may also like to read about:
- Theosophy, pages 270–271
- Channelling, pages 42–43
- Western Mystery Traditions, pages 184–185
- Freemasonry, pages 268–269
- Sacred Geometry, pages 250–251
- Archeoastronomy, pages 254–255

Ancient Egyptian civilization endured for over 3,000 years and achieved amazing architectural feats like the **pyramids** and the **Sphinx**, which are said to encode secret wisdom, and even to conceal a **Hall of Records** according to Edgar Cayce, the famous 'Sleeping Seer' of Virginia Beach, USA. Central to Egyptian religion were funerary rites and spells, such as those collected in the **Book of the Dead**.

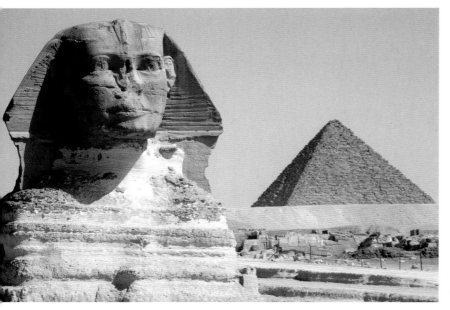

The Sphinx and the Great Pyramid *Many mysteries surround the origins, construction and age of the pyramids and the Sphinx at the Giza necropolis site in Egypt.*

The pyramids

Funerary monuments in ancient Egypt developed from flat-roofed mud-brick structures with slanting walls named *mastaba*, from the word for 'bench', which were built over burial pits to protect them from grave robbers, starting from the late fourth millennium BCE. Stacking *mastaba* atop one another gave a stepped pyramid form, and this was achieved most notably in the reign of King Djoser of the Third Dynasty (2667–2648 BCE), at the start of the Old Kingdom Period, with the construction of the stepped stone pyramid at Saqqara. This feat is attributed to the vizier Imhotep, who later became a semi-divine culture-hero figure, important to groups such as the Freemasons. It is speculated that pyramids were intended to mimic the form of the primeval mound from which life originally sprang.

True pyramids, with smooth sides culminating in a point, were constructed in the Fourth, Fifth and Sixth Dynasties (mid–late third millennium BCE), most famously by Khufu (a.k.a. Cheops; c. 2550 BCE), who constructed the Great Pyramid at Giza. Over 100 pyramids were eventually constructed in Egypt.

The Great Pyramid

Originally standing 146.59 m (481 ft) high, the Great Pyramid was the world's tallest building for almost 4,000 years, until the construction of Lincoln Cathedral, in eastern England, in the 14th century. Features such as its exact orientation to the cardinal points of the compass, the precise plane of its original surfaces (now denuded of their smooth facing) and the enduring mystery surrounding its construction have inspired beliefs that its makers had access to mystical wisdom. Theosophists and others, for instance, see the pyramid-builders as part of a chain of transmission of wisdom from Atlantis to the Western mystery tradition.

The Great Pyramid is believed by many to encode natural and mystical laws of nature in its measurements and proportions, and many esoteric properties have been attributed to it. It is claimed, for instance, that the King's Chamber inside the Great Pyramid has the same dimensions as the Holy of Holies in the Temple of Solomon, and that the height of the pyramid is precisely one billionth the distance of the Earth from the Sun (in fact, this calculation is roughly a million miles out). Sceptics dismiss such claims as 'pyramidiocy', and point out that if you compare enough numbers you will find some coincidences that are apparently meaningful.

The riddle of the Sphinx

To the south of the Pyramid of Khafre, in a shallow depression, sits a monumental statue with the head of a human and the body of a lion. Its Western name derives from a mythological creature of the ancient Greeks. Mainstream Egyptology claims that it was carved 4,500 years ago in the likeness of the pharaoh Khafre (2520–2494 BCE), and shaped around a natural limestone outcrop that had been quarried for stone for the Great Pyramid. The body of the Sphinx is 72.55 m (238 ft) long and 20.22 m (66 ft 4 in) tall, while its face is 4 m (13 ft) wide. It is surrounded by a headdress, and originally wore a ritual beard, a fragment of which is now in the British Museum in London.

The mystery surrounding the symbolism of the statue has been dubbed 'the Riddle of the Sphinx', but this risks confusion with the original such riddle, from the Greek tale of Oedipus. Contested dating of parts of the Sphinx has led to suggestions that it was originally carved many thousands of years before Khafre, and is therefore evidence that a prehistoric civilization flourished millennia before the accepted origins of civilization.

The Hall of Records

Mainstream Egyptology recognizes three passages underneath the Sphinx, but according to some, much greater secrets are concealed below. Edgar Cayce, known as 'the sleeping seer' for his trance readings, claimed there was an underground Hall of Records, a kind of 'hard copy' of the Akashic Record (a record of all knowledge and events, imprinted on the psychic ether and accessible by psychics). According to a reading Cayce made in 1933:

> 'A record of Atlantis… of the first destruction, and the changes that took place in the land… of the peoples and their varied activities in other lands, and a record of… the building of the pyramid of initiation… In position, [this record] lies – as the sun rises from the waters – as the line of the shadows… falls between the paws of the Sphinx; that was set later as the sentinel or guard and which may not be entered from the connecting chambers from the Sphinx's right paw until the time has been fulfilled… [it lies] between the Sphinx and the river.' [378–16; 29 October, 1933]

The Book of the Dead

Ancient Egyptians believed that the soul had several aspects, including the *ka* (equivalent to the life force), the *ba* (equivalent to the personality) and the *akh* (which could become a sort of ghost). Happiness in the afterlife depended on these components successfully negotiating the perils of the next world, and to help ensure this a complex system of prayers and magic evolved over the course of a thousand years.

Such spells first appeared inscribed on pyramids in the Fifth and Sixth Dynasties, and are known as Pyramid Texts. These later evolved into spells written on wooden coffins, known as Coffin Texts, and finally, c. 1450 BCE, into collections of spells written on papyri or painted on the walls of tombs, which are collectively known as the Book of the Dead.

Individual books were drawn from a repertoire of over 200 spells, which were intended to provision and protect the deceased. For instance, a copy might include a spell to animate *ushabti*, small figurines that would come to life in the spirit world and perform mandatory but monotonous tasks in place of the dead person's spirit, such as toiling in the Field of Reeds, where agricultural chores would be performed until the end of time.

The Book of the Dead *The group of wall paintings and papyri collectively known as the Egyptian Book of the Dead contains ancient spells and curses. This section has been dated to 1085–945 BCE.*

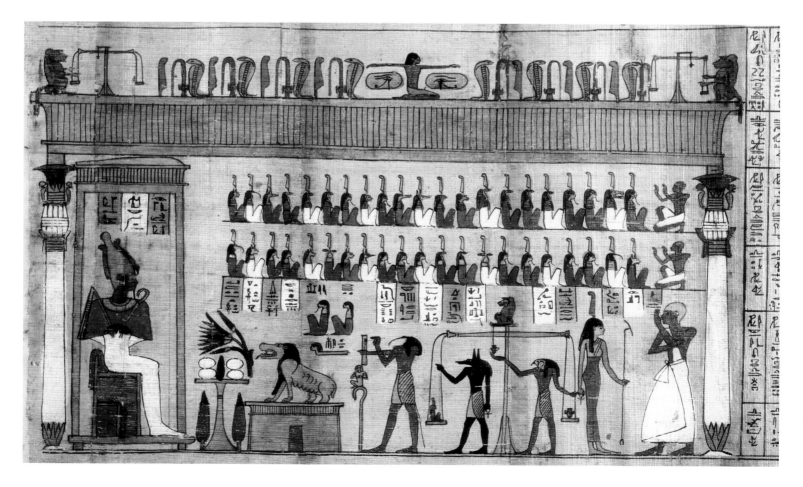

JUDAEO-CHRISTIAN MYSTERIES

The apparently monolithic nature of the major monotheistic religions of the West conceals an incredible diversity of mysticism, folklore and popular superstition. Mysteries that span 4,000 years of history, from the ancient Jewish enigma of the **Ark of the Covenant** and the legendary **Tomb of Jesus** dating back to the dawn of the Christian era, to the medieval mysteries of the **Turin Shroud** and the **Black Madonnas**, bear witness to the complex interplay of biblical dogma, localized cult beliefs and popular faith.

If you are interested in **Judaeo-Christian Mysteries**, you may also like to read about:

- **Judaism**, pages 186–187
- **Christianity**, pages 190–191
- **The Kabbalah**, pages 188–189
- **Western Mystery Traditions**, pages 184–185
- **The Gnostic Gospels**, pages 192–193
- **Knights Templar**, pages 264–265
- **The Holy Grail**, pages 282–283
- **The Goddess**, pages 294–295

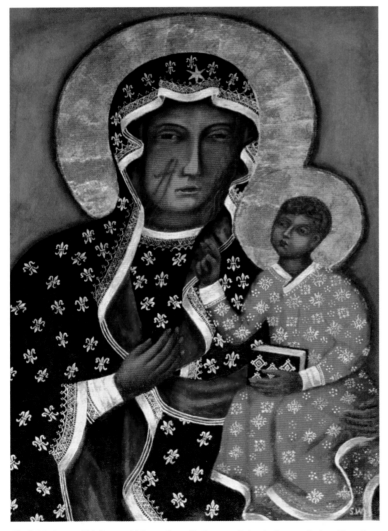

Black Madonna *This icon, which was found in Poznan, Poland, shows a dusky-skinned Madonna holding the baby Jesus.*

The Ark of the Covenant

In the Old Testament the Ark was a chest built to contain the Tablets of Law, inscribed by God with the Ten Commandments. It was made from rich wood and gold, and was probably about the size of a coffee table (1.3 m/4 ft 3 in long and 76 cm/2 ft 6 in wide and deep). It was fitted with golden rings through which poles could be inserted to make it portable, and it had a solid gold cover known as the Mercy Seat, upon which sat two cherubim – winged sphinx-like creatures. When the Israelites camped during their wanderings in the desert, they housed the Ark in an elaborate tent-shrine known as the Tabernacle, which provided the model for the Holy of Holies, the innermost sanctum of the Temple of Solomon in Jerusalem, where the Ark later resided.

Great power was attributed to the Ark. The divine presence, or *Shekinah*, would materialize between the outstretched wings of the cherubim, appearing as a sort of speaking cloud. The Ark could destroy opposing armies or city walls, bring plague and ruin to enemies and kill those who touched it or displeased it in some way, for it sometimes appears to have had a will of its own. One explanation for these powers is that the Ark and Tabernacle together constituted a potent electrical technology – a type of capacitor similar to a Leyden jar, which allowed huge static charges to be generated, stored and discharged.

Mystery surrounds the fate of the Ark. The last biblical reference places it at the First Temple in 623 BCE. Most historians believe it was looted and probably destroyed by the Babylonians in 586 BCE, or by one of the many other conquering armies that passed through Jerusalem. Other traditions about the fate of the Ark include that it was hidden within the Temple Mount or that it was stolen by the legendary Ethiopian king Menelik and still exists in a chapel in the Ethiopian town of Axum.

Black Madonnas

There are many statues and images of the Blessed Virgin Mary around the world that depict her with dark or black skin, and these are known as Black

Madonnas. Many of these images may have been created to reflect prevalent colouration in local communities, but there is a particular tradition in Europe, dating back to the very early medieval era, of intense popular veneration of dark-skinned statues and images that cannot be explained in this way. Famous examples include the Black Madonna of Montserrat (Spain) and the Black Madonna of Czestochowa (Poland).

One explanation is that the images were darkened to illustrate a line from the Song of Songs: 'Negra sum sed Formosa' ('I am black but beautiful'). Another is that the images represent Christianized pagan traditions and Earth and Mother Goddess figures, such as Isis (whose cult was spread across Europe by the Romans and who was often depicted as black). The Christian cults surrounding these images thus reflect very ancient traditions. Worship of Black Madonnas has also been linked to Gnosticism, the Cathars and the Templars, who were known especially to venerate them.

The Tomb of Jesus

According to orthodox Christian dogma, Jesus had no permanent tomb, as his body ascended to heaven after he rose from the dead. But legends of varying antiquity have suggested other fates. Ancient Hindu and medieval Islamic texts tell of a Christ-like figure named Isa or Yuz Asaf who journeyed to India to preach and study, and the influential 19th-century Muslim scholar Ghulam Ahmad popularized the claim that Roza Bal, a tomb and shrine in Srinagar in Kashmir, is the tomb of Jesus.

The bloodline of Christ mythology, popularized by *The Holy Blood and the Holy Grail* by Michael Baigent, Richard Leigh and Henry Lincoln (1982) and Dan Brown's *The Da Vinci Code* (2003), also holds that Jesus survived the Crucifixion but came to the West, founded the Merovingian dynasty and was buried in southern France, possibly near the village of Rennes-le-Château. Such heresies challenge mainstream Christianity and are often connected to Gnosticism and associated groups like the Cathars and Knights Templar, or to Marian/Goddess cults, and thus have spiritual significance beyond their status as archeological/historical curiosities.

The Turin Shroud

A bolt of linen imprinted on both sides with the full-length image of a bearded man is said to be the shroud used as the winding sheet for Jesus when he was taken down from the Cross. It is housed in Turin Cathedral, Italy, but was first attested in the historical record in France in 1353. Circumstantial evidence links it to the Mandylion, a cloth bearing the face of Jesus that supposedly dated back to 1st-century CE Jerusalem and was sacred to the Byzantines.

Interest in the Shroud exploded after it was photographed in 1898 and 1931, revealing a negative image far more impressive than the faint marks visible with the naked eye. The negative seems to show a man with injuries consistent with crucifixion. Sindologists — people who believe the Shroud is authentic — argue that the image is that of Christ, imprinted on the cloth through natural (sweat and blood), paranormal (a burst of radiation emitted at the moment of the Resurrection) or supernatural processes.

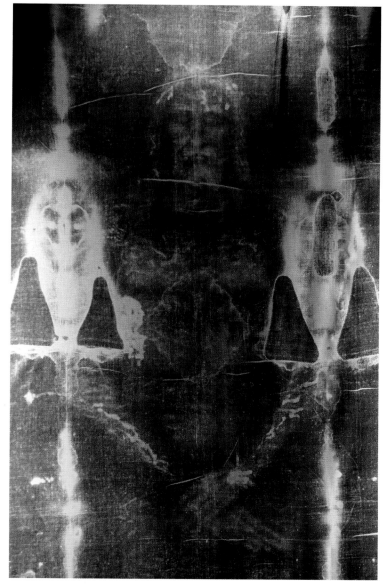

Turin Shroud *This photograph negative of the famous shroud held at Turin Cathedral, Italy shows far more detail than when the cloth is viewed normally.*

Sceptics point to a 1978 research project that dated the Shroud's linen to 1260–1390 CE, appearing to confirm that it was a medieval fake, although how such a sophisticated fake could be produced with medieval technology is a mystery in itself. Writers such as Nicholas Allen, Lynn Picknett and Clive Prince have suggested that it was created with a form of photographic technology, and have linked the Shroud to Leonardo da Vinci and heretical schools of Gnostic Christianity. The quality of the image on the shroud only becomes truly apparent when viewed in photographic negative, which poses substantial questions to those who believe it is a medieval fake. It is suggested that the image of the head (which some claim was produced separately from that of the body and is therefore not in proportion) is an actual photograph of da Vinci. Such theories must contend with evidence that dates the first appearance of the Shroud to before da Vinci was born.

THE HOLY GRAIL

If you are interested in **The Holy Grail**, you may also like to read about :
- Judaeo-Christian Mysteries, pages 280–281
- Knights Templar, pages 264–265
- The Gnostic Gospels, pages 192–193
- The Goddess, pages 294–295

Despite confusion over its true **nature**, the Holy Grail has become the most famous relic in Christianity, thanks to its association with **Arthurian legend** and the latter-day popularity of the **bloodline of Christ** mythology. Academic debate over the **sources of the Grail legend** obscures for many its role as inspirational spiritual allegory.

The nature of the Grail

In modern popular thought, the Holy Grail is the cup that was used to catch blood dripping from Christ's wounds during the Crucifixion. It is often conflated with the Holy Chalice, the cup Jesus used during the Last Supper. Powers attributed to this relic include the ability to heal wounds and grant immortality, produce inexhaustible food and drink and bring fertility and prosperity to the land.

The Grail is not mentioned in the Bible, however. The tradition of the Holy Chalice dates back to the 6th century CE, while the first written source for the Grail is Chrétien de Troyes' *Perceval, le Conte du Graal* (a.k.a. *Perceval, the Story of the Grail*), penned between 1180 and 1191. In its earliest appearances, the Grail is simply a dish or bowl, and the word is thought to derive from the medieval Latin *gradalis* or *gradale*, meaning a dish or platter used to serve delicacies at a feast.

In other accounts, the Grail is a stone that fell from heaven or even an emerald from the crown Lucifer wore before the Fall. A more recent interpretation is that the medieval Latin *San Greal* should actually be parsed as *Sang Real*, or Royal Blood. In this reading, the Holy Grail is Christ's bloodline – a secret lineage of descendants.

Real-life candidates for the Holy Grail can be found around the world. Examples include the Nanteos Cup in Wales, the Chalice of Antioch (in the Metropolitan Museum in New York, USA) and the *Sacro Catino* of Genoa Cathedral, Italy.

The Arthurian connection

The legend of the Grail is inextricably bound up with a cycle of medieval romances concerning the legendary King Arthur and his knights of the Round Table, of which Chrétien de Troyes' *Perceval* is the first. Other important instances are Robert de Boron's *Joseph d'Arimathie*, and Wolfram von Eschenbach's *Parzival*. All these date from the late 12th and early 13th centuries CE. Grail romances divide into Early History and Quest romances, which deal respectively with the origins and early history of the Grail, and the quest to obtain it.

The central narrative of this cycle is that the Grail was brought to Britain by Joseph of Arimathea and bequeathed to a line of royal descendants culminating in the wounded Fisher King, whose lameness blights his land.

Only the perfect knight can recover the Grail, and in doing so heal the Fisher King and restore prosperity to the land.

Perceval is the protagonist of the first Quest romances. As an innocent young knight he stumbles upon the Grail Castle and is vouchsafed a vision of the Grail, but fails to ask the right question. In later romances Perceval is superseded by Galahad, the perfect Christian knight. The illegitimate son of Lancelot, Galahad grows up in monastic fashion and becomes a pious, chaste, pure-hearted knight, who is able to sit upon the Siege Perilous – the magical seat at Arthur's court that is fatal to any but he who will achieve the Grail. Galahad leads the quest to seek the Grail and eventually achieves it, at which point he ascends to heaven.

The quest to achieve the Grail is often read as an allegory of spiritual growth and self-realization; in some versions of the tale, such as Mallory's *Morte d'Arthur*, this interpretation is made explicit. Alchemical and other esoteric readings of the legend are also possible – for instance, achieving the Grail becomes synonymous with creating the Philosopher's Stone; both feats require the alchemist/questing knight to undergo a process of spiritual transformation and purification.

Sources of the Grail legend

The Grail romances derive from oral folk traditions, and display many motifs and characters familiar from folklore, especially Celtic folklore, which features cauldrons of regeneration and plenty, and characters analogous to figures such as Arthur and Merlin. In the 19th century it was fashionable to emphasize these Celtic sources and view the Grail legend as a Christian gloss on pagan folk traditions, but more recent scholarship has focused on Christian inspirations for the tale, in particular attempts by the medieval Church to popularize the sacrament of Holy Communion.

The bloodline of Christ

The book *The Holy Blood and the Holy Grail* by Michael Baigent, Richard Leigh and Henry Lincoln (1982) was the primary inspiration for the popular belief that the Holy Grail is actually a metaphor for the bloodline of Jesus. It has spawned a mythology surrounding Jesus's supposed survival of the Crucifixion. In this narrative Mary Magdalene bore Jesus's child and the holy family came to live in the south of France or Britain, where their descendants

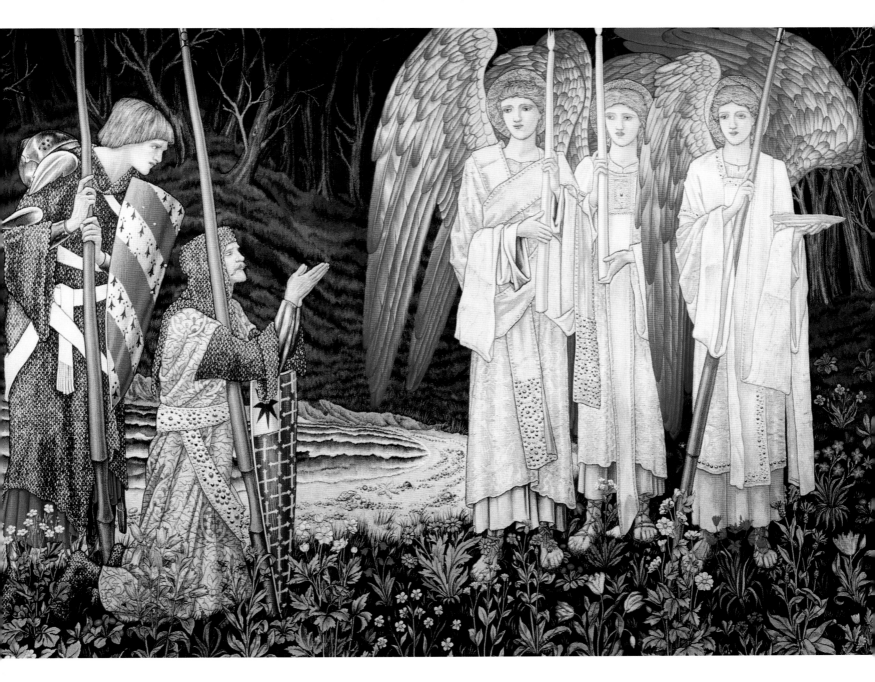

went on to found royal dynasties and embody a more personal, Gnostic brand of Christianity than that offered by the established Church. Its authority threatened, the Church and affiliated secular powers engaged in a long battle to suppress the truth.

In this reading the Holy Grail becomes an allegory for a secret tradition of spirituality that embraces direct personal access to the divine and takes in Gnosticism and pre-Christian mysticism, including Goddess worship and fertility cults. The Grail legend lies at the nexus of a host of related mysteries, including the Cathars, the Knights Templar, Black Madonnas and the Freemasons, and sacred sites such as Rennes-le-Château in southern France, Rosslyn Chapel near Edinburgh, Scotland, and Glastonbury Tor in Somerset, England (all purported, at one time or another, to be the home of the Grail).

The Holy Grail *This detail from a tapestry produced in the 1890s by Morris and Co. after a design by Edward Burne-Jones depicts the knights attaining the Holy Grail. It is part of a series based on Sir Thomas Malory's* Le Morte d'Arthur.

It is suggested, for instance, that the Holy Grail — either as an object or a secret (that is, knowledge or custody of descendants of Jesus) constituted the hidden treasure of the Cathars, the Knights Templar and the Freemasons, and that possession of this treasure lay behind the wealth and power of these sects and the animosity of the established Church towards them. Knowledge of the Grail is also said to have encouraged these sects to develop their unorthodox, heretical interpretations of Christianity. Clues to these mysteries are held to be incorporated into the structures and landscapes of Rennes, Rosslyn Chapel and Glastonbury.

PROPHECY AND NOSTRADAMUS

If you are interested in **Prophecy and Nostradamus**, you may also like to read about:
● **Western Astrology**, pages 56–57
● **Other Forms of Divination**, pages 72–73
● **Herbalism**, pages 152–153

The fame of Nostradamus and the alleged accuracy of his many **prophecies** form a sharp contrast to the controversy that has always surrounded him. Heated debate still rages about the success of his **quatrains**, and whether they were truly predictive or can only be validated with the benefit of hindsight and some inventive interpretation.

The prophecies

Michel de Nostredame was born in southern France in 1503. He worked as an apothecary and was celebrated for inventing a 'rose pill' that was considered to be effective against the plague. In 1550 he wrote an almanac under the name of Nostradamus, and its success encouraged him to write at least one almanac for each successive year. These almanacs are thought to contain over 6,000 prophecies. They were supplemented in 1555 by his famous *Les Propheties*, a collection of rhymed quatrains (four-line predictive poems) arranged in sections of 100 quatrains each, known as centuries. Allegedly in order to protect himself from religious persecution, but also to follow the fashion of the time, Nostradamus wrote the quatrains in a mixture of languages, with the further complication of obscure word games. This made them difficult to understand at the time, and unfortunately that is still the case. The quatrains are open to many interpretations, which means that their level of accuracy has been hotly disputed since their first publication. The manner in which Nostradamus made his predictions is also disputed. There are claims that he did so in a state of trance, based on a letter in which he wrote of seeing visions in a bowl of water set on a brass tripod, lit by a candle. However, some authorities claim this letter was mistranslated and that Nostradamus wrote it was 'as though' he did these things.

The quatrains

Detailed analysis of the quatrains has shown that many of them are based on apocalyptic predictions from the Bible as well as Latin historians such as Plutarch, so they describe events from the past in order to predict the future. The quatrains dwell on all manner of disasters, natural and man-made, as well as the arrival of the Antichrist, and were written at a time when many people feared the imminent end of the world.

The accuracy or otherwise of Nostradamus's quatrains is hard to quantify, since many of them have been poorly translated from the Old French in which they were written. Some of the translations have even been deliberately worded to fit the details of known world events. Another difficulty is that the descriptions of people, such as 'Heaven's great ruler', 'another Hannibal' or 'three great brothers' (sometimes believed to describe John, Robert and Edward Kennedy), are open to all sorts of interpretations, especially when applied in retrospect to disasters.

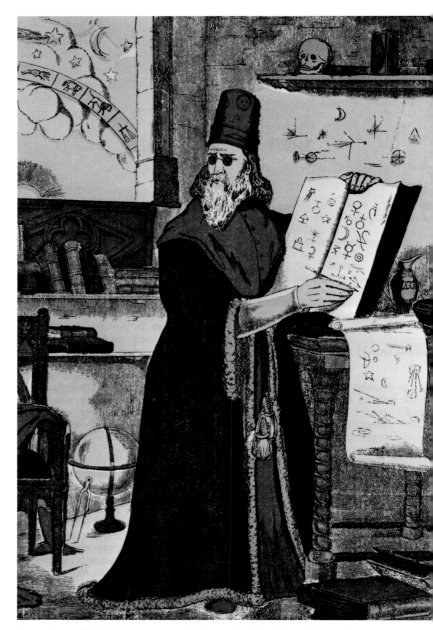

Nostradamus *This 19th-century engraving by Jean C. Pellerin depicts the astrologer Nostradamus. He was asked to draw up horoscopes for the children of Henry II of France.*

MAYAN PROPHECY

If you are interested in **Mayan Prophecy**, you may also like to read about:
- **Native American Spirituality**, pages 232–233
- **Landscape Lines**, pages 258–259

Mayan prophecy is based on the very complex calendar developed by the **Mayan civilization**. They believed that the end of one cycle within the **Great Year** and the start of the next heralds a time of outstanding evolution in the human psyche. It is thought that the next **cycle**, which begins in 2012, will take humans to a new world age.

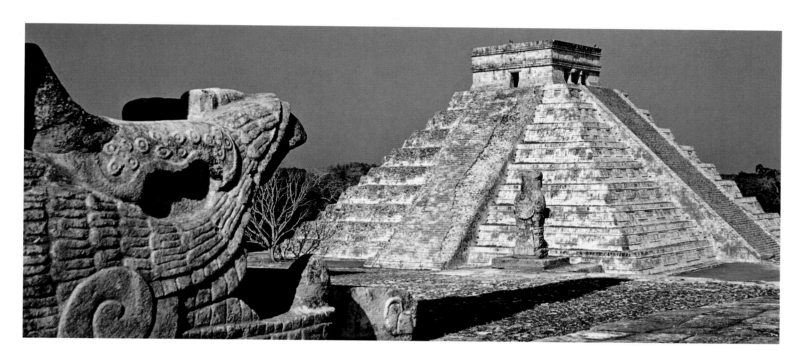

Kukulcan temple *At the equinoxes, the sun casts shadows that look like a serpent over the Kukulcan temple at Chichen Itza, Mexico.*

The Mayan civilization

The Mayans were a highly advanced Mesoamerican civilization, living in what is now Mexico and northern Central America between c. 1800 BCE and the 9th century CE. They created their own written language, which is believed to be the only one in the pre-Columbian Americas. One of their most astonishing feats was to build many stone monuments and pyramids that were aligned to record various astronomical events, including the Sun's solstices and equinoxes.

The Great Year

The Mayans, in common with many other ancient civilizations (including the Egyptians, Tibetans and Hopi), knew of the astronomical Great Year, which runs for approximately 26,000 years and is composed of 12 individual ages, each of which lasts for just over 2,100 years. This cycle always moves backwards. In Western astrological terms, at the present time we are emerging from the Age of Pisces and moving into the Age of Aquarius. The ancient Mayans were accomplished astronomers and recognized that the 26,000-year cycle corresponds with the Sun's orbit around Alcyone, the brightest star in the Pleiades constellation.

The cycles and the prophecies

The Mayans divided the Great Year into five lesser Creation Cycles. They calculated that the current Creation Cycle, which they called the Age of the Fifth Sun, began on 13 August, 3113 BCE and ends on 21 December, 2012 CE. This end date is believed to mark a major turning point in human evolution.

The Creation Cycles are divided into smaller cycles, known as the '13 baktun count' or 'long count'. The current baktun cycle began in 1618, and the Mayans predicted that it would be a period in which humans would become distanced from nature, with an over-emphasis on power. These imbalances, they said, will be corrected with the start of the new Creation Cycle, which in their view would constitute a collective rebirth for mankind.

MYTHICAL CREATURES

World mythology features many creatures that allegedly possess magical powers.

Such creatures may reflect ancient animistic traditions (see pages 230–231) in which all

living things are believed to be imbued with a spirit. Two in particular have captured the

imagination of millions of people around the world – the **unicorn** and the **dragon**.

If you are interested in **Mythical Creatures**, you may also like to read about:
- **Native American Spirituality**, pages 232–233
- **Channelling**, pages 42–43
- **Wicca**, pages 240–241
- **Landscape Lines**, pages 258–259

The unicorn

This creature is usually depicted with the body of a horse, but with a single, usually spiral, horn growing out of its forehead. Perhaps the earliest mention of the unicorn is by the ancient Greek writer and historian Herodotus, who in the 5th century BCE wrote of the 'horned ass' of Africa. Another mention from that period came in the writings of the Greek historian and physician

The unicorn This 15th-century tapestry, called The Lady and the Unicorn, *displays the traditional image of a unicorn being captured by a maiden.*

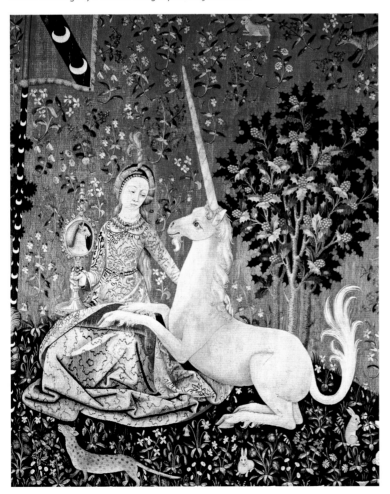

Ctesias, who visited Persia and brought back fantastic travellers' tales. He described the unicorn as fleet of foot with a body like an ass. Drinking cups fashioned from its horn could, it was claimed, prevent poisoning.

In late antiquity the unique symbolism of the unicorn was recorded in the *Physiologus*, one of the earliest forms of bestiary. Unicorns, it was said, could be captured only by a maiden. Upon seeing a maiden the unicorn was believed to lay its head in her lap and fall asleep, an image considered to represent Christ's incarnation. Unicorns are also found in Eastern traditions. The Chinese unicorn is called Ch'i lin and is considered a creature of great power and wisdom. Its appearance is a sign of good fortune and signals the birth of a great leader. Ch'i lin was said to appear before the mother of the great Chinese sage Confucius. Japanese unicorns are called Kirin or Sin-you. The Kirin is gentle and solitary, while the Sin-you is powerful and fierce and noted for its ability to distinguish right from wrong.

The dragon

This is another fascinating creature found throughout world mythology. Essentially, a dragon is a great snake and dragons are part of the widespread mythology associated with serpents. Creation myths from many ancient cultures feature a cosmic serpent that could have a range of roles, including symbolizing the first manifestation of spirit; a monster to be overcome before order can be achieved in the world; a fertility god; or the guardian of the underworld.

It is interesting that despite these ancient links between world cultures, the dragon took on very different guises in Eastern and Western mythologies.

Dragons of the West

In the West dragons are generally a negative force, evil and earthbound, cave-dwelling, fire-breathing and destructive. The serpent of the Garden of Eden represents one of the earliest references to dragons. Some writers have argued that the curse laid on the serpent in the Old Testament reflects an attempt to discredit serpent cults, which were seen as a threat to the emerging Jewish faith.

One of the most famous Western legends associated with the dragon is the story of St George, who was said to have encountered a dragon at a town in Libya. The dragon dwelt in a great lake, poisoned the air with his foul

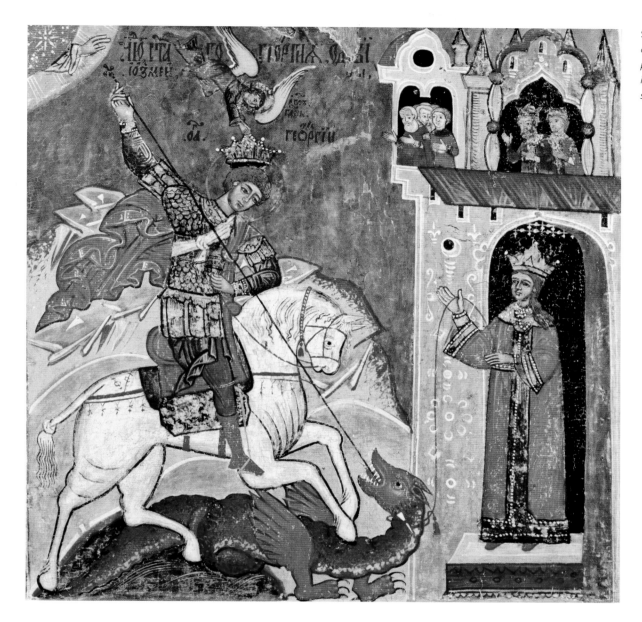

St George and the Dragon *This detail from a late 16th-century painting from the Ukraine illustrates the legend of St George slaying the dragon.*

breath and demanded sacrifices, including the king's own daughter. At this point St George arrived and pinned the advancing dragon with his lance, either killing it or leading it back to the city bound with the princess's girdle, according to different versions. St George persuaded the people that his strength had come from Christ and the entire city converted to Christianity. This myth is often interpreted as the dragon, symbolizing pagan belief, being overcome by Christianity. Despite its fearsome nature, it was believed that a dragon could be defeated by the power of the Cross, and an encounter with a dragon was an opportunity to prove the strength of one's faith.

Dragons of the East

By contrast, in the East dragons are almost always benevolent. In ancient China the dragon was regarded as a most sacred animal, and was the emblem of Chinese emperors. It is the first of the four Chinese Divine Creatures along with the unicorn, the phoenix and the tortoise. Unlike the evil, fire-breathing dragons of the West, the Chinese dragon is a beneficent and gracious creature and is worshipped as the divine ruler of lakes, rivers and seas. It is a powerful, yet gentle creature that brings rain to the earth, encourages crops and cools the toiling farmer.

Today the dragon is still thought to bring good fortune and abundance, and remains one of the most popular of Chinese art motifs, being sculptured on stone pillars of temples and embroidered on gold and silk tapestries. Those born in the year of the dragon are to be honoured and respected because these people are said to take on their characteristics of wisdom, long life, wealth and luck. Images and symbols of the dragon, in and around the home or work place, are said to bring prosperity and good fortune.

Interestingly, in both England and China dragons are often used to describe the energies that run in the earth. These are sometimes called ley lines or dragon lines and are akin to the Aboriginal songlines (see page 229) – recitations of spirit routes through the landscape.

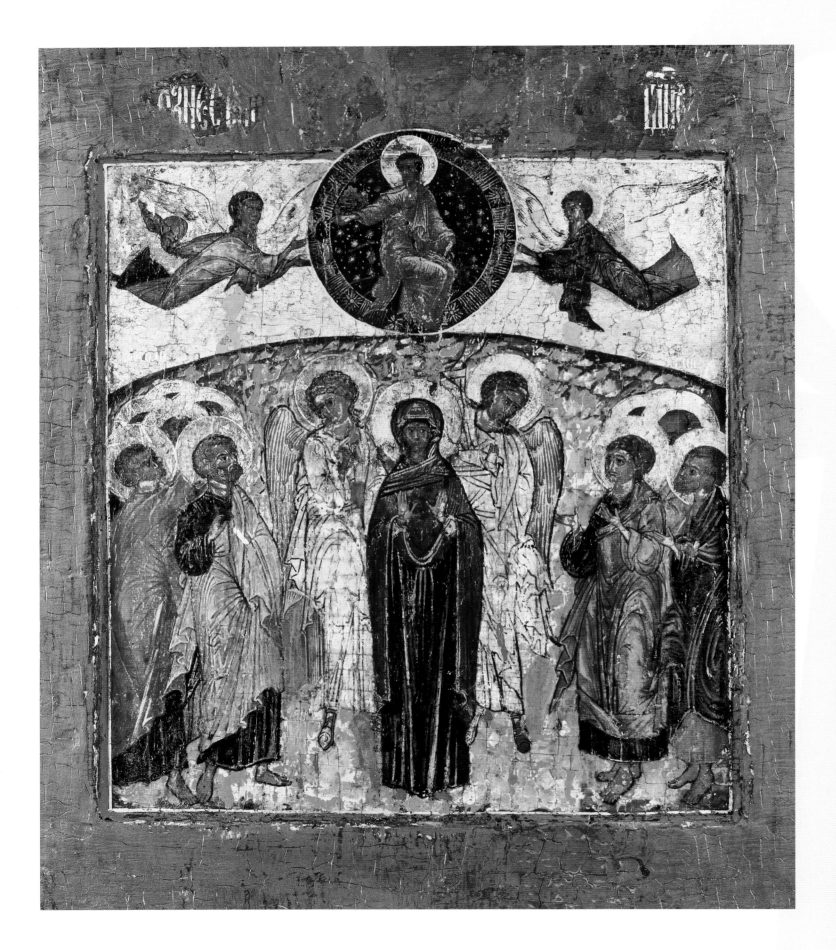

PATHS TO OTHER REALMS

Awareness of a higher plane of existence beyond the material world has been recognized by every culture and in every age. The greatest artists, writers and mystics of each country have attempted to convey the concept of the spiritual dimension throughout history. But how are we to make contact with this spiritual plane? World religions have provided organized structures for the expression of spiritual yearning, but there are other, more personal paths to the divine. These might include belief in the assistance offered by spirit entities such as angels and fairies, the practice of rituals like pilgrimage and retreats or the guidance of spiritual leaders. This section explores these alternative roads to greater awareness.

Blake's exploration of the spiritual world

The experiences of artists and mystics have inspired many in the quest for a more direct experience of the mystical and otherworldly. Perhaps one of the most famous visionaries was the 19th-century English poet William Blake (1757–1827), whose poetry, art and personal letters record his special awareness of the spirit world. Blake claimed to have experienced visions from an early age; at the age of eight he reported having seen 'a tree filled with angels, bright angelic wings bespangling every bough like stars', and he believed archangels directly inspired much of his creative work. Blake rejected the conventional views of religion; instead he believed in the innate spirituality of all humanity. In his book *The Marriage of Heaven and Hell*, produced in the 1790s, Blake wrote: 'men forgot that All deities reside in the human breast'. His life was a testament to his personal quest to communicate his understanding of the world of spirit – through his art, letters and creative writing. Today Blake's faith in the insights provided by angels is shared by hundreds of thousands of people around the world who are finding their own deep sense of connection to angels. Seeking angelic guidance and inspiration is currently one of the most popular paths to spiritual awareness and growth.

Ascension of Christ *This late 17th-century Russian icon shows the Christian representation of the ascension of Jesus Christ to heaven.*

The power of spiritual guidance

Peruvian-born American Carlos Castaneda (1925–1998) was one of many writers to describe the profound influence of a personal guide or guru in their spiritual development. Castaneda described in a series of books the teachings of a shaman, Don Juan Matus, a Yaqui Indian. Castaneda claimed that Don Juan guided him through a series of transforming experiences, including visionary meetings with gods and taking on the spirit body of a crow. Although the reliability of Castaneda's experiences has been questioned, his writing reveals a profound personal awakening that has inspired millions of people around the world.

The role of retreat and pilgrimage

For many it is retreat from the everyday, busy world that brings about deeper levels of awareness. Isolation and retreat have been important breakthrough experiences in virtually every major religion and faith throughout the centuries. Pilgrimage has also been recognized as an important transformative path, not just as a means of connecting with holy and sacred places, but in order to experience the trials and revelations provided by the journey. While the Muslim pilgrimage to Mecca, the Hajj, is perhaps the best-known pilgrimage practised today, other routes have been rediscovered, such as the Christian pilgrimage to Santiago de Compostela in Spain, one most famously described by American actress and writer Shirley MacLaine.

A universal goal

Whatever form our path to spiritual awareness may take, the goal remains the same: a sense of connection with the ultimate reality of all things. The nature of this reality is perhaps best conveyed by the Eastern concept termed Brahman by Hindus and the Tao by Taoists. Brahman is an all-pervasive, powerful energy described in the sacred texts, the Upanishads, as follows:

> *'Tranquil, let one worship it*
> *As that from which he came forth,*
> *As that into which he will be dissolved,*
> *As that in which he breathes.'*

ANGELS

Most familiar to us today as winged spiritual beings of grace and protection, the historical **origin of angels** is complex. The concept of deathless **beings of light** and pure love, not limited by the boundaries of time and space, is common to a number of different cultures and traditions from around the world. The word 'angel' is derived from the Greek *angelos*, meaning messenger, and the name refers to their most important function, which is to act as an intermediary between earth and heaven, delivering messages or **intervening during times of crisis**, according to the divine will.

If you are interested in **Angels**, you may also like to read about:
- **Judaism**, pages 186–187
- **Christianity**, pages 190–191
- **Islam**, pages 196–197
- **Channelling**, pages 42–43

The origin of angels

Angels have fascinated humans for centuries, but their origins in history is complicated due to the fact that they, or similar spirit beings, can be found within many cultures and religions around the globe. The Western concept of angels has been shaped by the Hebrew and Christian scriptures, which include archangels such as Michael the warrior angel, who leads his legions of light against the forces of evil, and the cherubim and seraphim or highest order of angels. Angels are also recorded in the Koran, where it is written: 'You shall see the angels circling around the throne, giving glory to their Lord.'

Angels, or divine helpers, are found within ancient Sumerian, Babylonian, Persian, Egyptian and Greek writings. An ancient Sumerian stone column depicts a winged being pouring the water of life into the king's cup, while in Egyptian mythology the goddess Isis uses her wings to breathe life into her dead husband and brother Osiris. In addition, spirit beings similar to angels can be found in all the world's religions, mythologies and folk lore. From the shamanic cultures of isolated tribes through to the great world religions of Islam, Buddhism, Hinduism and Islam, these multidimensional beings play a key role in protecting and supporting the healthy development of all people. Their roles include guardian angels, spirits of the home, healing angels, muses and many more.

Beings of light

Angels are commonly described as 'beings of light' and sometimes 'fearful to behold' due to their tall stature, purity and sheer power. They are considered to exist in the spirit realm, but have the ability to assume human form and are often described as beautiful, graceful beings with wings and a halo. It is generally considered by New Age writers and thinkers that the angelic mission is to remind us of the good we carry within us, the good that we truly are.

Artists typically depict angels as having wings and often halos, although it is probable that these images originated through ancient religions and mythology as a symbolic way to convey the idea of angels crossing forth from the spirit world to Earth and then back again. For example, many ancient gods were depicted as birds or as having wings. In the Bible angels appear to be men and are described as such. The name given to the archangel Gabriel means 'Man of God'.

Prior to the Enlightenment that took place in the late 17th and 18th centuries angels were believed to play a magical role in spiritual life. Writers and mystics such as the Italian St Thomas Aquinas (1225–1274) and the poet Dante (1265–1321) described angelic visions and inspiration. However, after the scientific revolution interest in the role of angels declined, with some notable exceptions, including the famed Swedish mystic Emanuel Swedenborg (1688–1772). He called the spirits of dead humans 'angels' and claimed to visit them often in the spirit world through trance states. The English poet William Blake (1757–1827) was one of the most famous writers to describe angelic visions and the inspirational and guiding role angels played in both his writing and his art.

But what exactly are these beings of light? Some traditions, including the New Age movement, suggest that angels are beings of energy that exist in the spirit realm and can only be encountered when we tune into them during prayer or ritual. Other traditions hold that each person has a guardian angel watching over them and that this angel will respond when help is requested, while some believe contact should only be initiated from the angelic side.

Intervention in times of crisis

Today angels have gained renewed popularity due in part to a widespread hunger for spiritual reassurance and guidance. More and more people are looking to angels for assistance or even intervention, not only during times of crisis, but also in times of safety and stability. Typical descriptions of angels can be found in numerous stories of supportive, yet mysterious strangers who come to a person during a time of need, providing help of some kind, and

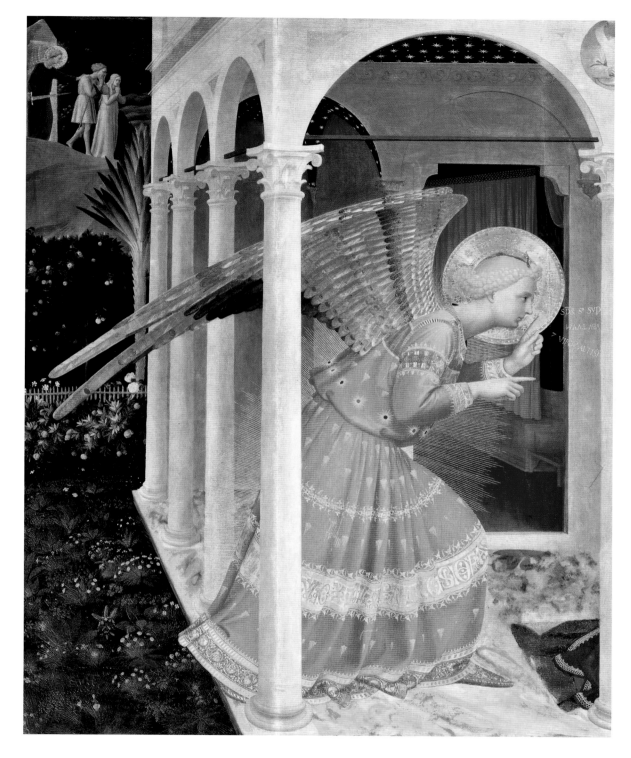

Angel Gabriel *Gabriel is perhaps the best-known angel of the Christian tradition. This detail from* The Annunciation *by Fra Angelico (1395–1445) shows a traditional winged and haloed Angel Gabriel.*

then disappear in an unexplained way. Similarly, stories of spirits who come to comfort and lead dying people through the transition from this world are often described as angels, but are sometimes discovered to be deceased family members or friends of the person about to pass. One famous angel sighting occurred during the First World War when the so-called Angels of Mons were thought to have saved retreating French and British soldiers from the Germans in the battle of Mons, Belgium, in 1914.

There are elaborate rituals for calling upon the presence of angels, but most people consider there to be no special words or mystic phrases that must be learned; rather, a simple and sincere focusing of heart and mind may be all that is necessary. Those who believe in angels record that when they ask for angelic help, paths open to them that they could not see before. The voice of their intuition begins to speak more clearly, angelic calling cards such as white feathers mysteriously appear and dreams become more meaningful.

FAIRIES

Fairies are elusive, magical and ethereal beings associated with the elements of nature: earth, water, fire and air. Although common to many cultures, the term 'fairy' is particularly associated with **northern European traditions**. Fairies are said to be immortal earth spirits with magical powers who occupy a limbo **land** between Earth and the world of spirit.

If you are interested in **Fairies**, you may also like to read about:

- Hinduism, pages 204–205
- Shinto, pages 236–237
- Angels, pages 290–291
- Mythical Creatures, pages 286–287
- Native American Spirituality, pages 232–233

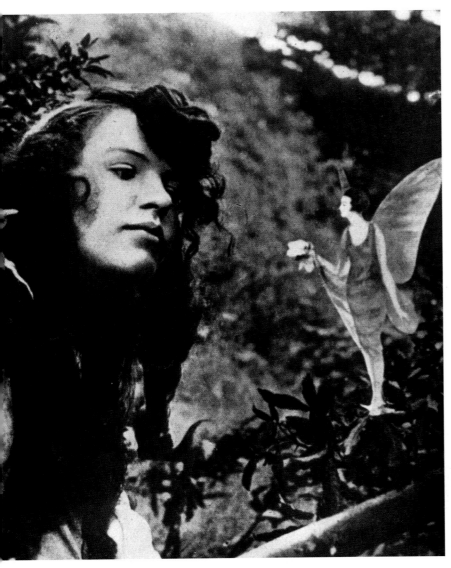

The Cottingley fairies *Elsie Wright with fairies, photographed by Frances Griffiths at Cottingley Glen, West Yorkshire, England, August, 1917. Although now admitted as a hoax, the Cottingley photographs were a sensation in the interwar period in Britain.*

Nature spirits

These are beings thought to be specifically associated with the natural world, and because nature is composed of the basic elements – earth, water, fire and air – they are said to be from the 'elemental realm'. Virtually every culture features ancient traditions of spirits associated with the natural world. The Hindu tradition incorporates such elemental deities as Varuna, who presides over the sky and rain, and Rudra, who presides over the wind and storms, while the Shinto tradition of Japan recognizes *Kami* or spirits of place. In the West nature spirits are most often referred to as fairies, but they can have many other names, including brownies, devas, dryads, elves, gnomes, leprechauns, nymphs, pixies and sprites.

Northern European traditions

The popular concept of fairies as tiny winged creatures with magical powers is mainly associated with northern European cultures, especially the Celtic folklore of Ireland, Wales, Brittany and Cornwall. In Ireland they are known as *Tuatha de Danaan*, or people of the goddess Danu, a divine race that once ruled Ireland. The Tuatha were thought to be strong and beautiful as well as skilled in magic, and pre-Celtic mythology is rich with accounts of their heroic and magical deeds.

There are numerous ideas about how fairies originated. One is that they are descendants of the children of Eve; another is that they are fallen angels, not sufficiently evil to be dismissed from heaven, but not sufficiently good to remain in heaven. A third idea is that stories about fairies arose to explain misfortunes and disasters, while another suggests that they are spirits of the restless dead, and yet another that they are simply small human beings.

Regardless of the origins of fairies, interacting with them is never considered to be straightforward. They can be helpful to people, especially those who respect animals and nature, but numerous superstitions also suggest a darker side. For example, it is said that fairies can snatch babies, or curse a person to ill health or a household to poverty. In order to stay in favour with the fairies, some folk tales suggest that humans should leave out food, drink and gifts for the fairies. In return the fairies will bestow wealth and health on a family.

Fairy life and land

Fairies come in all shapes and sizes, but in the traditional Western view they are tiny and resemble humans with wings. It is said that they are only visible to those with clairvoyant sight, but if they wish they can make themselves visible to anyone. Some are said to be fearsome creatures with awesome powers, while others such as leprechauns and brownies are more friendly and lovable by nature. Whatever their appearance, fairies are thought to have a great affinity with nature. They are said to live in the Land of Fairy or Elf Land, which is believed to exist in a timeless underground world. At night they step out from Elf Land to dance, sing, travel and have fun or make mischief.

Some traditions claim that certain types of fairies belong to a fairy clan or kingdom, while others are individual, exalted beings very close to the angelic kingdom. The fairy clan honours a fairy queen who serves as their spokesperson. Other traditions emphasize the immortality of fairies, and in consequence they are reputed to have a different perception of time than humans. One folk tale, for example, tells of a young Welshman who entered a fairy ring to dance with the nature sprites. He was instantly transported to the world of the fairies and spent many happy years there. However, upon his return to the world of mortals he found only a few minutes of earthly time had elapsed, suggesting that fairies live in a different time dimension.

The disappearance of fairies

From the 18th century onwards folklore has recorded the departure of fairies from our world. Explanations for this disappearance include the decline in human belief in fairies, pollution, urbanization and technological advances. Despite this, belief in fairies still lingers and reports of sightings still occur.

Today many people believe that fairies and other elementals are making themselves known through visions and natural signs in order to urge us to treat the natural world more kindly. Most recently, the emergence of what has been termed eco spirituality has led to a new recognition of the importance of honouring the spirits of place as a metaphor for respecting and honouring nature.

Fairies at a Window *This 1860s watercolour and gouache painting by John Anster Fitzgerald (1832–1906) is an example of the perceived nature and look of fairies; ethereal, feminine and winged.*

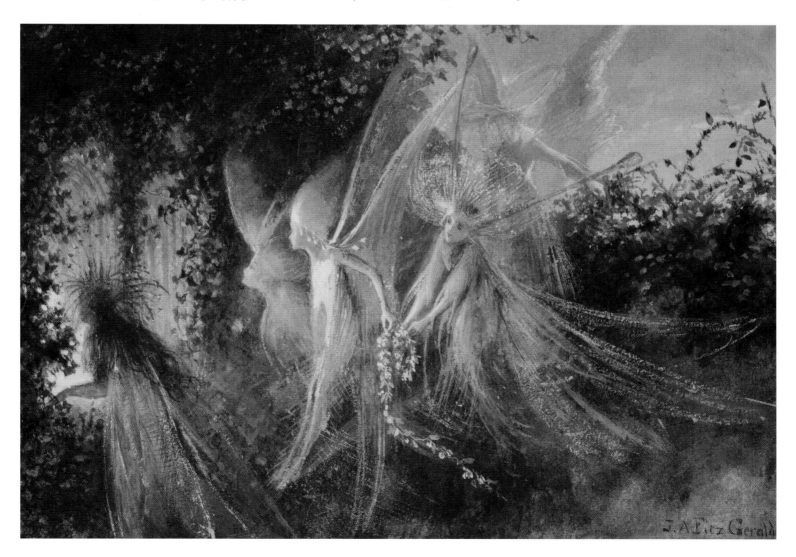

THE GODDESS

A universal symbol of fertility and the divine feminine, **the cult of goddess worship** dates back some 30,000 years. Throughout the centuries the goddess has assumed **many thousand faces** and names, but she has most often represented Mother Nature. In recent years the symbol of the goddess has been recognized as a powerful embodiment of female archetypes that can inspire and enlighten both women and men.

If you are interested in **The Goddess**, you may also like to read about:

- **The Collective Unconscious**, pages 20–21
- **Green Spirituality**, pages 260–261
- **Sacred Land**, pages 246–247
- **Hinduism**, pages 204–205
- **Christianity**, pages 190–191
- **Paganism**, pages 238–239
- **Wicca**, pages 240–241

The cult of goddess worship

Opinion is divided, but some experts believe that worship of the goddess or divine feminine force is as old as the Stone Age and may actually predate worship of masculine deities. The importance of fertility for crops, domesticated animals, wild animals and for the tribe itself was of paramount

Venus of Willendorf *One of the better-known examples of a possible prehistoric 'goddess statue'. Measuring 11.5 cm (4½ in) tall and carved from limestone, its origin and original purpose are still widely debated.*

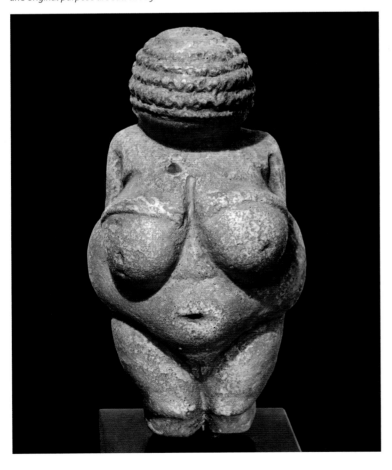

significance to the survival of our primitive ancestors, so it is no surprise that the female life-giving principle may have been considered divine. Some goddess statues such as the Venus of Willendorf (c. 24,000–22,000 BCE) survive from this era.

Many academics believe that the suppression of goddess worship in Western Europe occurred around 3000 BCE, when the Indo-Europeans invaded Europe from the east. They brought with them some of the elements of modern civilization: the horse, war, belief in male gods, exploitation of nature and knowledge of the male role in procreation. Goddess worship was gradually combined with worship of male gods to produce a variety of pagan polytheistic religions among the ancient Greeks, Romans and Celts.

Even though the rise of male-centred religions from about 4000 BCE led to a subordination of the goddess cult, her influence lingered and remains an important part of many belief systems in the world today, in particular Hinduism, the cult of the Virgin Mary in Christianity, Paganism and Wicca, where the goddess is given primacy.

The rediscovery of female divinity in the West was in part triggered by archeological finds in the 1960s and 1970s of the so-called Venus figurines – carvings of females with exaggerated belly and breasts – which appeared to be votive objects. These and other research findings suggested that in the distant past matriarchal societies that honoured the feminine had dominated Europe. Such discoveries coincided with the emergence of feminism and encouraged women to celebrate feminine principles embodied in goddesses from various traditions around the world. Jungian psychologists such as Jean Shinoda Bolen have explored the feminine archetypes embodied in Greek goddesses such as Artemis, the huntress, considered to personify independence, and Demeter, the maternal archetype. In this approach women are encouraged to examine the archetypes they may identify with most strongly and to question the positive as well as negative aspects of each archetype.

Many thousand faces

The goddess appears universally as the symbol for fertility and she is also the ruler of truth, wisdom, nature, the earth, the home, justice, healing, love, birth, death and those aspects of life that cannot be explained by logic or science,

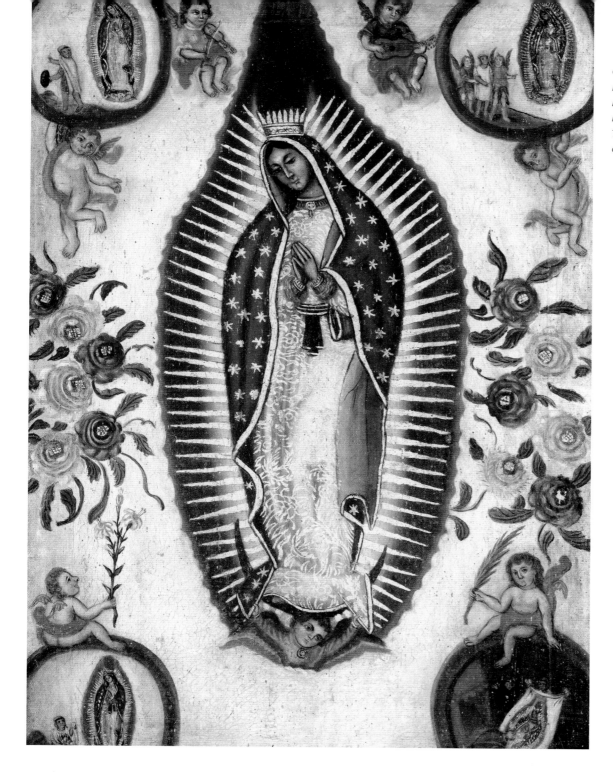

namely emotion, intuition and psychic power. She has numerous different facets to her nature and is often described by writers and academics as having many thousand faces.

In many neo-pagan traditions the goddess has three forms – Maiden, Mother and Crone – corresponding to the story of a woman's life cycle and the waxing, full and waning phases of the Moon. The Maiden represents youth, emerging sexuality and the huntress running with her hounds. The Mother symbolizes feminine power, fertility and nurturing. The Crone is wisdom, the compassion that comes from experience and the one who guides us through the death experience. As Mother Nature, the Moon, Creator, Destroyer, the Queen of the Heavens and the primary source of magic and inner power, the goddess embodies, for all those who believe in her, the very essence of modern witchcraft.

Modern witchcraft

In recent years a renaissance of goddess worship occurred with the re-emergence of Wicca, a neo-pagan Celtic religion of nature and goddess worship popularized in 1954 by Gerald Gardner (1884–1964).

ALCHEMY

If you are interested in **Alchemy**, you may also like to read about:

- **Uncovering the Unconscious,** pages 18–19
- **Mystical and Transcendent States,** pages 34–35
- **Western Astrology,** pages 56–57
- **Numerology,** pages 66–67

Commonly accepted to refer to attempts to change **base metal into gold**, the term **alchemy** also describes the art of converting that which is base in a spiritual sense into something that aspires to perfection. Carl Jung's work in psychology prompted a revival of interest in the spiritual dimension of alchemy and **the quest for spiritual perfection**.

Base metal into gold

The term alchemy, in its widest spiritual as well as material sense, covers a vast range of topics, from the discovery of a single cure for all diseases to the quest for immortality; from the creation of artificial life and straightforward descriptions of scientific techniques to the search for spiritual enlightenment through a variety of mystic techniques, such as astrology and numerology.

From a spiritual perspective, alchemy is the mystical art of human spiritual transformation into a higher or more evolved being. The spiritual teachings of alchemy are based on the age-old idea that humans have a spirit or soul as well as a physical body. Centuries ago alchemists believed that if a way was found to compress or concentrate the spirit, the secret of changing one aspect of nature into another could be discovered. The elusive catalyst that allowed this change to take place became known over time as the philosopher's stone.

The philosopher's stone was a legendary substance, not actually a stone, but a powder or liquid that could turn base metal into gold and, if swallowed, give everlasting life. For a long time it was the most sought-after goal in Western alchemy. In the view of spiritual alchemy, making the philosopher's stone was also thought to bring enlightenment upon the maker. Harry Potter aside, in recent years the philosopher's stone has been the subject, inspiration or plot feature of innumerable artistic works, novels, comics, films, animations and even musical compositions. It is also a popular item in many video games.

Alchemy through the ages

Alchemy probably first emerged in ancient Egypt, where the methods of transmuting base metals into gold were kept secret by temple priests, and also in China, where the gold thus produced was thought to have the ability to cure disease and prolong life. Western alchemy can be traced back to the work of those ancient Egyptian priests, but it also has its basis in Eastern mysticism and the Aristotelian theory of the composition of matter. The Greek philosopher Aristotle (384–322 BCE) taught that all matter was composed of four elements: earth, water, fire and air. Different materials found in nature contained different ratios of these four elements, and so by proper treatment a base metal could be turned to gold.

In the 8th and 9th centuries, Chinese, Greek and Alexandrian alchemical lore entered the Arab world, where alchemists postulated that all metals were

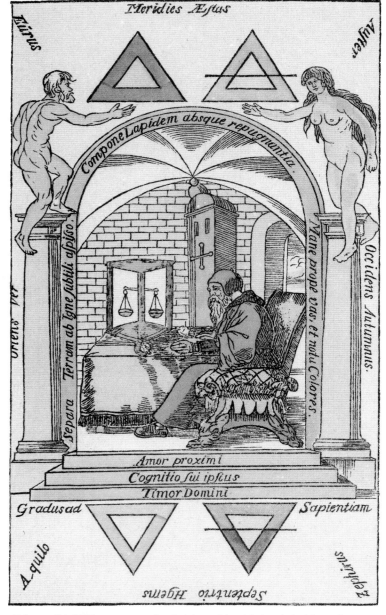

Alchemy *This 1785 copper engraving depicts an alchemist at work studying and weighing materials on a set of scales.*

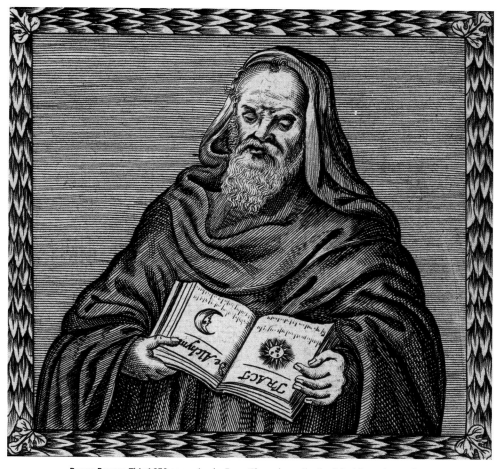

Roger Bacon *This 1650 engraving by Franz Cleyn shows the English philosopher and scholar Roger Bacon reading from a book of astrology.*

composed not of four elements, but of two: sulphur and mercury. They also adopted the Chinese alchemists' concept of a philosopher's stone – a medicine that could turn a sick (base) metal into gold and act as the El or elixir of life – and so began a never-ending quest for this elusive catalyst. Indirectly, via Arabic, Greek manuscripts were translated into Latin, and alchemical explanations of the nature of matter can be found in the treatises of such European scholars as Albertus Magnus (c. 1200–1280) and Roger Bacon (c. 1214–1294).

Arab alchemical treatises were held in high regard in the Middle Ages, but they fell from favour in the 18th century following the advent of the scientific revolution. Previously, alchemists had been respected figures on the European scene, and kings and nobles often supported them in the hope of increasing their revenue. But among the sincere followers of alchemy there were also charlatans and swindlers, and their fraudulent activities led to alchemy falling into disrepute. Even as late as 1783 a chemist called John Price claimed he had turned mercury into gold. When he was asked by the Royal Society to perform the experiment in public, he reluctantly agreed. On the appointed day, however, he poisoned himself to death in front of the audience.

In the 16th and 17th centuries many practical alchemists, such as Paracelsus (1493–1541), the first in Europe to mention zinc and use the word 'alcohol', turned from trying to create gold towards preparing medicine. The story is told of a 17th-century chemist who claimed he had found the elixir of life in the waters of a mineral spring. This substance has since been identified as the laxative sodium sulphate.

After the scientific revolution in the late 17th and 18th centuries, alchemy became less popular and interest in transmutation became limited to astrologers and numerologists. Nevertheless, the scientific facts that had been accumulated by alchemists in their search for gold became one of the foundations of modern chemistry and medicine.

The quest for spiritual perfection

In the West interest in the spiritual dimension of alchemy was rekindled in the mid-20th century through the work of Swiss psychologist Carl Jung (1875–1961). Today scientists have finally discovered how to change base metals into gold, but the process is uneconomical and so modern alchemy has become a spiritual rather than a practical quest, and the search for spiritual perfection and the study of the mystic arts have taken precedence over the quest for easy riches. The symbolism of turning base metal into gold represents exactly what they are trying to do within, with practices such as meditation and visualization, which is to refine themselves spiritually.

PILGRIMAGE AND RETREATS

If you are interested in **Pilgrimage and Retreats**, you may also like to read about:
● **Meditation**, pages 78–79
● **Christianity**, pages 190–191
● **Buddhism**, pages 208–209
● **Islam**, pages 196–197

A pilgrimage is a **sacred journey** to a place or shrine of great importance to a person's beliefs and faith, and an individual who makes such a journey is called a pilgrim. With a **history** dating as far back as civilization itself, pilgrimages and retreats offer someone **respite** and a chance to **reflect** on what is really important in their lives.

Sacred journey

A pilgrimage is a journey or quest of great moral and spiritual significance, and one that is inward as well as outward in nature. Pilgrims seek to strengthen and renew their faith through travel. The working definition of pilgrimage is a transformative journey to a sacred centre, and that is what distinguishes a pilgrim from being a tourist. For a tourist, travel is an end in itself. For a pilgrim, travel is a means to an end. Pilgrims travel with a clear intention, to draw closer to God, and they make their journey with a heightened expectation. English writer John Bunyan (1628–1688) famously described the pilgrim and his spiritual progress in *The Pilgrim's Progress* (1684) as follows:

'There's no discouragement
Shall make him once relent
His first avowed intent
To be a pilgrim.'

Pilgrimage is therefore sacred travel and the pilgrim expects to return transformed, changed or converted from the person they were before they began their journey.

The history of pilgrimage

Since civilization began, humans have been making pilgrimages and some of these pilgrimages have changed the course of history. Clearly the pilgrimage fulfilled, and continues to fulfil, a basic human need.

Religious pilgrimages to sacred places have the longest history. The earliest-known pilgrimage site is Abydos in Egypt where people gathered each year at the place where Osiris, the King of the Dead, died and was reborn. This dates the practice of religious pilgrimage to at least c. 3000 BCE, and all the major world religions have pilgrimage sites. For centuries, Muslims have journeyed to Mecca, home of the beloved prophet Muhammad and the place where Islam came into being; Jews and Christians to Jerusalem, the spiritual birthplace of Judaism and a highly significant place in the historical life of Jesus for Christians; and Hindus to Vrindavan, their most sacred and holy place. Several of the Psalms, notably 120–134, are called the 'Psalms of Ascent', songs sung by the faithful as they made their pilgrimage upward to Jerusalem. Buddhism offers five sites of pilgrimage: the Buddha's birthplace at Kapilavastu; the site where he attained enlightenment, Bodh Gaya; where he first preached at Benares; where he achieved Parinirvana (final nirvana) at Kusinagara; and Mount Tai Shan, considered a deity itself and venerated by the Chinese since at least the third millennium BCE.

The common thread with most religious pilgrimages is spiritual growth. Although there are a number of other reasons why people take a religious pilgrimage – some in hope of a cure, some for penance and others to connect themselves with their community – for most the journey is one of inspiration and fulfilment.

Today pilgrimage is a term used in a more general sense than the strictly religious. People also make pilgrimages to sites of death and disaster. Where the World Trade Center once stood in New York, USA, has become a site of pilgrimage for many. Influential British scientist Richard Dawkins, who disavows any kind of religious stand, subtitled one of his books: 'Pilgrimage to the dawn of evolution'. For Dawkins, a pilgrimage is something that returns or connects him to his roots. But however the term pilgrimage is used, it is still a means of connecting or finding meaning by joining parts to make them whole.

Respite and reflection

Instead of making a journey to a specific site or shrine, a retreat is where a person removes themselves from the world for a period of time for the purpose of contemplation. It can be a solitary or a community experience. Some retreats are held in silence, while others involve extensive conversation. Retreats are often conducted at private or remote locations, or at a retreat centre such as a monastery.

Retreats are considered important for Buddhists, having been a common practice since the Vassa, or rainy-season retreat, was established by the founder of Buddhism, Prince Gautama Siddhartha Buddha (c. 560–483 BCE). Retreats are also popular in many Christian churches, where they are seen as mirroring Christ's 40 days in the desert. However, as retreats are principally an opportunity for reflection, someone need not be religious to go on one.

Mecca *The 27th night of Ramadan, 'Laylet al-Qadr' (Night of Power), is one of the holiest nights of the Islamic calendar, the night when the Koran began to be revealed to the Prophet Muhammad. Almost one million pilgrims visit Mecca from all over the world and pray throughout the night.*

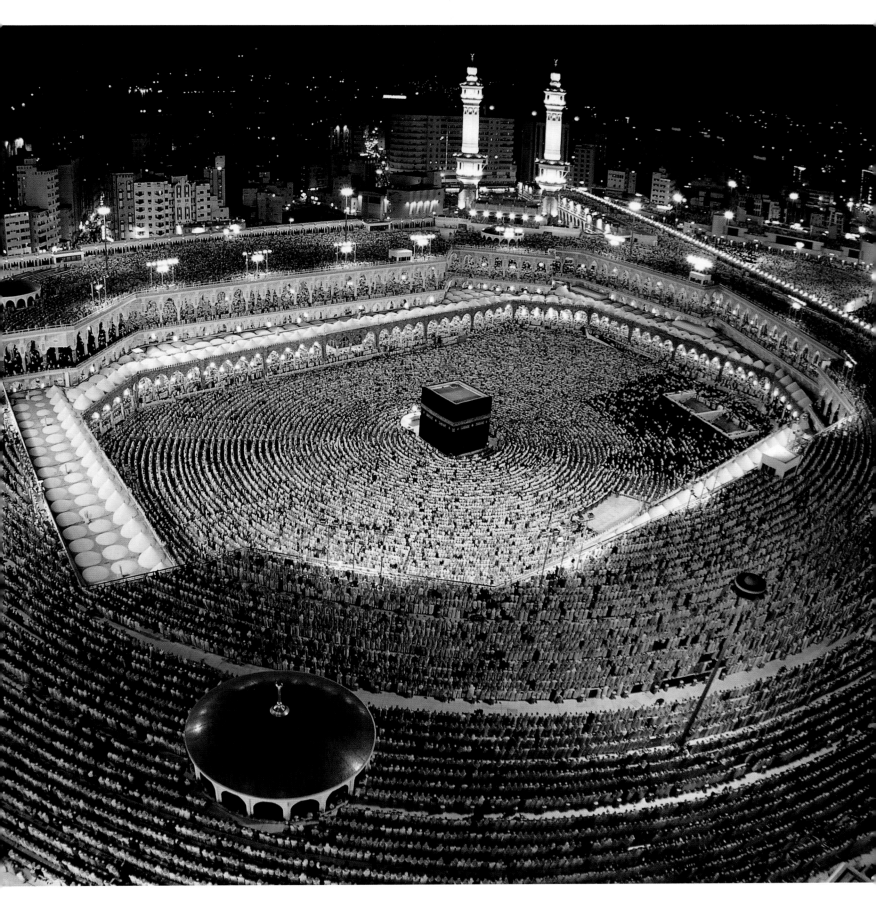

SPIRITUAL LEADERS

A spiritual leader is any person who inspires others to seek out and live a more spiritual life. Jesus, Buddha and Muhammad were great spiritual leaders and the example they set as spiritual teachers has been followed down the centuries. Every major religion has its spiritual leaders, but in the Hindu tradition the concept of the teacher or **guru** is considered vital in assisting individuals on the path to spiritual growth. Among the notable **spiritual leaders of other traditions** is the Dalai Lama, but there are some contemporary spiritual leaders whose message is not tied to any particular religion.

If you are interested in **Spiritual Leaders**, you may also like to read about:
- Channelling, pages 42–43
- Hinduism, pages 204–205
- Christianity, pages 190–191
- Buddhism, pages 208–209
- Tibetan Buddhism, page 212
- Zen Buddhism, page 213
- Tantra, pages 214–215
- Theosophy, pages 270–271

The guru

In the Hindu tradition a guru is a teacher or guide who belongs to a sect or order focused on a deity. The guru is considered to have a lineage stretching back to the founding father of the sect, and sometimes even to the deity itself. The guru is considered to be the authentic guardian of the sect's teachings, and in some traditions is seen as the actual embodiment of the divine. Hence devotion to one's guru is a means to spiritual enlightenment.

Bhagavan Shree Rajneesh *The Indian guru and his followers settled on a vast ranch in Oregon, USA, in the hope of spreading the message of religious enlightenment.*

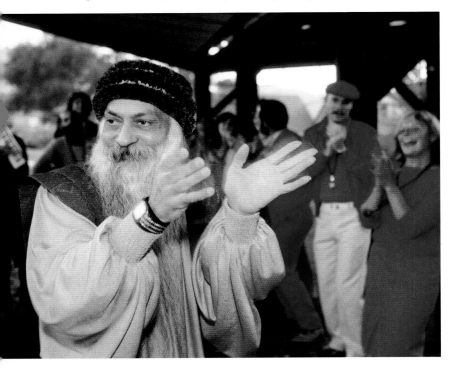

Within the tantric tradition, the guru is particularly important and is the vehicle by which secret spiritual truths are revealed to the initiate.

Initially inspired by Madame Blavatsky (1831–1891) and the Theosophy Society in the 19th century, the concept of the guru has been embraced by many in the West, and numerous Hindu spiritual leaders have attracted widespread followings. Jiddu Krishnamurti (1895–1986) was trained by the Theosophist Annie Besant (1847–1933) to become a world spiritual leader. Although he rejected this role, he remained an influential figure until his death, teaching a doctrine of pure awareness. Aurobindo Ghose (1872–1950) was involved in the Indian independence movement and jailed for terrorist activities as a young man. He underwent a spiritual transformation while in prison and, once released, founded an ashram where he developed a system of spiritual development called 'integral yoga'. Tamil mystic Ramana Maharshi (1879–1950) taught a form of meditation based on considering the question of one's own identity; in that way, he believed, a person's various roles and personae can be removed to reveal the pure consciousness at the heart of the self. Ramana's teachings about self-enquiry, the practice he is most widely associated with, have been classified as the Path of Knowledge (*Jnana marga*) among the Indian schools of thought.

More recent examples of influential leaders include Indian philosopher and spiritual leader Osho (1931–1990), previously known as Bhagavan Shree Rajneesh, who fused Eastern meditation with Western psychotherapies; Maharishi Mahesh Yogi (1917–2008), the founder of the Transcendental Meditation movement; and Swami Sivananda (1887–1963) from the holy town of Rishikesh, who inspired the development of Western yoga centres.

Osho, who rose to prominence in the 1960s and 1970s, continued teaching and guiding devoted followers up until his death. Many of his techniques were controversial, but they have been preserved by the Osho Foundation, which continues to practise and spread Osho's teachings, despite the collapse of the ashram. Osho taught a form of monism, that God is in everything and everyone and that there is no division between 'God' and 'not-God'; people, even at their worst, are divine. Osho's teachings emphasize the importance of meditation, awareness, love, celebration, creativity and humour – qualities that in his view are suppressed by adherence to static belief systems, religious tradition and socialization.

Sai Baba is an Indian guru who goes by the name of Bhagavan Sri Sathya Sai Baba. Although highly revered by many, he remains a controversial figure and some people claim his apparent miraculous abilities are simply tricks. However, his message of love and the unity of all world religions continues to inspire. Sai Baba advocates the five basic human values: *sathya* (truth), *dharma* (appropriate conduct, living in accord with natural law), *ahimsa* (non-violence), *prema* (love for God and all his creatures) and *shantih* (peace).

Mother Meera, born Kamala Reddy in 1960 in India, is believed by her devotees to be an embodiment (avatar) of the Divine Mother. She is reputed to have experienced her first *samadhi*, or state of intense spiritual concentration, as a child, lasting an entire day. Today she receives thousands of visitors of all religions for *darshan*, conducted in total silence at no cost, which consists of a ritual in which she touches a person's head and then looks into their eyes. During this process, she reportedly 'unties knots' in the person's subtle energy system and permeates them with spiritual light.

Spiritual leaders of other traditions

Although the guru is of particular importance in the Hindu tradition, other influential leaders have emerged from different faiths and movements. One of the most influential leaders worldwide, the Dalai Lama is the spiritual and political leader of the Tibetan people, according to Tibetan Buddhism. He is believed to be the current incarnation of a long line of Tulkus, or Buddhist Masters, and is respected by millions of people for his advocacy of non-violent resistance and compassionate awareness of the sufferings of others.

In 1962, Eileen Caddy (1917–2008), born in Alexandria, Egypt, went to live in a caravan near Findhorn on the windswept shores of the Moray Firth in Scotland with her husband Peter and a friend, Dorothy Maclean. The spiritual community they established grew into the Findhorn Foundation, dedicated to 'planetary service, co-creation with nature and attunement to the divinity within all beings', and now has 100 residents and 14,000 visitors a year. The community has no formal doctrine or creed and offers a range of workshops and events in the environment of a working ecovillage.

Amma *Mata Amritanandamayi was born in 1953 and is recognized as a universal representative of the Divine Mother. She is also known as the 'hugging saint' and is said to have hugged at least 30 million people in the past 30 years.*

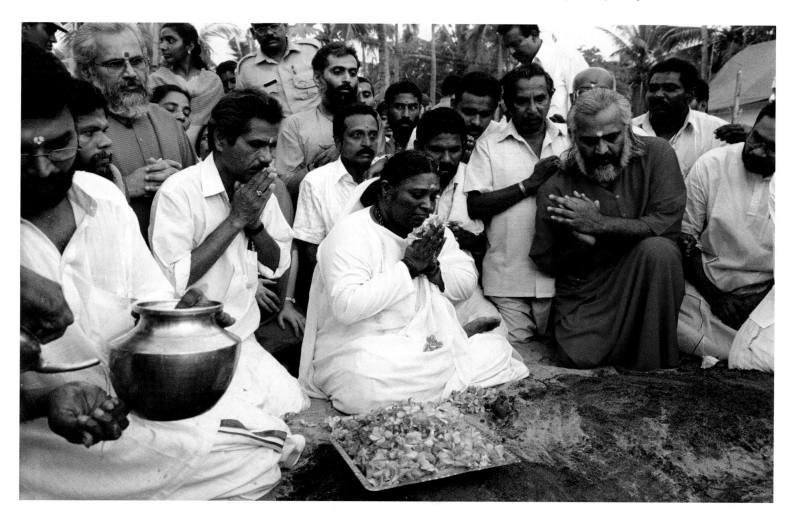

ENERGY

Energy is the vital life force thought to transcend time and space and permeate all phenomena. Every ancient, traditional and indigenous spiritual and healing system in the world recognizes and uses the concept of vital energy, also known as **the universal life force**, but it has found its strongest expression in Eastern mysticism. In India it is called prana, in China chi or qi and in Japan ki. In the last few decades, striking parallels have been discovered between **quantum physics** and the concept of a universal life force, and the New Age movement has embraced the more recent theory of invisible **energy fields**.

If you are interested in **Energy**, you may also like to read about:

- **Breathwork**, page 81
- **Ayurveda**, pages 94–95
- **Traditional Chinese Medicine**, pages 98–101
- **Acupuncture**, page 126
- **Acupressure**, page 127
- **Energy Psychology Therapies**, page 87
- **Hinduism**, pages 204–205
- **Hindu Sacred Texts**, pages 206–207
- **Buddhism**, pages 208–209
- **Taoism**, pages 216–217

The universal life force

The existence of a universal life force has been widely acknowledged since ancient times, and is found in all the different cultures and belief systems across the globe. Modern physics has also recognized the principle of energy underpinning the nature of our world. According to 'quantum field theories', developed in the main by German-born American theoretical physicist Albert Einstein (1879–1955), there is no distinction between the solid particles we term matter and the space surrounding them. Matter and space are seen as both part of the quantum field, matter simply being local concentrations of energy within the field.

Quantum physics and mysticism

A groundbreaking book by Austrian-born American physicist Fritjof Capra called *The Tao of Physics: An Exploration of the Parallels Between Modern Physics and Eastern Mysticism*, published in 1975, explored the connection between modern physics (quantum theory) and Eastern mysticism/philosophy. Of most significance was the shared understanding between physics and Eastern mysticism that the universe is a dynamic interconnected unity with all living things in a constant energy exchange. Capra noted the similarity of the Chinese sage Chang Tsai's (1020–1077) description of the nature of chi with the description of the quantum field: 'When the chi condenses, its visibility becomes apparent so that there are then the shapes [of individual things]. When it disperses its visibility is no longer apparent and there are no shapes.'

Capra further noted links between the quantum field and the Eastern view of the Great Void – the underlying reality that lies behind all phenomena. This is termed the Brahman by Hindus, the Dharmakaya by Buddhists and the Tao by Taoists. The Brahman is described as formless or a 'Void' because it defies description or specification. However, the Void is not 'nothingness', but rather is the source of all life. In the sacred Hindu texts known as the Upanishads, it is described as follows:

'Brahman is life. Brahman is joy. Brahman is the Void…
Joy, verily, is the same as the Void.
The Void, verily, that is the same as joy.'

Austrian physicist Walter Thirring described the quantum field as follows: 'The field exists always and everywhere; it can never be removed. It is the carrier of all material phenomena. It is the 'void' out of which the proton creates the pi-mesons [subatomic particles]. Being and fading of particles are merely forms of motion in the field.' In a striking parallel view, Chang Tsai notes: 'The Great Void cannot but consist of chi; this chi cannot but condense to form all things; and these things cannot but become dispersed so as to form (once more) the Great Void.'

Energy fields

The parallels between modern science and theories of a vital force or energy have recently been developed and once again brought to public attention by the English biologist Rupert Sheldrake. Sheldrake suggests that all organisms have an invisible energy field around them, which carries the history of that organism and which communicates to the energy fields of other organisms. This theory has been embraced by the New Age movement for a number of important reasons. First, it questions a survival-of-the-fittest theory of evolution based on chance and circumstance and replaces it with something more deep and purposeful. Second, it helps reclaim an understanding of life that acknowledges the existence of other dimensions. And finally, it indicates that the energy surrounding every organism may actually be alive and conscious in some form. Taking this last point one step further, many in the New Age movement theorize that these energy fields could be the realm where non-material beings, such as angels and other spiritual guides, reside.

T'ai chi *Outdoor group t'ai chi exercise is very popular in China and is often performed in parks and other open spaces in the early morning.*

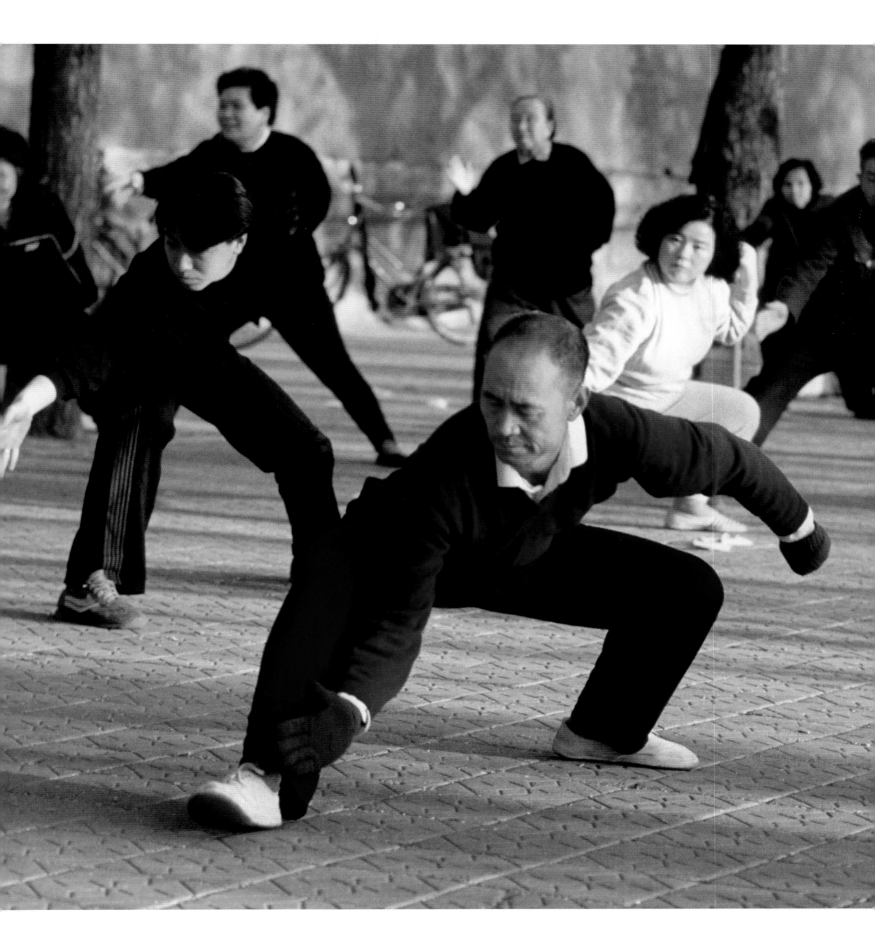

CONTEMPORARY SPIRITUALITY

If you are interested in **Contemporary Spirituality**, then all entries in this book are relevant, because they all build to create a modern understanding.

Contemporary spirituality emerges from all the diverse traditions in our **global village**. It approaches spirituality with a multicultural and **interfaith attitude**, and recognizes the difference between spirituality and religion. It is centrally concerned with **individual spiritual experience** as the starting point for exploration and development.

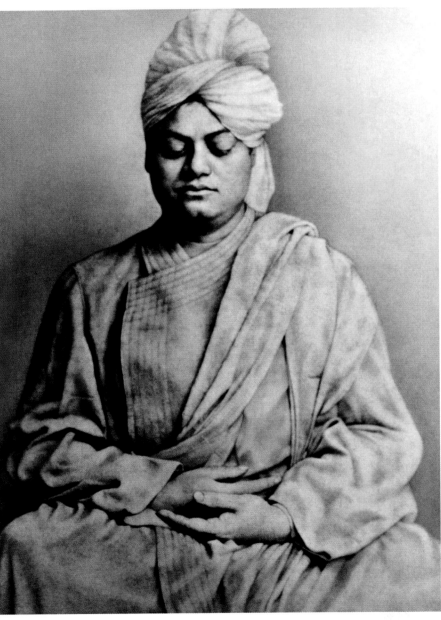

Swami Vivekananda *This picture of the Hindu spiritual leader Swami Vivekananda was taken at the Ice House in Chennai, South India.*

Global village and interfaith

Two hundred years ago the world's spiritual traditions existed in isolation from each other. Today travel, mass communications and literacy give everyone access to what was previously unknown. The writings of all the world's religious traditions are universally available, and in most schools modern children learn about different beliefs and worship, preparing them for citizenship in a global community.

The *World Values Survey*, which is the most reliable contemporary survey of beliefs across the globe, suggests that there has been a substantial cultural change. In modernized and free societies, where people have access to diverse views, up to 70 per cent of the population has moved away from a single-faith tradition. These people have not become atheistic, but have adopted a more general and inclusive approach to spirituality.

One of the earliest examples of this inclusive approach was the 1893 World Parliament of Religions in Chicago, USA; there is now a World Parliament every two years. One of the most significant moments of that first gathering was when the Hindu teacher, Swami Vivekananda, told the story of a frog that lived in a well. This frog then met another frog that lived in the ocean. The frog from the small well refused to believe that there was anything more special than his well. Vivekananda suggested that traditional religions were sometimes like that frog in the well – they needed to appreciate the greater ocean.

There is now a worldwide interfaith movement, which encourages dialogue between the faiths, and its logo is a circle containing the symbols of the major faiths.

The difference between spirituality and religion

Contemporary spirituality suggests that there is a difference between spirituality and religion. Religion can be described as an organized set of beliefs and customs practised by a group. Spirituality, on the other hand, is an individual and personal experience.

Ofsted, the major government body concerned with children's education in the UK, describes spirituality as 'that aspect of inner life through which pupils acquire insights into their personal experience which are of enduring worth. It is characterized by reflection, the attribution of meaning to experience, valuing a non-material dimension to life and intimations of an

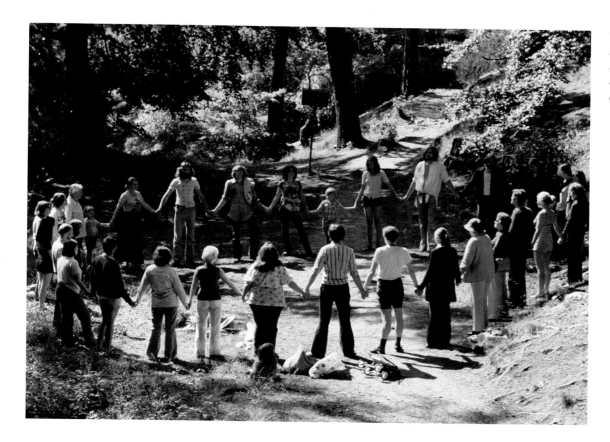

The Findhorn Foundation *This ecovillage in northern Scotland is Europe's biggest and most well-established holistic community, working with spirituality and environmental harmony.*

enduring reality. "Spiritual" is not synonymous with "religious"; all areas of the curriculum may contribute to pupils' spiritual development.'

Most religions, however, originate in spiritual experience, and people within religions also have individual spiritual experiences. Contemporary spirituality tends to support the development of the individual and be suspicious of any faith that claims a monopoly on truth.

One contemporary definition of spirituality developed by the Foundation for Holistic Spirituality states that it is 'the natural human connection with the wonder and energy of nature, cosmos and all existence; and the instinct to explore and understand its meaning'.

Beliefs and values – a holistic approach

Contemporary spirituality takes a holistic approach that is open-hearted and open-minded, seeking to understand all the many different aspects of existence. It honours the essence of traditional faiths. It also seeks to understand and include the crucial relationships between spirituality and health, social justice, environmental issues and citizenship.

Drawing on the essence of traditional spiritual practice, it suggests that there are three major components to spirituality, which people can choose to practise on a daily basis:

- **Connect** Everyone benefits from regularly pausing to connect with and experience the wonder and energy of life.
- **Reflect** Through regular self-assessment we choose suitable next steps to develop our love and consciousness.
- **Serve** There is a moral imperative to do no harm and be of service.

Individual spiritual experience

At the core of contemporary spirituality is the idea that every individual can connect with and experience the wonder, energy and spirit of life. The Alister Hardy Research Foundation collects data on spiritual experience. It suggests that it is 'an aspect of natural human experience. It can come in on us, or arise in us, suddenly, at any time, in any place, and can affect and even change our lives. It can happen to anyone, whether religiously inclined or atheist, spiritually inclined or materialist, and regardless of age, sex, nationality or culture.'

It can be triggered by many types of situation, and the following is a short list of just a few keywords:

Ecstatic	Devotional	Meditative	Studious
Dance	Arts	Landscape	Pilgrimage
Drumming	Prayer	Music	Ritual
Pain	Trauma	Suffering	Crisis
Parenting	Angels	Gardening	Caring
Hermit	Evangelical	Extrovert	Introvert
Chanting	Psychic	Healing	Sacred spaces

Although there are many different triggers, the actual nature of the experience is generally the same, beneficial and life-enhancing. People report a change in how they feel and think. They use words such as: oneness with all creation, heightened awareness, love and fulfilment. But in general explaining the experience to others is not easy because it can often be hard to express in words. The important thing is the experience itself and how it changes a person's perception of the spiritual world.

INDEX

Page numbers in *italics* refer to captions/illustrations.

A

ABC Technique of Rational Beliefs 28
abhyanga 97
abundance 52
Abydos 298
acceptance and commitment therapy 29
acid foods:
　in food combining 148
acid reflux 148
acne 94, 101, 157
　causes 148
acupressure 87, *100*, 127
　research 127
　seated 127
　self-help treatment 127
acupuncture 87, 90, *100*, 101, 126, 145
　acupoints *104*
　Chinese 126
　research 126
　therapeutic treatment 126
　Western 126
acute illnesses 93
Adamski, George 256
addictions 87
Adi Granth 223
Advaita 206
Aetherius Society 271
Africa:
　beliefs 234–5
　Voudoun 238
aggression:
　learning 26
agriculture:
　innovations in 272
agrimony essence 159
aikido 117
Akashic Record 271, 279
Aksakof, Alexander N. 41
alchemists 263, *296*
alchemy 296–7

alcoholism 86
Alexander, Frederick 118, *119*
Alexander III, Pope 264
Alexander technique 82, 105, 118–19
　research 119
Alexandrian Wicca 240
Alister Hardy Research Foundation 305
Allen, Nicholas 281
allergies 94, 161
allopathic medicine 75, 132
Alpert, Richard (Ram Dass) *34*, 35
alphabets:
　ancient 64
alpine mint bush essence 159
altered state of consciousness 30
Amana 225
Amaterasu 236–7, *236*
American Medical Association (AMA) 132
American School of Osteopathy 133
amethyst 167
Amma *301*
amygdala 84
anaemia 153
anaesthesia:
　effect of herbs on 152
Anasazi people 259
anatomy:
　Tibetan painting *103*
ancestral spirits 234
ancestral traditions 230–1
Ancient Druid Order 243
ancient mysteries 245, 275–87
angels 290–1, *291*
　intervention from 290–1
　origins 290
Angels of Mons 291
anima 19, 20
animals:
　power 233
animism 225, 230, 232, 236, 238
animus 19, 20
Ankmahor *128*
anmo 124
anomalous experiences 48
anthropology 245
Anthroposophy 50, 263, 266, 272–3

anti-inflammatories 157
antioxidants 147
anxiety 118
　causes 28
　reflex points *131*
　relieving 79, 152, 157
anxiety disorders 87
Apache 246
Apollo programme *261*
apples 147
applied kinesiology (AK) 168, *168*
　research 168
archaeology 245
archeoastronomy 245, 254–5
archetypes 20
　psychology 21
architecture:
　innovations in 272, 273, *273*
　of monuments 250–1
Aristotle 296
Arjuna 206
Ark of the Covenant 280
aromatherapy 156–7
art therapy 15, 32
Artemis 294
　cult of 243
arthritis 153, 156, 163
　rheumatoid 177
Arthurian legend 282
asanas 106
ascended masters 42–3
asclepion *23*
Asclepius *23*
Aserinsky, Eugene 22
Ashmole, Elias 268
Ashtanga yoga 205
asparagus 153
Assagioli, Roberto 32, *32*
assumptions:
　irrational 28
asthma 79, 86, 87, 94, 161
astral projection 46, 47
astrologers 37
astrological charts 56–7, *57*
astrology 55, 263
　Chinese 58
　forms of 56–7

Great Year 285
　Vedic 60–1
　Western 56–7
astronomy 56, 245
　Chinese measurements 255
　Great Year 285
　megaliths and 254
　Native American 255
Aswang 231
Atlantis 43, 245, 275, 276–7, *277*
Atlantologists 277
attachment theory 26
attainment 37
attraction, laws of *53*
Aubrey, John 243
Aur Ain Soph 188
aura 172, 173, *173*
　healing through 171
Aurobindo, Sri 204
Australian Aboriginal people 225
　Dreamtime 225, 228–9, *228*, 246
　rock painting *247*
　sacred sites 228, 229
　songlines 228, 229, 287
　spirituality 228–9
Australian Bush Flower Essences 158, 159
autogenic training 80, 84
autointoxication 151
autosuggestion:
　optimistic 30
Avalon, Arthur 172
Avebury 252, 253
Awa 235
awakened mind 16
awareness:
　heightened 81
Ayers Rock 225, 228, 229, *229*
ayurveda 75, 93, 94–7, 171
　diagnosis 97
　herbal therapies 97
　key concepts 93, 94
　practitioners 94
　precautions 97
　treatments 97
Aztecs:
　temples 255

Bab 200
Babylonians 52
Bach, Dr Edward 158
Bach Flower Remedies 158, 159
back pain 163, 165
backache:
    reflex points 131
Bacon, Sir Francis 43
Bacon, Roger 297, 297
Baha, Abdul 200, 201
Bahai 200–1
    Lotus Temple 201
    spiritual beliefs 200, 201
Baha'u'llah 200–1
Baigent, Michael 281, 282
Bailey, Alice 38, 173, 195
Bali:
    spiritual culture 230
Bandler, Richard 31
Bandura, Albert 26
Bards, Ovates and Druids, Order of 243
Barruel, Abbé Augustin de 267
basil oil 156
Bassui, Master 213
Bates method 83, 105, 141
    precautions 141
    research 141
    techniques 141
Bates, Dr William 141
Bathela 231
Bayly, Doreen 129
Beatles 205
Beck, Aaron T. 28, 52
Bede, Venerable 48, 49
beech essence 159
Beecher, Henry 75
behavioural modification 103
behavioural therapy:
    cognitive 28–9, 32
    dialectical 29
    rational emotive 28
behaviourism 15, 26
beings of light 290
Beltane 241
Benares 298
Benveniste, Dr Jacques 164
bereavement:
    coping with 33

Bernard of Clairvaux 264
Bernheim, Hippolyte 30
Besant, Annie 43, 43, 270, 271, 271, 272, 300
beta brain waves 17
beta-endorphin 80
Bhagavad Gita 207
Bhakti yoga 205
Bhutan:
    monastery 212
Biame's Cave 229
Bible 52, 183, 186, 190, 284
Binu 235
biodynamic farming 272
bioenergetics 82
biofeedback 86
Black Madonnas 274, 275, 280–1, 280, 283
black pepper oil 156
black streams 256
black-eyed Susan essence 159
Blackmore, Dr Susan 46
    OBE vision 46
Blake, William 289, 290
Blavatsky, Madame Helena Petrovna 43, 203, 270, 270, 271, 277, 300
bleeding disorders:
    contraindications 152, 164
bloating 148
blood cells:
    white 77
blood clots:
    contraindications 164
blood pressure 177
    high (hypertension) 79, 80, 86, 87, 94, 177
Bloom, William 80
Blot 239
Blue Beryl 102
Blue Lagoon, Iceland 165
Bodh Gaya 298
Bodhidharma 213
Bodhisattvas 43, 210
body:
    re-educating 118
    separation of spirit from 171
    spirit and 171–7
body work 105–14
    mental benefits 105
    spiritual benefits 105

body-centred therapies 82–3
body-mind interactions 16, 155
body-mind therapy 82
Boirac, Emile 39
Bolen, Jean Shinoda 294
bones:
    casting 55
Book of Changes see I Ching
Book of the Dead 278, 279, 279
    Tibetan 35, 210, 211
book of spells 241
Bord, Janet and Colin 245
Boron, Robert de 282
Bowen, Tom 138
Bowen technique 105, 138, 138
    health benefits 138
    research 138
    treatment 138
Bowlby, John 26
Brahma 60, 205
Brahman 206, 289, 302
Brahmanas 206
Braid, James 30
brain:
    cortex 84, 85
    functions 16
    hemispheres 16
    limbic system 84, 85
    magnetic stimulation 46
    mind and 16–17
    MRI scan 84
    parts 16, 17
    right hemisphere 38, 41
    structure of 16, 17
brain-wave synchronization 46
breast cancer 103
breast-feeding:
    contraindications 152
breath of life 225
breathing:
    cleansing technique 45
breathwork 81, 84
Brentor Church, Devon 258
Briggs, Katherine Cook 24
Brigit 239
Brittany:
    standing stones 252, 252
bronchitis 94, 157
Brown, Dan 275, 281
Buchanan, Rhodes 41

Budapest, Zsuzsanna 241
Buddha 21, 202, 208, 209, 209
    meditating 79
Buddhism 16, 34, 37, 43, 52, 114, 208–9
    Dharma 208
    Four Noble Truths 208, 210
    jewels of 208–9
    and medicine 102
    monks 209, 209
    Noble Eightfold Path 208, 210
    origins 203
    philosophy 93
    pilgrimage sites 298
    retreats 298
    sacred texts 210
    Sangha 208, 209
    spiritual aspirations 203
    Tibetan 50
    traditions 208, 209, 212–13
Buitani 230
Bulwer-Lytton, Edward 275
Bunyan, John 266, 298
burial mounds 252
Burne-Jones, Sir Edward 283
    Astrologia 36
bush gardenia essence 159
Byrne, Rhonda 52, 53

C

Caddy, Eileen 301
Cade, Cecil Maxwell 16–17
Cahokia, Illinois 255
Calina people 225
Callahan, Roger 87
Callahan technique see Thought Field Therapy
Campbell, Joseph 21, 226
Camphill Communities 272
cancer 143
    breast 103
    contraindications 121
Cannon, Walter 75
Capra, Fritjof 203, 302
Caraka Samhita 94
Caravaggio, Michelangelo Merisi da:
    Fortune Teller 69

carbohydrates:
  in food combining 148
cardamom oil 157
cardiovascular diseases 87, 143
Carnac:
  standing stones *252*
Carson, Rachel 260
Casa Grande 255
Castaneda, Carlos 289
Castillo 255
Castlerigg stone circle 251
  ground plan *251*
cataracts 141
Cathars 281, 283
Catholicism 190, 191
  suppression of Gospels 192
Cayce, Edgar 37, 277, 279
CBT *see* cognitive behavioural therapy
Cebuano peoples 231
Celtic belief system 238
central nervous system (CNS) 76
cerebral hemispheres 16
Cernunnos *239*, 241
chakras 45, 106
  associations 172
  blockage 82
  channelling energy through 174
  crystals and 166, 167
  earth 261
  healing through 171
  polarity therapy and 169
  positions *83*, *172*
  sound related to 163
  theory 172–3
chamomile oil 157
Chandranandana 102
Chang San-Feng 112
Chang Tsai 302
channelling 39, 42–3, 44
chanting 35
character armour 82
*Chemical Wedding of Christian
  Rosenkreuz* 266
Cherokee people 232
cherubim 290
chi (*ki*) 37, 98, 155
  channelling for healing 174
  congested 98
  controlling 248
  excess 98

flow of 126
restoring balance of 174
stagnant 98
chi kung 101, 112, 114–15
  breathing 114
  energy or breath work 114
  focusing mind 114
  health benefits 114
  Moving the Rainbow *115*
  posture 114
  practice 114
  research 114
Ch'i lin 286
Chichén Itzá 255, *285*
chilblains:
  precautions 164
China:
  archaeological measuring devices
    255
  Cultural Revolution 114
  Divine Creatures 287
  Han Dynasty 149
Chinese astrology 58–9
Chinese medicine *see* Traditional
    Chinese Medicine
chirognomy 68
chiromancy 69
chiropractic 75, 132–5
  branches of 135
  conditions treated 134
  origins 132, 133–4
  research 135
  techniques 134–5
  treatments 134–5, *135*
chlorine 164
Choi Hong Hi, General 117
choleric personality 15, *15*
cholesterol:
  lowering 94, 147
Chou, Duke of 70
Chrétien de Troyes 282
Christ 21, 43, 183, 184–5, 190–1, 192
  ascension *288*
  bloodline 282–3
  fasting 150
  heritage 183
  tomb 280, 281
Christian Community 273
Christianity 43, 52, 190–1
  communion/Mass *190*, 191

Holy Grail 282–3
  meditation 78
  overcoming paganism 287
  pilgrimage 289, 298
  retreats 298
  sacraments 191
  sacred texts 183, 190
  spiritual traditions 183, 190, 273
  symbol 250
  tomb of Jesus 281
chronic conditions:
  treating 93, 94
chronic venous insufficiency 152
Chuang Tzu 203, 218, 219
Chun Quoit, Cornwall *257*
Church Universal and Triumphant
    271
cinchona bark 160
circulatory disorders 80
  contraindications 164
citrine 167
clairalience 40
clairaudience 40
claircognizance 41
clairgustance 40
clairsentience 40
clairvoyance 37, *39*, 40
cleansing techniques 44, 45
clematis essence 159
client-centred psychology 27
closing down 44, 45
Cloud Hands *113*
CNS *see* central nervous system
Co-Masonry 271
Cocharelli of Genoa *265*
Coffin Texts 279
cognitive behavioural therapy (CBT)
    15, 28–9, 32
coherence 86
coincidence:
  meaningful 20
coins:
  throwing *71*
colds 153
collective unconscious 15, 18, 20–1
colonics 150, 151
  precautions 151
colour therapy 162
  precautions 162
  research 162

colours:
  of crystals 166, 167
Columbus, Christopher 43
complex 20
concentration:
  increasing 80
  poor 148
conditioning 26
Confessio Fraternitatis 266
Confucianism 220–1
  as religion 221
  sacred texts 220–1
  Sokchonje 221
Confucius 58, 70, 220, *220*, 286
consciousness 18
  altered state of 30
  definition 16
  levels of 16–17
  luminous 34
  multi-dimensions of 35
  study of 15
conspiracy theories 267
constellations 56, 61
constipation 151
  acupressure for *127*
  reflex points *131*
constitution (*prakriti*) 94
continuity hypothesis 23
Control Cycle *99*
Cooke, Grace 195
core strength 110
Corpus Hermeticum 185
cosmic consciousness 171
cosmic ordering 52, 53
Coué, Emile 30
Course in Miracles 195
Cousins, Norman 77
Covenant of the Goddess 241
Coyote 232
Craig, Gary 87
cranial osteopathy 135
craniosacral therapy 105, 136, *136*
  diagnosis 136
  research 136
  treatment 136
Creation Cycles 285
Creation myths 286
creative visualization 33
creativity 16
  boosting 80

creator gods 234

Crete:

    palace-temples 246

Critchlow, Keith 250–1, *251*

Crowley, Aleister 240, 263

crystal therapy 166–7, *166*

    precautions 167

    research 167

crystalline grid 43

crystals 44

    and chakras 166, 167

    colours 167

    forms 167

    gem essences 166, 167

    meditating 166, 167

    wearing 166, 167

Ctesias 286

Cultural Revolution 114

curanderos 227

cursuses 253

cymatics 163

    imaging *163*

cytokines 76, 77

Czestochowa:

    Black Madonna 281

D

Da Vinci Code 263, 281

Dalai Lama 203, 212, 300, 301

Damarri 229

Däniken, Erich von 245, 259

Dante Alighieri 290

Dao De Jing 218

Darling Scarp 229

Darwin, Charles 271

Dawkins, Richard 298

decumbiture charts 57

Deep Ecology movement 261

defibrillators:

    contraindications 164

déja senti 39

déjà vécu 39

déjà visité 39

déjà vu 39

Delphic Oracle 42, *42*, 55

Dement, William C. 22

dementia 152

Demeter 21, 294

depression 18, 87, 152, 153, 161, 175

    causes of 148

    overcoming 29

    severe: causes 28

dermatitis:

    precautions 164

dermatoglyphics 68, 69

dervishes 35, *78*, *198*, 199

Descartes, René 12

Destruction Cycle 99, *99*

detoxification 93

detoxing 150–1

    precautions 151

    research 151

Dev, Guru Arjan 223

Devas 204, 205, 292

Devereux, Paul 256

Dhammapada 210, 212

Dhanwantari *95*

Dharma 208

Dharmic Hinduism 204

diabetes 87, 94, 143

    contraindications 121

dialectical behaviour therapy 29

Dianic Wicca 241

dietary changes 143

dietary supplements 143

dietary therapy 97, 101, 103

digestive disorders 94, 153

    causes 148

digestive system 156

    resting 150

Dila 231

diuretics:

    foods 151

divination 37, 55–73

divinational trance 39

Djabugay people 229

Djanggawul 228

Djoser, King 278

dog rose essence 159

Dogon 225, 226

    calendar 235

    dancer *224*

    rock painting *235*

    spiritual beliefs 234, 235

Dokuon, Master 213

dolmens 252, 256, *257*

Domhoff, William 23

Domnu 239

Donne, W. 39

Donnelly, Ignatius 276

doshas 93, 94, 96–7, 102

Dossey, Larry 171

Dougans, Inge 130

dowsing:

    energy 256

    pendulum 72

    traditional 256

Dowth 252

dragon lines 229, 287

Dragon Project 256

dragons 286–7, *287*

    Eastern 287

    Western 286–7

drama therapy 15, 32

dreaming sleep 16

dreams 16, 22–3

    definition 22

    deprivation 22

    future seen in 39

    importance of 22

    interpreting 22, 55

    lucid 23, 46, 48

    phases 22

    reasons for 22–3

    recurring 23

    unconscious and 18

Dreamtime 225, 228–9, 246

dreamwork 32

drugs:

    hallucinogenic 35, 46

    from herbs 152

    interaction with herbs 152

    psychedelic 35, 226

Druidry 225, 238, 242–3

    beliefs 242, 243

    original 242, 243

    practice 242, 243

    revival of 243, 245

    rituals 243

    symbols 243, *243*

Druids *242*

    levels 243

    orders 242, 243

Dryades (dryads) 243, 292

Duisburg-Marxloh:

    mosque *197*

Dvaita 206

E

Earth:

    'body' of 260–1

    curvature: calculating 255

    healing by 261

    seen from Space *261*

    self-regulation 260

earth energies 245, 256–7

Earth Mysteries 245–61

    origins 245

    present-day 245

earthworks 252–3, 255

Easter island:

    carvings *230*, 231, *231*, 252

Eastern faiths 203–23

    influence on West 203

    origins 203

    spiritual aspirations 203

Eastern medicine 93–103

Eastern Orthodox Church 190, 191

Eastern spirituality 78

Ebbinghaus, Hermann 15

ECG *see* electrocardiogram

Eckankar 271

Eclectic Wicca 241

Eclectics 132

eco-paganism 260

ecology 261

ecopsychology 260, 261

ecstasy 34

eczema 79, 80, 86, 161, 177

    precautions 164

Eddas 238

education:

    teaching methods 272

EEG *see* electroencephalogram

effigy mounds 253, *253*

effleurage *121*

ego 18

Egyptians 52

    Ancient Egyptian wisdom 278–9

Ehrsson, Henrik 46

Eight Principles 98–9

Einstein, Albert 27, 37, 38, 302

Eitel, Ernest J. 249

Elder Futhark 53

electional astrology 57

electrocardiogram (ECG) *86*

electroencephalogram (EEG) *86*

electromagnetic energy spectrum 155

elements 56
  Five Elements Systems 99
  in Tibetan medicine 103
Eliade, Mircea 226
Eliot, T.S. 39
elixir of life 297
Ellis, Albert 28, *28*, 52
embodied psychology 82
EMDR *see* Eye Movement
  Desensitization and Reprocessing
Emerald Tablet 52, *53*
Emotional Freedom Technique 87, *87*
emotional healing 160
emotional response:
  components of 84
emotion(s):
  negative 158
  neurobiology of 84–5
  repressed 15, 81
Emoto, Dr Masaru 164
emWave Personal Stress Reliever 86
endocrine system 76, 173
Endorphin Effect 80, 84
enemas 151
energy 155
  balance of 169
  bodily: theory of 82
  channelling for healing 174
  flow of 37, 82, 87
  applied kinesiology 168
  blockages in 155
  harmonising 124–5
  polarity therapy 169
  restoring balance to 87, 105
  healing 176
  kundalini 172, 215
  life force 155, 234, 302
  low levels of 148
  psychokinetic 39
  as therapy 155
energy dowsing 256
energy fields 55, 302
energy lines *258*
energy meridian regulation 87
energy psychology 12
energy psychology therapies 87
energy therapies 155–69
  principles 155
Enkai 234
enlightenment 203, 204, 210

Enlightenment, Age of 75, 245, 290
Enneagram 15, 24, 25, *25*
Enochian magic 240
Enthusiast 25
enzymes:
  digestive 148
epilepsy 86
  contraindications 121
  controlling 16
Erickson, Milton 30, 31, *31*
Escamilla, Isidra:
  Our Lady of Guadelupe 295
Eschenbach, Wolfram von 282
esoteric societies 263–73
ESP *see* extra-sensory perception
essential oils:
  absorption 157
  characteristics 157
  diluting 157
  effects of 156
  precautions 157
  research 157
  uses 157
  in water 164
Ethiopia:
  standing stones 252
eucalyptus oil 157
Eucharist 191
exceptional human experiences 16,
  48–9
exercise 144
exploitive type 24
extra-sensory perception (ESP) 38–9,
  40, 41
extroverts 24
Eye Movement Desensitization and
  Reprocessing (EMDR) 84, 85, 87
eyes:
  examination of 140
  iris: study of 140
eyesight:
  improving: Bates method 141, *141*

F

face reading 72, 73
fairies 292–3, *292*, *293*
  disappearance 293

faith healing *194*
faiths:
  Eastern 203–23
  Western 183–201
false memory syndrome 39
family therapy 32
Farr, Florence 263
fasting 150
  precautions 151
Fateh Ali Khan, Nusrat 199, *199*
father-figure types 21
fatigue 153
fears:
  irrational 19
Feeling Triad 25
feeling types 24
feet:
  reflex points *129*, *131*
Feldenkrais, Moshe 137
Feldenkrais method 82, 105, 137, *137*
  health benefits 137
  research 137
Felkin, Dr Robert 273
female psyche:
  male side 19, 20
feng shui 245, 248–9
  Compass School 249
  disciplines 248–9
  Form School 248–9
  modern 248, 249
Fenwick, Dr Peter 49
fertility:
  problems 153
  symbol of 294
Fibonacci progression *250*
fight or flight 75, 77, 80
Findhorn Foundation 301, *305*
fingerprints 69
first aid:
  reflexology 130
Fisher King 282
Fitzgerald, John Anster:
  Fairies at a Window 293
Fitzgerald, Dr William 128–9
Five Classics 220
Five Elements System 98, 99
flavonoids 147
flotation therapy 164
flower essences 158–9
  research 158

fly agaric *161*
focusing 82, 83
food combining 148
  precautions 148
  research 148
food supplements 143
foods:
  acid: in food combining 148
  functional 143
  superfoods 147
  yin and yang 149
Ford, Henry 50
forebrain 16, *17*
Fortune, Dion 258
Four Noble Truths 208, 210
Four Tantras 102
Four Valleys 200
Fourth Way 25
fractures 163
  contraindications 164
France:
  standing stones 252, *252*
Frazer, Sir James 240
free association 18
  origins 268
free will 27
Freemasonry 243, 263, 266, 267, 268,
  278, 283
  degrees 268
  lodge *262*
  orders 268
  rituals 268
  and Templars 264
Freud, Sigmund 15, 18, *19*, 22, 26, 30
friction (massage) *121*
Fromm, Erich 24
fruit 149
  in food combining 148
Fu Hsi 70
functional foods 143
funerary monuments 278
Funk, Casimir 146

G

Gaba(a) 231
Gabriel, Angel 196, 290, *291*
Gaia Hypothesis 260
Galen 75

Gandhi, Mahatma 222
Ganesha 205
ganzfeld experiments 41
Gao cheng zhen 255
Gardner, Gerald Brousseau 240, 245, *248*, 295
   High Magic's Aid 240
garlic 153
Gattefossé, René-Maurice 156
Gautama Siddhartha 52, 298
Gayatri Yantra *214*
Geller, Uri 41, *41*
gem essences 166
Gendlin, Eugene 83
Generation Cycle 99, *99*
geometry:
   sacred (canonical) 245, 250–1, *250, 251*
geopathic stress 256
George, St 286–7, *287*
Germain, St 43
German Pagan Reconstructionism 238
Gestalt theory 29
Ghose, Aurobindo 300
ghosts 41
GI *see* glycaemic index
ginkgo biloba 151
ginseng 152
Giotto di Bondone:
   Flight into Egypt 191
Glastonbury Tor 246, 283
glaucoma 141
global village 304
glue ear 135
glycaemic index (GI):
   low 147
gnomes 292
Gnosticism 183, 184–5, 281
   gospels 192, *193*
God 183
Goddess Spirituality 225, 238, 239
goddess worship 294–5
godhis 239
gods:
   creator 234
Goethe, Johann Wolfgang von 272
Goetheanum 273, *273*
gold:
   changing base metal into 296–7
Golden Dawn 245, 263, 266, 273

golden proportion 250, *250, 251*
Golding, William 260
Goodheart, George J. 168
gorse essence 159
Gospel of Philip 192
Gospel of Thomas 192
Gospel of Truth 192
Govinda, Anagarike 214
Grahamists 132
Grail 282–3, *283*
grain 149
granite 256
Granth Sahib *223*
Graves, Tom 256, 261
Great Departure 208
Great Pyramid 278, *278*
   King's Chamber 256, 278
Great Void 302
Great White Brotherhood of Secret
   Masters 271
Great Year 285
Greeks 52
green spirituality 245, 260–1
Greer, John Michael 243
'grid' 42, 43
grief 161
   coping with 33
Grinder, John 31
Grof, Stanislav 81
growth spiral 250, *251*
Guadalupe:
   Black Madonna *274*
   Our Lady of *295*
guided imagery *see* creative
   visualization
gunas 94, 97
Gundestrup cauldron *239*
Gurdjieff, G.I. *24*, 25, 198
gurus 204, 205, 300–1
Gyushi 102

H

Hachiman 237
haemorrhoids:
   contraindications 151
Hahnemann, Dr Samuel 160, *160*
Hajj (pilgrimage) 197, 289, 298
Hakomi method 82, 83

Hall, Calvin S. 22–3
Hall, Judy 50
hallucinations 81
hallucinogens 35, 46
Hamon, Count Louis 68
hands:
   reflex points *131*
Hannukah 186
harmony 163
hatha yoga 106, 204
Hatha Yoga Pradipika 106
Hawaii:
   spiritual culture 230
Hawkins, Gerald 254
Hay, William Howard 148
hay fever 161
head-shrinking 225
headaches 134, 135, 153
   reflex points *131*
healing:
   emotional 160
   physical 160
heart disease:
   contraindications 152
heart rate 175
Heart Sutra 210
HeartMath system 86
heathenry 225, 238–9
Heindel, Max 273
Hellerwork 105
Helper 25
herbal nutrients 143
herbal remedies 97, 101, 103
   precautions 97
herbalism *142*, 144, 145, 152–3
   health benefits 153
   precautions 152
   research 152
   traditions 152
herbs:
   ayurvedic 94
   burning 233
   collecting *153*
   drugs from 152
   interaction with drugs 152
Hermes Trismegistus 52, 185
Hermetic Order of the Golden Dawn
   245, 263, 266, 273
Hermetic philosophers 266
Hermetic tradition 53

Hermeticism 184, 185
Herodotus 286
hexagrams 70–1, *70*
high blood pressure *see* hypertension
Hill, Napoleon 52
Hillman, James 21
hindbrain 16, *17*
Hinduism 34, 37, 50, 52, *95*, 204–5
   Devas 204, 205
   eclecticism 204
   Enlightenment 204
   evolution 203
   gurus 204, 205, 300–1
   origins 203
   pilgrimage *204*, 298
   sacred texts 203, 204, 206–7
   spiritual aspirations 203
   yogas 204–5
Hip Rolls *111*
hippocampus 84
Hippocrates *15*, *23*, *74*, 75, 76, 160
Hitler, Adolf 187
hoarding type 24
Hohokam people 255
holistic approach 105
holly essence 159
Holocaust 187
Holotropic Breathwork 81
Holt, Henry 41
Holy Blood and the Holy Grail, The
   263, 281, 282
Holy Grail 282–3, *283*
Holy Spirit *182*
homeopathy 75, 90, 132, 160–1, 272
   precautions 161
   research 161
   symptom picture 161
Hoomi, Koot 270, 273
Hopewell peoples 259
horary astrology 57
hormonal imbalance 152
horoscopes *see* astrological charts
houses:
   astrological 56, 61
Huang Ti (Huangdi), Emperor 58
Hugues de Payen 264
Human Potential Movement 41
humanistic psychology 27
humours 15, *15*, 75, 102, 171
   balancing 93

Hund, Baron Gotthelf von 268
Huxley, Thomas 15
Hydropaths 132
hydrotherapy 144, *145*, 164–5
    precautions 164
    research 165
Hygienists 132
hypertension (high blood pressure) 79,
    80, 86, 87, 94, 177
hyperventilation 81
hypnogogic state 16
hypnopompic state 16
hypnosis 30
    undergoing 30
hypnotherapy 15, 30
    development of 30

I

'I AM' movement 271
I Ching 55, 70–1, 98, 220–1
    trigrams 249
Ichazo, Oscar 25
id 18
illnesses:
    acute 93
    chronic 93, 94
    prevention 93
    psychosomatic 16
Iluminati 267
Imbolc 241
Imhotep 278
immune system:
    boosting 77
    effects of CNS on 76
    effects of stress on 77
immunization 161
impatiens essence 159
Incas 149
incontinence 86
India:
    healthcare 94
Indian head massage 123, *123*
    research 123
indigestion:
    acupressure for *127*
Individualist 25
individuation 18

Indonesia:
    spiritual culture 230
infections 135
infertility 152, 161
Infinite Life Sutra 210
inflammation:
    treatment of 163
inflammatory bowel diseases:
    contraindications 151
information:
    processing 31
information-processing model 84–5
Ingham, Eunice 129
inner eye 40
Innocent II, Pope 264
insomnia 80, 87, 175
Instinctive Triad 25
Integrative Body Psychotherapy 82, 83
intellect 16
interfaith movement 304
introverts 24
intuiting types 24
intuition 16, 38
Iranaeus 192
iridology 140
    charts *140*
    diagnosis 140
    research 140
irrational assumptions 28
irritable bowel syndrome 79, 80, 86,
    101, 161
    causes 148
Isis 290
Islam 52, 196–7
    five pillars 196–7
    Hajj (pilgrimage) 197, 289, 298
    heritage 183
    mosque *197*
    sacred texts 183, 196, 198
    Sharia law 196, 197
    spiritual traditions 183, 196, 198–9
Ixchel 225
iyengar 106

J

Jackson, Hughlings 22
Jainism 222
    five vows 222

sculptures *222*
    spiritual aspirations 203
Jains 222
jamais vu 39
Java:
    spiritual culture 231
Jenny, Dr Hans 163
Jerusalem 298
Jesus Christ *see* Christ
jet lag 80
Jewish-Masonic conspiracy 267
Jivaroan people 225
Jnana yoga 205
Joseph of Arimathea 282
ju-jitsu 117
Judaeo-Christian mysteries 280–1
Judaism 52, 186–7
    fasting 150
    festivals 186
    heritage 183
    Holocaust 187
    observances 186
    pilgrimage 298
    principles of faith 186
    sacred texts 183, 186
    spiritual traditions 183
    see also Kabbalah
Judge, William Q. 270
judgement types 24–5
judo 117
Jung, Carl 38, 55, 62, 203, 210, 214,
    296, 297
    psychological types 24
Jung, Carl Gustav 15, 18–19, 20–1, *20*,
    22
juniper oil 156
Juok 234

K

Kabbalah 183, 188, 240, 263
    divine emanations 188
    sacred texts 188
    Tree of Life 188, *189*
Kagura 236, 237, *237*
Kailash, Mount *244*
Kama Sutra 215
Kami 236, 292

Kangaroo Dreaming 229
kangaroo pine essence 159
kapha dosha 96–7, 102
Kapilavastu 298
karate 116–17
karma 50, 60, 204
    harmful 222
karma yoga 106
kebatinan 231
Keleman, Stanley 82, 83
Kelly, Aidan 240
Kelly, Charles 83
Kemetism 238
Khafre, pharaoh 278
Khufu (Cheops) 278
Khunrath, Heinrich *53*
ki see chi
kidney cleanse 150, 151
Kin Wên 70
kinesiology 168
Kirin 286
Kirlian, Semyon 173
Kirlian Photography (KP) *154*, 173
Kleitman, Nathaniel 22
Knapp, J. Augustus:
    Atlantis 277
Kneipp, Sebastian 144, *144*
Knight, J.Z. 42
Knights Templar 263, 264, 281, 283
    downfall 264, *265*
    and Freemasonry 264, 268
    myths 264
Knossos 246
Koans 213
Kogi Indians 259
Koran 183, 196, 198, 290
kosher 186
Krieger, Dolores 176
Krishna 206
Krishnamurti, Jiddu 271, *271*, 272, 300
kriya yoga 106
Kronos 21
Kukulcan 255, *285*
kum nye 103
kundalini 172, 215
kung fu *116*, 117
Kunz, Dora 176
Kuriyama, I. 147
Kurtz, Ron 83
Kusinagara 298

L

Lakota people 233
landscape lines 245, 258–9
landscapes:
    divination 248–9
    imbued with meaning 246
Lao Tzu 58, 216, 218, *218*
laughter therapy 77
lavender oil 156, 157
Lawton, Arthur 256, 258
laying-on of hands 133, *177*
Leadbetter, Charles W. 43, 172–3, 203,
    271
Leader 25
learning:
    process of 15
learning curve 15
Leary, Timothy 34, 35, *35*
Lebe 235
Leigh, Richard 281, 282
Leih Tzu 218
Lennon, John 50
Lenormand, Marie Anne Adelaide 68
lentils 149
Leonardo da Vinci 281
leprechauns 292, 293
Leslie, Desmond 256
Lévi, Eliphas 263
levitation 37
    self- 41
Lévy-Bruhl, Lucien 246
ley lines 245, 256, 258, 287
    and UFOs 256
Liberal Catholic Church 271
Liébeault, Ambroise-Auguste 30
life force(s) 155, 234, 302
    balancing 93, 94, 96–7
life-between-lives regression 50–1
light 155
    beings of 290
    therapeutic applications 162
lights:
    strobe 162
limbic system 84, *85*
Lincoln, Abraham 27
Lincoln, Henry 281, 282
Lindlahr, Dr Henry 144
Lindlahr, Victor 143, 144
Ling, Per Henrick 120
Lisina, Maya Ivanovna 86

liver cleanse 150–1
liver infusion pumps:
    contraindications 164
Lockyer, Sir Norman 254
Lotus Sutra 210, 246
Lotus Temple *201*
Lovelock, James 260, *260*
Lowen, Alexander 82
Loyalist 25
lucid dreaming 23, 46, 48
Lughnasadh 241
luminous consciousness 34
luopan *249*

M

Maasai 234
Mabon 241
McElroy, Margaret 42
MacFadden, Bernarr 144
MacLaine, Shirley 289
Maclean, Dorothy 301
macrobiotics 149
    diet 149
    holistic approach 149
    origins 149
    precautions 149
    research 149
McTimoney, John 135
McTimoney chiropractic 135
Madhyamika Karika Vritti 37
Magellan, Ferdinand 230
magic circle *44*
magnesium sulphate 164
magnetic healing 133
magnetic resonance imaging (MRI)
    15, 30
Magnus, Albertus 297
Mahabharata 206
Maharshi, Ramana 300
Mahatmas 43
Mahavir, Shri 222
Mahayana Buddhism 208, 209
Mahesh Yogi, Maharishi 79, 205, *205*,
    300
Major Arcana 62
male psyche:
    feminine side 19, 20

Malory, Sir Thomas *283*
Mamma 234
Man Mound, Baraboo 253
mana 230
mandalas 214, *214*
Mandylion 281
mansika prakriti 94
mantras 214
Maori people 225
    sacred places 231
    spiritual culture 230–1
maps:
    mental 31
Margulis, Lynn 260
Marindi 228
marketing type:
    Myers-Briggs Type indicator 24
Marquardt, Hanne 130
martial arts 105, 112, 114, 116–17
    research 117
    styles 116
Maslow, Abraham 27
mass media 275
massage:
    deep-tissue 139
    Indian head 123
    Swedish 105, 120–1
    Thai 122
mastaba 278
materialization *195*
Matus, Don Juan 289
Maui 230
Mayan paganism 238
Mayan prophecy 285
Mayans 225, 285
    saches 259
    temples 255
Mayari 231
MBII *see* Myers-Briggs Type Indicator
meaningful coincidence 20
Mecca 197, 298, *299*
meditation 34, 35, 78–9, 93
    autogenic 80
    crystal 166, 167
    essential characteristics 78
    focal points for 172
    therapeutic benefits 78–9
    transcendental (TM) 79
    upon mantras 214
    upon yantras 214

meditative state 16
mediums 37, 194–5, *195*
mediumship 39
    channelling 42–3
Meera, Mother 301
megalithic monuments 252
megaliths:
    and astronomy 254
Mehta, Narendra 123
melancholic personality 15, *15*
Melanesia:
    spiritual culture 230
memory:
    effects on 175
    study of 15
memory loss 152
menhirs 252
menopausal problems 153, 161
menorah *187*
menstrual problems 153, 161
mental attitude 94, 97
mental maps 31
mercury 297
meridians *100*, 101, 124, 126, 129
    channelling energy through 174
    energy 87
Merlin 43
Merovingian dynasty 281
mesmerism 30
mesopaganism 238
Meta Model 31
Metamorphic technique 130
metaphysics 12
Michael, Archangel 290
Michell, John 245, 251, 254, *258*, 261
Micronesia:
    spiritual culture 230
midbrain 16, *17*
Midsummer 241
migraine 86, 87, 135, 161
milk thistle *150*, 151
Miller, Neal 86
Milton Mode 31
mimulus essence 159
mind:
    brain and 16
    definition 16
    dimensions of 37–53
    philosophy of 37
    power of 33

re-educating 118
  study of 15
mind-body interactions 16, 155
mind-body therapies 75–87
mindfulness 28, 29, 80
minerals 143, 146
  daily intake 146
  precautions 146
  research 146
Minor Arcana 62
Minzoku-Shinto 237
Mississippian Indians 255
Mitchell, Edgar 41
Moai 231, *231*, 252
modelling 31
modes 56
Mohawk, Professor John 232
Mohr, Bärbel 53
Monks Mound 255
monoliths 252
monomyths 21
Mons:
  angels of 291
Montserrat:
  Black Madonna 281
monuments:
  architecture 250–1
  megalithic 252
Moon 295
moonstone 167
moral sense 18
Morgan, Annie *195*
Morya, Mahatma 270
Moses 21, 183
mother 21
Mother Nature 295
Motivator 25
mountain devil essence 159
movement practices 93
Moving the Rainbow *115*
moxibustion 101
MRI *see* magnetic resonance imaging
Msoura 252
Muhammad, Prophet 183, 196, 198, 298
Muldoon, Sylvan 46
mundane astrology 57
muscle strength 168
muscular injuries 163
Myers, Isabel Briggs 24

Myers, W.H. 41
Myers-Briggs Type Indicator (MBTI) 15
myofascial system:
  realigning 139, *139*
mysteries:
  ancient 275–87
mystery traditions:
  Western 184–5
mystical state 34–5
mysticism:
  quantum physics and 302
mystics 37
mythical creatures 286–7
mythology 20, 21

N

Nabulwinjbulwinj *247*
Nadi-sodhana pranayama *81*
Naess, Arne 261
Nag Hammadi 192
Nanak, Sri Guru 223, *223*
Nancy School of Psychotherapy 30
Naranjo, Claudio 25
natal chart 56–7, *57*
Native American Spirituality 225, 232–3
  power animals 233
  rituals 232
  smudging 233, 256
  spirit guides 233
  sweat lodge 233
  totems 232, *232*
  vision quests 233
Native Americans 50
  astronomy 255
  shamans 42, 47
Native Cat Dreaming 229
nature:
  patterns of 250
  spirit of 232
Nature Cure movement 143, 144
nature worship 238
naturopathy 143, 144–5, 150
  diagnosis 145
  key principles 144–5
  nutrition 145
  research 145
  therapies 143

Nauri peoples 230
nautilus shell *251*
Navajos 232
Nazca lines 245, 258–9, *259*
Nbbana Sutta 34
near-death experiences 16, 48–9
neck tension:
  reflex points *131*
negative emotions 158
negative thoughts:
  challenging 28–9
  combating 29
neo-paganism 238, 245, 260
nerve ganglia 173
nervous system 76, 175
  autonomic *76*
  central (CNS) 76
  channelling energy through 174
  effects on immune system 76
neuro-hypnotism 30
neuro-linguistic programming (NLP) 15, 31
neurobiology of emotion 84–5
neuropathy:
  contraindications 164
neuroscientists 15
neutral spine 110, 111
  finding 111
New Age Atlantis 276–7
New Age movement 271, 275, 302
New Age notions 260–1
New Age shamanism 226, 227
New Testament 183, 190
Newgrange 252, 253
Newham, C.A. 254
Newton, Joseph Fort 268
Nez Perce people 232
Nikhilananda, Swami 214
Ninigi 237
ninjitsu *117*
Nirvana 34
Nirvana Sutra 34
NLP *see* neuro-linguistic programming
Noble Eightfold Path 208, 210
Nommo 225, 235
Noongar people 229
Norse paganism 238–9
Nostradamus 37, 284, *284*
  prophecies 284
  quatrains 284

Nourlangie Rock *247*
numerology 66–7
nutrients 146
nutrition:
  connection with health 143
  pH balance 145
nutritional therapy 143–53
  assessments 143
  evolution 143
  treatments 143
nymphs 292

O

OBE *see* out-of-body experiences
obesity 143
object deformation 41
objective psyche 20
occult:
  meaning 263
occult societies 263–73
Oceania:
  spiritual culture 230–1
Odinism 238
Ofsted 304–5
Ohsawa, George 149, *149*
Olcott, Henry Steel 270
olfactory nerve 156
Olorun (Olodumare) 234–5
Omaha people 232
Ono, Yoko 50
operant conditioning 26
optimistic autosuggestion 30
Order of Bards, Ovates and Druids 243
Order of the Star of the East 271, *271*
Order of the Strict Observance 268
Ordo Templis Orientis (OTO) 273
Oresme, Nicolas 18
orgasm 82
orgone 82
orisha tradition 234–5, *234*
Orr, Leonard 81
Orthodox Christianity 190, 191
Osho (Bhagavan Shree Rajneesh) 300–1, *300*
Osiris 21, 290, 298
Osmond, Humphrey 35
Ostara 241

osteopathy 90, 132–5
  branches of 135
  conditions treated 134
  origins 132–4
  research 135
  techniques 134–5
  treatments 134–5, *134*
osteoporosis 143
  contraindications 121, 164
OTO *see* Ordo Templis Orientis
out-of-body experiences (OBE) 23, 44, 46–7, 48
  induced 46
Oxyrhynchus 192

P

pacemakers:
  contraindications 164
paganism 225, 238–9, 294
  beliefs 238–9
  categories 238
pain:
  chronic 177
  management 33, 177
  treatment of 163
pain relief:
  essential oils 157
Paleolithic era 246
paleopaganism 238
Palmer, Daniel David 133, 134
palming 141
palmistry 68–9
panchakarma 93, 94, 97
  precautions 97
panic attacks 80
pantheism 238, 241
Paracelsus 18, 297
Paramahansa Yogananda 38, *38*
paramnesia 39
parapsychology 39
Parashar, Maharishi 60
Parnia, Dr Sam 49
Passover 186
past lives 50–1
past-life astrolgy 57
past-life readings 50, 51
past-life regression 50

past-life therapies 50–1
Patanjali 106
Patton, General George S. 50
Paul, St 171, *184*, 185
Pavlov, Ivan 15, 26
Payen, Hugues de 264
Peacemaker 25
Peale, Norman Vincent 52
pectin 147
Peczely, Ignatz von 140
Pellerin, Jean C. engraving *284*
pendulum dowsing 72
pentagonal geometry *250*
pentagram 241
peppermint oil 157
perceptive types 24–5
Perfection of Wisdom Sutra 212
Perls, Fritz 22, 31
Persephone 21
Persinger, Michael 46
persona 19
personality:
  effect of unconscious on 18
  elements of 18
  psychological types 24–5
  types 15, *15*
PET scans *see* positron emission topography
Peters, Roberta *110*
petrissage *121*
petroforms *233*
pH balance 145
Philip IV of France 264, *265*
Philippines:
  spiritual culture 231
Philosopher's Stone 282, 296, 297
philosophy of mind 37
phlegmatic personality 15, *15*
phobias 26, 87, 161
physical healing 160
physical therapies 103
physics 37
Physiologus 286
physiomedicalists 132
pi 251
Picknett, Lynn 281
Pilates 105, 110–11
  core strength 108
  Hip Rolls *111*
  instruction 111

movements 111
  research 111
Pilates, Joseph 110, *110*
pilgrimage 223, 298
  Buddhist 246
  definition 298
  Hindu *204*
  history of 298
  importance of 289
  Islamic (Hajj) 197, 289, 298
  to Mount Kailash *245*
pitta dosha 96, 102
pixies 292
placebo effect 16, 75
placebos 77
planets:
  in astrology 56, 60–1
Platearius, Mattheaus *143*
Plato 24, 49, 276, *276*, 277
Pleiades 285
PNI *see* psychoneuroimmunology
polarity therapy 169
  precautions 169
  research 169
poltergeists 41
polycystic ovary syndrome 101
Polynesia:
  spiritual culture 230
polytheism 225, 238, 241
Poor Knights of Christ and the Temple of Solomon *see* Knights Templar
popular culture 275
positive attitude 44
positive thinking:
  power of 52–3
positron emission topography (PET scans) 15
post-operative healing 163
post-traumatic stress disorder (PTSD) 85
posture:
  natural 118
postures (*asanas*) 106
potentization 161
power animals 233
power yoga 106
Poznan:
  Black Madonna *280*
prakriti 94
prana 7, 155, 225

pranayama 81, *81*, 97, 106
prayer:
  benefits of 171
prayer flags 212
precognition 38, 39, 127
pregnancy:
  contraindications 121, 122, 125, 126, 151, 152, 164
premonition 38, 39
Price, John 297
Priessnitz, Vincent 144
Prince, Clive 281
proinflammatory cytokines 76
Prometheus 21
prophecy 284
prophets 37
prostate:
  hyperplasia 152
protective light bubble 45, *45*
proteins:
  in food combining 148
Protestantism 190, 191
Psalms 298
pschological conditioning 26
Psilocybe Project *34*, 35
psoriasis 101, 161
psyche:
  exploration of 15
  objective 20
  study of 18–19
psyche versus *soma* 75
psychedelic drugs 35, 226
psychiatric conditions:
  contraindications 177
psychic abilities 16
psychic influences 55
psychic powers:
  attaining 37
psychic protection 44–5
psychic sense 37
psychic skills 37–53, 40–1
psychic strengthening 44
psychics 37
psychoanalysis 32
psychokinesis 40, 41
psychokinetic energy 39
psychological types 24–5
psychology:
  approaches 15–35
  humanistic 27

psychometry 40, 41

psychoneuroimmunology (PNI) 75, 76–7

psychosomatic illnesses 16

psychosynthesis 32

psychotherapies 15

  body-centred 82–3

Ptolemy 56

PTSD *see* post-traumatic stress disorder

pulses 149

punishment 26

Pure Land Sutra 210

Puthoff, Harold 47

pyramid of needs 27

Pyramid Texts 279

pyramids 251, 278

  radiation anomalies 256

  stepped 255

Pythagoras 66, *67*, 184, *185*, 267

Pythagorean system 66

Pythagoreanism 184

Pythia 37, *42*

Q

Qawali 199, *199*

qigong *see* chi kung

qualities:

  unacceptable 19

quantum physics 37, 53, 203, 302

quartz 167

quinine 160

Qu'ran *see* Koran

R

Ra:

  priests of 37

radiation:

  at megalithic sites 256, *257*

radiesthesia 256

radio waves 155

Radix 82, 83

Rainbow Snake 228, *228*

raja yoga 106

rajas 97

Rajneesh, Bhagavan Shree (Osho) 300, *300*

Rakozi, Master 43

Ram Das (Richard Alpert) *34*, 35

Ramadan *298*

Ramayana 206, *207*

Ramsay, Andrew 264

rapid eye movement (REM) 22

rapture 34

Rapu Nui 231

rasayana 97

rational emotive behavioural therapy 28

Raynaud's disease:

  precautions 164

reality:

  nature of 16

realms:

  other: paths to 289–305

reasoning 16

Rebirthing Breathwork 81

receptive type 24

red lily essence 159

Redfield, James 52

reflexology 128–31

  Egyptian 128, *128*

  health benefits 130

  reflex points 128, 129–30, *129*, *131*

  research 130

  techniques 130

  variants 130

  Vertical Reflex Therapy (VRT) 130

Reformer 25

Reich, Wilhelm 82

reiki 171, 174–5

  origins 174

  practitioners 174–5

  precautions 175

  research 175

  treatment 175, *175*

reincarnation 50, 204

relativity 37

relaxation 79

religion 21

  interfaith movement 304

  link with transcendence 34

  spirituality and 304–5

religious devotion 35

REM *see* rapid eye movement

remote viewing 46, 47

Rennes-le-Château 281, 283

repression 32

Rescue Remedy 159

resonant frequency 163

respiratory tract infections 161

retreats 289, 298

Reuss, Theodor 273

revisitation 81

rheumatism 153, 163

rheumatoid arthritis 177

Rhine, Joseph B. 39, *40*, 41

Rhine, Louisa 39

Richet, Charles 38

Rite of Memphis and Misraim 273

Rivdan, Festival of 200

Roberts, Jane 42

Robison, John 267

rock paintings *235*, 246, *247*

Rogers, Carl 27

Rolf, Dr Ida 139

rolfing 82, 105, 139, *139*

  research 139

  treatments 139

Rollright Stones 256

romantic movement 245

Rose Cross *266*

rose quartz 167

rosemary oil 156

Rosenberg, Jack 82, 83

Rosenkreuz, Christian 266

Rosicrucianism 263, 266, 267

  and Freemasons 268

  manifestos 266

Rosslyn Chapel 283

Rubenfeld, Ilana 83

Rubenfeld Synergy Method 82, 83

Rumi 198, *198*, 199

runes 64–5

  alphabet *65*

  casting 64

  interpreting 64

  stones 253

'Running Man' *13*

S

Sacred Ecologists 238

sacred geometry 245, 250–1, *250*, *251*

sacred land 246

sacred places 246

Sagas 238

Sahba, Farborz:

  temple designed by *201*

Sai Baba 301

saints 43

Salah 196

salt:

  in diet 151

Samanta-Laughton, Dr Manjir 12

Samhain 241

samurai *117*

sand paintings 212, *212*

Sanders, Alex 240

Sangha 208, 209

sangoma 226

sanguine personality 15, *15*

Santana Dharma 204

Santiago de Compostela 289

Saqqara 278

sareerika prakriti 94

Satir, Virginia 31

sattva 97

Sawm 196

Scandinavia:

  rune stones 253

  standing stones 252

scents:

  treatment using 156

schizophrenia:

  contraindications 177

School of Analytical Psychology *20*

Schroth, Anton Victor 144

Schrotkur regime 144

Schucman, Dr Helen 195

Schultz, Johannes 80

Scientology 50

Scott-Ellis, William 277

scrying 72

sea water:

  treatment with 164, *165*

seaweeds 149

seclusion 35

second sight 40

secret societies 263–73

Sect Shinto 237

seers 37

self-actualization 27

self-awareness 29

self-confidence:
boosting 80
self-esteem:
loss of 87
self-healing 105
acupressure 127
reflexology 130
self-levitation 41
self-realization 32
Selye, Hans 75
sema 35
sen (energy lines) 122
Senegambia:
stones 252
sensing types 24
sensory deprivation 46
sensory overload 46
sensory perception 16
seraphim 290
Serpent Dreaming 229
serpent lines 229
Serpent Mound, Ohio 253
serpents 286
sexual desire 18
sexual dysfunction 86
sexual energy 82
shadow self 19, 20, 22
Shah, Idries 198
Shahadah 196
Shakti 215
Shaktism 172
Shakyamuni Buddha 102
shamanism 225, 226–7, 238, 245
New Age 227
worldwide 226–7
shamans 35, 37, 227, 259
identifying 226
initiation 226
transformation 226
work of 226
Shambhala 211
shape shifting 41
Shapiro, Francine 85
Sharia law 196
Shavout(h) 186
Shekinah 280
Sheldrake, Rupert 55, 302
Shia Muslims 196
shiatsu 124–5, 124, 125
precautions 125

techniques 124–5
therapeutic treatment 125
Shilluk peoples 234
Shinto 225, 236–7, 292
Kagura 236, 237, 237
kami 236
practices 236, 237
styles of 236, 237
Shiva 21, 205, 215
Shrine Shinto 237
Siddhartha Gautama 208
siddhis 37, 41
sidereal zodiac 60
sigils:
as talismans 64
Sikhism 223
gurus 223
spiritual aspirations 203
spiritual beliefs 223
Silbury Hill 253
silence 35
Silva, José 41
Silva Method 41
Singh, Gobind 223
Sinnett, A.P. 270
sinus congestion:
reflex points 131
sinusitis:
chronic 135
Sioux people 232
sirodhara 96
Sivananda, Swami 300
sixth sense 38–9, 40
Skalds 238
skin disorders 153, 175
Skinner, B.F. 26
sleep:
dreaming 16
REM stage 46
smudging 233, 256
sodium sulphate 297
Sokchonje 221
solar systems:
emergence 155
solstices:
measuring 255
soma:
versus psyche 75
Somatic Emotional Therapy 82, 83
songlines 228, 229, 287

soul 21
sound therapy 163
research 163
spells:
book of 241
Spence, Lewis 243
Sphinx 278–9, 278
spinach 147
spine:
neutral 110
finding 111
spirit:
body and 171–7
healing power of 171
separation of body anad 171
spirit guides 42, 233
spirits 41
ancestral 234
comforting dying 291
of nature 292
worshipping 225
spiritual development:
yoga 106
spiritual guidance 289
spiritual healing 171, 176, 194
precautions 177
research 177
spiritual leaders 300–1
spiritual practices 93, 223
exploration of 289
goals 34
spiritual realm 289–305
spiritual regression 51
spiritual societies 263
Spiritualism 50, 194–5
churches 194–5
healing 194
materialization 195
mediums 194–5
spirituality 144
contemporary 304–5
Eastern 78
healing power of 171
holistic approach 305
individual experience 305
religion and 304–5
splashing 141
sprites 292
Stahl, G.E. 225
standing stones 252, 252

Star of the East, Order of the 271, 271
Stargate Project 47
stars:
emergence 155
Steiner, Rudolf 50, 263, 266, 272–3, 272, 277
Steiner Schools 272
Stella Matutina 263, 273
Still, Andrew 132–3, 133, 134
stomach ache 148
Stone Age 56, 246
Stone, Dr Randolph 169, 169
stone circles 246, 250–1
Stonehenge 242, 243, 252, 253, 254, 254
stonemasons 268, 269
Strabo 243
straightness 259
Strassman, Rick 49
stress:
acupressure for 127
effects on immune system 77
geopathic 256
management 29, 30, 77
reduction of 33, 80
relieving 79, 152
stress-related conditions 175
Strict Observance, Order of the 268
strobe lights 162
subtle protection 44
succussion 160
Sufism 35, 50, 183, 198–9
drumming and chanting 180
Mehlevi Order 199
philosophy 198–9
practices 199
Qawali 199, 199
sacred text 198
Sukkot(h) 186
sulphur 297
Sumerians 56
Summer Solstice 241
Sun Salutation (Surya Namaskar) 108–9
Sunni Muslims 196
superconscious 32
superego 18
superfoods 147
research 147
supernatural powers 41

surgery:
    Western 93
Surya Namaskar (Sun Salutation) 108–9
Susano 236, 237
Sushruta Samhita 94
sushumna nadi 172
Sutherland, Dr William 136
Sutras 34, 106, 210, 212
Swatmarama 106
Swazi people 234
sweat lodge 233
swedana 97
Swedenborg, Emanuel 290
Swedish massage 105, 120–1, 120
    history 120
    precautions 121
    research 121
    techniques 121
    therapeutic benefits 120
swinging 141
symbel 239
synastry 57
synchronicity 20, 55
Szent-Györgyi, Albert 146

T

Tabernacle 280
tae kwan do 117
Tagalog people 231
t'ai chi 93, 101, 112–13, 112, 303
    benefits 112–13
    Cloud Hands 113
    movements 112
    origins 112
    practice 112–13
    research 113
    symbol 98
Tai Shan, Mount 298
talismans:
    sigils as 64
tamas 97
Tampaku, Tamai 124
Tane 231
Tangaroa 225, 230, 231
Tangatu manu 231
Tantra 214–15

beliefs 214
practices 214–15, 215
sexual rites 215
tantras 212
Tao 216, 289
Tao Te Ching 217, 218
Taoism 78, 98, 114, 149, 216–17
    origins 203
    ritual 217
    sacred texts 217, 218–19
    spiritual aspirations 203
    wu wei 216–17
Tapirape people 226
tapotement 121
Targ, Russell 47
tarot 55, 62–3
    card designs 62, 63
    reading 54, 62
    spreads 62
tasseomancy 72, 73, 73
TCM see Traditional Chinese Medicine
tea leaves:
    reading 72, 73, 73
tea tree oil 157
telepathy 37, 40, 41
teleportation 37, 41
tension:
    dispelling 105
        neck: reflex points 131
        treating 86
Teotihuacan 255, 255
Teresa of Avila, St 34
TFT see Thought Field Therapy
Thai massage 122, 122
    precautions 122
    research 122
thalassotherapy 164
thangkas 102
Theodism 238
Theophrastus 15
Theosophy 43, 203, 245, 263, 270–1, 272, 275, 277, 278, 300
Thera 277
therapeutic touch 176
Theravada Buddhism 208, 209
Thetford, Dr William 195
Thinking Triad 25
thinking types 24
third eye 40
Thirring, Walter 302

Thom, Alexander 254
Thomas Aquinas, St 290
Thompsonians 132
Thor 225
thought 16
Thought Field Therapy (TFT) 87
thought-form projection 41
thought-transference 41
thoughts:
    negative:
        challenging 28–9
        combating 29
thrombosis:
    contraindications 121
thyroid problems:
    contraindications 121
Tibetan Book of the Dead 35, 210, 211
Tibetan Buddhism 208, 209, 212, 301
    customs 212
    religious iconography 212
    Vajrayana 212
Tibetan medicine 102–3
    Buddhism and 102
    humours 102
    key concepts 93
    practice 102
    precautions 103
    research 103
    traditions 102
    treatments 102, 103
    tree of health and disease 92
Tibetan Secret Masters 271, 273
tinnitus 86
Tirawa 232
Tirthankaras 222
tjukuba 246
TM see transcendental meditation
Toland, John 243
Tomlinson, Andy 50
Torah 183, 186
totems 232, 232
trace elements 146
Traditional Chinese Medicine (TCM) 75, 93, 98–101, 124
    diagnosis 101
    Eight Principles 98–9
    Five Elements System 98, 99
    key concepts 93
    meridians 98, 100, 101, 129
    pharmacy 101

precautions 101
research 101
treatments 98, 101
use of herbs 152
Tragerwork 105
trances:
    channelling 42
    divinational 39
transcendent state 34–5
transcendental meditation (TM) 79
transpersonal 32
transpersonal psychology 32
Trascendental Meditation 300
trauma:
    resolution of 81
travel sickness:
    acupressure for 127
tree of health and disease 92
Tree of Life 188, 189
tribal traditions 225
trigrams:
    in feng shui 249
Tripitaka 34, 210
triskelion 243, 243
Tuatha de Danaan 292
Tucano people 226
tui na 101, 124
Turin Shroud 280, 281, 281
'two attentions' 18
Tylor, Sir Edwward Burnett 225

U

UFOs 49, 245, 256
    ley lines and 258
Uluru (Ayers Rock) 225, 228, 229, 229
unconscious:
    collective 15, 18, 20–1
    influence of 18
    study of 18–19
unconscious collusion 19
unconscious drives 118
Underwood, Guy 256
Ungarinjin people 228
unicorn 286, 286
universal life force 302
Unkulunkulu 234
Unwaba 234

Upanishads 50, 172, 204, 206, 289, 302
Urarina people 225, 226
Usai, Dr Mikao 174, *174*

V

vacuflex reflexology 130
Vajravahara 246
Vajrayana Buddhism 212, 215
Valentinus 185, 192
Varuna 292
vata dosha 96, 102
Vatsayana 215
Vedanta 206
Vedas 203, 204, 206
Vedic astrology 60–1
vegetables 149
venous insufficiency:
    chronic 152
Venus figurines 294, *294*
Venus of Willendorf 294, *294*
Verbiest, Father Ferdinand *59*
Vertical Reflex Therapy (VRT) 130
vertigo 161
vesica piscis 250, 251
vibration (massage) *121*
vibrational therapy 163
vibrations:
    disordered 166
    plant 158, 159
Viking Age paganism 225, 238–9
Villeneuve, Arnaud de *269*
Virgin Mary 43, 294
Vishishtadvaita 206
Vishnu 205
vision quests 22, 233
visualization 32, 44
    techniques 33
vitamins 143, 146
    daily intake 146
    discovery of 146
    precautions 146
    research 146
Vivekananda, Swami 304, *304*
Voudoun 238
Vrindavan 298
VRT *see* Vertical Reflex Therapy

W

Wakan Tanka 225, 232
waking state 16
Waldorf Schools 272
Walton, K.G. 77
Warnbach, Helen 50
water:
    gazing into 55
    memory 164
water therapies 144, *145*, 164–5
    precautions 164
    research 165
Wati-Kutjara 228–9
Watkins, Alfred 258
Watson, John 26
weaknesses:
    repressed 19
Wedd, Tony 258
Weishaupt, Adam 267, *267*
Weiss, Brian 50
Western astrology 56–7
Western faiths 183–201
Western medicine 93
Wheel of Life *51*
Wheeler, John C. 49
White, Ian 159
White, JKohn B. 254
White, Rhea A. 48
White Eagle 195
Whitman, Walt 27
wholeness 21
    striving for 19
Wicca 225, 238, 240–1, 245, 294, 295
    ceremonies 241, *241*
    forms of 240–1
    magic rituals 241
    magical tools 241
    texts 241
    worship of God/Goddess 241
Wilhelm, Richard 70
witchcraft 295
Wolger, Roger 50
Wondjina 228
Woodroffe, Sir John 172
World Parliament of Religions 304
Worora people *228*
Wright, Elsie *292*
wu wei 216–17
Wundt, Wilhelm 15
Wyrd 239

X

X-rays 155

Y

Yaburara people 229
Yahweh 186
yang 58, 98, 112, 216
    foods 149
    in landscape 248
yantras 214, *214*
Yeats, W.B. 263
Yeshe, Thubten 212
yin 58, 98, 112, 216
    foods 149
    in landscape 248
yoga 34, 35, 78, 97, 105, 106–9, *170*
    asanas 106
    benefits 108
    branches 106
    ethics 106
    practice 108
    pranayama 81, 106
    precautions 108
    research 108
    Sun Salutation (*Surya Namaskar*) *108–9*
Yoga Sutras 106, 204
yogas (Hindu) 204–5
yogi *107*
yogurt:
    probiotic 143
Yoruba:
    traditions 234–5
Yule 241

Z

Zakat 196
Zazen 213
Zen Buddhism 208, 209, 213
    Koans 213
    masters 213
    monks *213*
    Zazen 213
Zener, Karl 40

Zener cards *40*, 41
zodiac:
    Chinese 58
    Indian *61*
    sidereal 60
    tropical 56
Zohar 188
Zulus 226, 234

ACKNOWLEDGEMENTS

akg-images 296, 153, 283, 288; British Library, London 48, 74, 297; Erich Lessing 230, 236; **Alamy** Adrian Sherratt 162; Alex Bramwell 229; Ali Kabas 198; ArkReligion.com 223; Barry Lewis 305; Bildarchiv Monheim GmbH 273; Bubbles Photolibrary 30, 136; David Chapman 257; David Lyons 243; dbimages 304; Gavin Hellier 204; Iain Masterton 248; Icelandic photo agency 165; imagebroker 2, 244; Interfoto 54, 205; Jeff Morgan health 138; Jeremy Horner 212; Jochen Tack 97, 197; Jon Arnold Images Ltd 231; Kathy deWitt 260; Martin Harvey 247; Mary Evans Picture Library 14, 39, 42, 43, 47, 150, 200, 220, 267; Masa Uemura 237; Miguel A Munoz Pellicer 134; Mike Goldwater 158; North Wind Picture Archives 195; Oliver Benn 177; Pat Behnke 217; Paul Prince Photography 258; Pavel Filatov 181; Pictorial Press Ltd 26, 35; Radius Images 233; Ruby 213; Sherab 102; Skyscan Photolibrary 254; Steve Allen Travel Photography 222; Steve Skjold 280; The London Art Archive 182, 269; The Print Collector 51; Tim Gainey 170; Westend 61 GmbH 168; Wolfgang Kaehler 303; **American Polarity Therapy Association** 169; **American Museum of Natural History** Anthropology Collection 5, 92; **Bernard Jensen** permission granted by Dr Ellen Tart-Jensen 140; **Bridgeman Art Library** Bibliothèque des Arts Decoratifs, Paris 227; Bibliothèque Nationale, Paris, France/Archives Charmet 132; British Library, London 265; British Museum, London 59; Dreamtime Gallery, London 228; Louvre, Paris 69; Monasterio Real, Guadalupe 274; Musée Guimet, Paris 211; Musée National du Moyen Age et des Thermes de Cluny, Paris 286; National Library, St Petersburg 142; National Museum of India, New Delhi 207; National Palace Museum, Taipei 218; Private Collection/Agnew's, London 36; Private Collection/Ancient Art and Architecture Collection Ltd 219; Private Collection/Dinodia 95, 214; Private Collection/The Maas Gallery, London 293; Private Collection/Richard and Kailas Icons, London 287; Wien Museum Karlsplatz 262: Camera Press Aufdembrinke/Schorr 41; Corbis Adam Woolfitt 242; Bettmann 19, 20, 28, 49, 270, 276, 284; Blue Lantern Studio 185, 277; Brooklyn Museum 295; Carl & Ann Purcell 278; Charles & Josette Lenars 235; Dave Bartruff 187; Fancy/Veer 151; Floris Leeuwenberg/The Cover Story 241; Frederic Soltan ¿Gao Shanyue/Xinhua Press 116; Geoffrey ⸗s 184; Gianni Dagli Orti 279; Historical

Picture Archive 21; Hugh Sitton 224; Hulton-Deutsch Collection 61; Image Source 145; Jeff Albertson 34; Jeremy Horner 202, 255; Jim Zuckerman 201; Jose Luis Pelaez Inc/Blend Images 8; Kazuyoshi Nomachi 299; Keren Su 101; Kerim Okten/epa 78; Leonard de Selva 79; Lester Lefkowitz 84, 86; Luca Tettoni 96, 122, 166; Marilyn Angel Wynn/Nativestock Pictures 232; Michele Westmorland 285; Nathan Benn 221, P Deliss/Godong 281; Pascal Deloche/Godong 190; Richard A Cooke 253; Rungroj Yongrit 209; Stapleton Collection 60, 68; Strauss/Curtis 126; Visuals unlimited 77; Walter Geiersperger 294; **cymatics.org** courtesy Dan Blore & Jan Meinema 163; **DK Images** Russell Sadur 141; **Fotolia** Jean-Yves Foy 249; **George Ohsawa Macrobiotic Foundation** 149; **Getty Images** 24; Andrea Pistolesi 112; Astromujoff 261; Hulton Archive 271; Joe Cornish 252; Matthew Naythons 300; Michael Rougier 110; Pablo Bartholomew/Contributor 199; **Institute for Antiquity and Christianity** 193; courtesy **Istituto di Psicosintesi, Florence** 32; **Kneippbund** http://www.kneippbund.at 144; **Lo Scarabeo** 63; **Lonely Planet Images** Chris Beall 259; **New Forest Observatory** (c) Greg Parker and Noel Carboni 13; **Octopus Publishing Group Ltd** 72, 108, 111, 115, 120, 121, 123, 124, 125, 127, 131, 147, 148, 157, 172, 173, 161, 167; Mike Good 81; Paul Bricknell 29; Peter Pugh-Cook 113; Russell Sadur 44, 45, 71; **Photolibrary Group** Botanica/Matthew Wakem 175; **Photoshot** WpN 52; **Picture Desk** The Art Archive/Ragab Papyrus Institute Cairo/Gianni Dagli Orti 128; The Art Archive/Private Collection/Gianni Dagli Orti 100; Scala photo Scala, Florence 191; Diocesan Museum, Cortona, photo Scala, Florence 291; British Library, London 107; **Science Photo Library** 133; Adam Gault 135; Alex Grey/Peter Arnold Inc 91; Garion Hutchings 154; Mauro Fermariello 137; Pasieka 80; **Shutterstock** Katrina Brown 159 above; letty17 159 below; Marie C Fields 146; Yan Vugenfirer 23; IKO 33; **Society of Teachers of the Alexander Technique** Photograph of F M Alexander © 2009 119; **The Milton H Erickson Foundation, Inc** 31; **Thomas Laird** 215; **TopFoto** 194; Alan Hart-Davis/Fortean 40; Charles Walker 53, 73, 266; Dr Susan Blackmore/Fortean 46; Fortean 272, 292; The Granger Collection 67, 83, 189; **Wellcome Institute Library, London** 103, 104; **Werner Forman Archive** National Museum, Copenhagen 239; Ninja Museum, Uemo 117; Tishman Collection, New York 234

Executive Editor Sandra Rigby
Senior Editor Charlotte Macey
Executive Art Editor Mark Stephens
Designer Janis Utton
Senior Production Controller Amanda Mackie
Picture Researcher Claire Gouldstone